Volume 3

Shoulder

EUROPEAN FEDERATION OF NATIONAL ASSOCIATIONS
OF ORTHOPAEDICS AND TRAUMATOLOGY

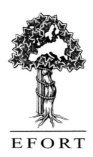

EFORT

SURGICAL TECHNIQUES
in
Orthopaedics and Traumatology

Coordinated by Professor Jacques Duparc
Honorary Chairman, Orthopaedic Department, Hôpital Bichat, Paris, France

Volume 3
Shoulder

Associate Editors
Mario Randelli - Jon Karlsson

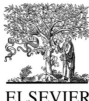

ELSEVIER
Paris, Amsterdam, New York, Oxford, Shannon, Tokyo

SURGICAL TECHNIQUES
in
Orthopaedics and Traumatology

Coordinated by Professor Jacques Duparc

In this collection:

1. General Knowledge   ISBN 2-84299-414-0

2. Spine   ISBN 2-84299-415-9

3. Shoulder   ISBN 2-84299-416-7

4. Arm, Forearm and Elbow   ISBN 2-84299-417-5

5. Wrist and Hand   ISBN 2-84299-439-6

6. Pelvic Ring and Hip   ISBN 2-84299-440-X

7. Femur and Knee   ISBN 2-84299-441-8

8. Lower Leg, Ankle and Foot   ISBN 2-84299-442-6

8 volume collection (full set)   ISBN 2-84299-443-4

Also available: the prestigious 4 volume Hardbound Package. Attractive loose-leaf binders allow continual updating. Includes quarterly updates and Internet access to the full text articles. For further information, please contact Editions Scientifiques et Médicales Elsevier or see: www.surgical-techniques-efort.com or www.elsevier.fr.

© 2003 Éditions scientifiques et médicales Elsevier SAS. Tous droits réservés. All rights reserved
23, rue Linois, 75724 Paris cedex 15, France
http://www.elsevier.fr – http://www.surgical-techniques-efort.com

Printed by SGIM, 10, rue du Parc, Parc Industriel Euronord, 31150 Bruguières, France

Bookbinding by Atenor, 11, rue de Lutèce, 78500 Sartrouville, France

Imprimé par SGIM, 10, rue du Parc, Parc Industriel Euronord, 31150 Bruguières, France

Façonnage par Atenor, 11, rue de Lutèce, 78500 Sartrouville, France

Dépôt légal N° : 03-557 - Janvier 2003   ISBN : 2-84299-416-7

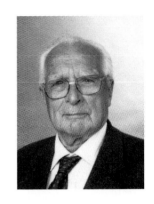

Preface

First and above all, this collection dedicated to surgical techniques in orthopaedics and traumatology is truly European.

It is published under the auspices of the European Federation of National Associations of Orthopaedics and Traumatology (EFORT), which at present groups 35 national associations. The creation of EFORT in 1992 resulted from the wish to form a European orthopaedic community. This has been made all the more important by the need to organise and standardise the training and qualifications of all European orthopaedists, according to the requirements and advice of the orthopaedic section of the European Union of Medical Specialists (UEMS).

Over the past 30 years, Europe has reclaimed its position among the leaders in the development of orthopaedics and traumatology. There has been a great deal of creativity. Among the many new contributions, we can mention the progress in osteosynthesis techniques due to the intramedullary nailing developed by Küntscher and the methods of internal fixation for fractures invented and developed mainly in Switzerland. The development of total joint replacement in the United Kingdom has revolutionised our field. Mention must also be made of the original ideas of Ilizarov, which were introduced and developed by the Italian School. We should add the Swedish National Survey of Hip and Knee Arthroplasties, initiated by the late Goran Bauer and continued by Peter Herberts, and the contributions to treatment of spinal pathology by R. Roy Camille and J. Dubousset of France. The above list is far from complete and will grow as new advances are made.

There is no doubt that Europe has an important role to play in the future of orthopaedics and traumatology.

This extraordinary growth and the development of increasingly sophisticated techniques in our field has made teaching and training more arduous. It has been suggested that the knowledge required by a general orthopaedic surgeon has increased 40 times over the past 40 years.

For all these reasons, EFORT decided to publish a collection covering the surgical techniques for all aspects of locomotor pathology in adults and children, without excluding non-operative treatment.

Thanks to the Editorial Board of EFORT, I have the honour - and also the very heavy responsibility - to be Editor of this work. For such a task, a large team was necessary, the members of which are listed at the end of this preface.

The collection is divided into eight sections, each under the responsibility of one or more Associate Editors. They have played an important part in selecting and contacting the contributing authors, in reviewing and coordinating the manuscripts. I must warmly thank these Associate Editors, who have accepted to undertake this additional work along with their surgical practice. They have played an essential role in its creation and publication.

The first section, "General Knowledge", is devoted to the general problems encountered in the practice of orthopaedic surgery: anaesthesia, prevention of deep venous thrombosis and infection, bone grafts, etc. The seven sections that follow concern the anatomical sites: the spine; shoulder; arm, elbow and forearm; hand and wrist; hip and pelvis; femur and knee; lower leg, ankle and foot.

It must be emphasised that this collection does not represent the work of a single group, school or institution, but rather results from the contributions of specialists and leaders in their fields throughout Europe. This explains its diversity. This collection is naturally written in English, which, as John Goodfellow put it, is the "new Esperanto" permitting scientific communication.

Each article must be considered as a separate entity and can be read without referring to the others. This has lead to some unavoidable overlapping, which we have tried to reduce to a minimum.

Most of the articles are devoted mainly to the surgical techniques themselves, which are described step by step and copiously illustrated. Variations of the techniques are discussed, as well as complications and clinical results. Some articles devote more discussion to the indications when this is necessary for the choice of treatment.

In general, the articles largely cover current orthopaedic practices. Most of these have already been widely tested by the orthopaedic community. Nevertheless, some articles discuss newer techniques, such as meniscal allograft transplantation, computerised pedicular screw fixation, video-assisted anterior approach to the spine, etc. It seems appropriate to include these new techniques which are already known to a large public but which have not yet been tested by time.

There are now two presentations of this collection. The first is the prestigious 4-volume, loose-leaf Hardbound Package which includes quarterly updates and access to the articles on Internet. The second, this edition, is divided into eight paperback volumes which may be purchased separately, allowing the specialised orthopaedic surgeon to select those parts of the collection devoted to his daily activities.

Many thanks to the editorial team at Elsevier - Sylvie Vercken, Agnès Brunel, Evelyne Lambert and Annabel Courage. I cannot too deeply express my appreciation to Gregg Colin for her assistance in the preparation of the manuscripts. Without her help, this publication would not have been possible.

Most of all, I would like to thank the authors and the Associate Editors who have contributed their time and their expertise to create this publication.

Jacques Duparc
Editor

The aim of EFORT, the European Federation of National Associations of Orthopaedics and Traumatology, is to promote science and education in the field of orthopaedics and traumatology.

The EFORT collection "Surgical Techniques in Orthopaedics and Traumatology", first published in 2000, was therefore a major step forward in demonstrating the great variety of European orthopaedic techniques.

Thanks to the unstinting work of Professor J. Duparc and the entire editorial board, in the short time since this collection has been launched it has attained a place in all the major European libraries. The next important step is the introduction of the new paperback edition. This will allow our orthopaedic colleagues who have specialised in a specific field to focus on one or several topics in which they are particularly interested.

On behalf of EFORT, I also want to thank the publisher, Elsevier, who accepted to join us in this editorial adventure to enhance orthopaedic operative techniques in Europe.

Nikolaus Böhler
President
European Federation of National Associations
of Orthopaedics and Traumatology (EFORT)

Patronage Committee

EFORT   Jacques Duparc, Michael A R Freeman, Erwin Morscher, Otto Sneppen, Paolo Gallinaro, Nikolaus Böhler

UEMS   Rafael Esteve de Miguel, Marc Speeckaert

Scientific Committee

Jacques Duparc, George Bentley, Henri Dorfmann, John Kenwright, Roger Lemaire, Frantisek Makai, Antonio Navarro, Panayotis N Soucacos, Nikolaus Böhler, Joachem Eulert, Frantz Langlais, Lars Lidgren, Pier Giorgio Marchetti, Wolfhart Puhl, Tibor Vízkelety

Editor

Jacques Duparc, MD, Professor
Honorary Chairman of Orthopaedic Department
Hôpital Bichat
Paris, France

Associate Editors

1. General Knowledge

Roger Lemaire, MD
Professor and Chairman
Department of Orthopaedic and Trauma Surgery
University Hospital
Liège, Belgium

2. Spine

Claus Carstens, MD
Head of Department
Paediatric Orthopaedics
Orthopaedic Hospital, University of Heidelberg
Heidelberg, Germany

Alain Deburge, MD
Professor, Department of Orthopaedics and Traumatology
Hôpital Beaujon
Clichy, France

3. Shoulder

Mario Randelli, MD
Professor
Istituto Clinico Humanitas
Milan, Italy

Jens-Ole Søjbjerg, MD, Professor
Department of Orthopaedics
University Hospital of Aarhus
Aarhus, Denmark

Jón Karlsson, MD, PhD
Department of Orthopaedics
Sahlgrenska University Hospital/Östra
Göteborg, Sweden

4. Arm, Forearm and Elbow

Norbert Gschwend, Prof Dr med
Orthopaedic Department
Schulthess Klinik
Zurich, Switzerland

Piet M. Rozing, MD
Department of Orthopaedic Surgery
Leiden University Medical Center
Leiden, The Netherlands

5. Wrist and Hand

Jean-Yves Alnot, MD, Professor
Chief of Orthopaedic Department
Upper Limb and Nerve Surgery Unit
Hôpital Bichat
Paris, France

Panayotis Soucacos, MD, FACS
Professor and Chairman
Department of Orthopaedic Surgery
University of Ioannina School of Medecine
Ioannina, Greece

6. Pelvic Ring and Hip

André Kaelin, MD
Paediatric Orthopaedic Unit
Hôpital des Enfants
Geneva, Switzerland

Erwin Morscher, MD, Professor
Felix Platter Hospital
Basel, Switzerland

Pär Slätis, MD, Professor
Orthopaedic Hospital of the Invalid Foundation – Helsinki
Grankulla, Finland

Roberto Giacometti Ceroni, MD
Istituto Galcazzi
Milan, Italy

7. Femur and Knee

Paul Aichroth, MD, MS FRCS
Emeritus Consultant Orthopaedic Surgeon
Knee Surgery Unit, The Wellington Hospital
London, United Kingdom

John Fixsen, MA, M.Chir, FRCS
Department of Orthopaedic Surgery
Great Ormond Street Hospital for Chidrren
London, United Kingdom

René Verdonk, MD, PhD
Department of Orthopaedic Surgery
Ghent University Hospital,
Ghent, Belgium

Ate Wymenga, MD
Knee Reconstruction Unit
Sint Maartenskliniek
Nijmegen, The Netherlands

8. Lower Leg, Ankle and Foot

Tomás Epeldegui Torre, MD, PhD
Hospital Nino Jesus
Madrid, Spain

Nikolaus Wülker, MD, Professor
Orthopaedic Department
Orthopädische Klinik und Poliklinik
Tubigen, Germany

Table of Contents
Volume 3 - Shoulder
Surgical Techniques in Orthopaedics and Traumatology

Preface

Table of Contents - Volume 3

Participating authors

The shoulder: anterior approaches (L Neumann,
IA De Almeida Filho) 55-160-A-10

The shoulder: superior and posterior approaches
(D Goutallier, JM Postel, P Leguilloux, L Petitclerc) 55-160-B-10

Shoulder arthroscopy (F Gòmez-Castresana Bachiller,
J Tena Arregui, FA Peña Gòmez) 55-160-C-10

Fractures of the clavicle (P Wiger, J Karlsson) 55-160-D-10

Acromioclavicular dislocations (J Eulert, TD Böhm) 55-160-E-10

Sternoclavicular dislocations (M Vastamäki). 55-170-A-10

Osteosynthesis of intra-articular fractures of the proximal
humerus (H Resch, P Povacz, R Schwaiger). 55-170-B-10

Shoulder prostheses: generalities and main designs
(F Duparc, J Duparc). 55-170-C-10

Hemi-arthroplasty (PM Rozing). 55-170-D-10

Total shoulder arthroplasty (IG Kelly) 55-170-E-10

Prosthetic treatment of fractures of the proximal humerus
(M Randelli). 55-180-A-10

Recurrent anterior shoulder instability: the Bankart procedure
(SA Copeland, R Emery) 55-180-B-10

Treatment of recurrent anterior instability: Latarjet-Bristow
procedure (G Walch, P Boileau) 55-180-C-10

Recurrent anterior instability: the arthroscopic techniques
(R Minola, G Zambonin) 55-180-D-10

Recurrent anterior instability of the shoulder:
the capsuloplasties (M Mansat) 55-180-E-10

Multidirectional instability of the shoulder (PP Symeonides). 55-190-A-10

Chronic posterior dislocations of the shoulder (M Randelli,
PL Gambrioli) 55-190-B-10

Arthroscopic subacromial decompression (ASAD)
(U Jonsson-Lillkrona, B Salomonsson). 55-190-C-10

Open anterior acromioplasty (F Postacchini, S Gumina) 55-190-D-10

Rotator cuff tears: the arthroscopic techniques (JF Kempf,
F Bonnomet). 55-190-E-10

Rotator cuff tears: the open technique (DF Gazielly) 55-200-A-10

Rheumatoid arthritis of the shoulder (JF Loehr, N Gschwend) 55-200-B-10

Massive rotator cuff tears: the musculo-tendinous transfer
(A Schneeberger, C Gerber) 55-200-C-10

Shoulder arthrodesis (B Wittner, U Holz). 55-200-D-10

Late sequelae at the shoulder in obstetrical palsy in children
(R Birch) 55-200-E-10

Early sequelae of the shoulder in obstetrical palsy (A Gilbert) 55-210-A-10

Paralytic shoulder in the adult (L Celli, C Rovesta,
MC Marongiu, A Celli) 55-210-B-10

Nerve entrapments around the shoulder (M Vastamäki). 55-210-B-40

Congenital elevation of the scapula (Sprengel's deformity)
(J Le Saout) 55-210-C-10

Conservative surgery for oncological pathology
of the shoulder (A Taminiau) 55-210-D-10

Forequarter amputation (W Winkelmann) 55-210-E-10

Index - Volume 3

Participating Authors
Volume 3 - Shoulder
Surgical Techniques in Orthopaedics and Traumatology

Birch R	55-200-E-10	Gschwend N	55-200-B-10	Povacz P	55-170-B-10
Böhm TD	55-160-E-10	Gumina S	55-190-D-10	Randelli M	55-180-A-10
Boileau P	55-180-C-10	Holz U	55-200-D-10		55-190-B-10
Bonnomet F	55-190-E-10	Jonsson-Lilkrona U	55-190-C-10	Resch H	55-170-B-10
Celli A	55-210-B-10	Karlsson J	55-160-D-10	Rovesta C	55-210-B-10
Celli L	55-210-B-10	Kelly IG	55-170-E-10	Rozing PM	55-170-D-10
Copeland SA	55-180-B-10	Kempf JF	55-190-E-10	Salomonsson B	55-190-C-10
De Almeida Filho IA	55-160-A-10	Le Saout J	55-210-C-10	Schneeberger A	55-200-C-10
Duparc F	55-170-C-10	Leguilloux P	55-160-B-10	Schwaiger R	55-170-B-10
Duparc J	55-170-C-10	Loehr JF	55-200-B-10	Symeonides PP	55-190-A-10
Emery R	55-180-B-10	Mansat M	55-180-E-10	Taminiau A	55-210-D-10
Eulert J	55-160-E-10	Marongui MC	55-210-B-10	Tena Arregui J	55-160-C-10
Gambrioli PL	55-190-B-10	Minola R	55-180-D-10	Vastamäki M	55-170-A-10
Gazielly DF	55-200-A-10	Neumann L	55-160-A-10		55-210-B-40
Gerber C	55-200-C-10	Peña Gómez F	55-160-C-10	Walch G	55-180-C-10
Gilbert A	55-210-A-10	Petitclerc L	55-160-B-10	Wiger P	55-160-D-10
Gómez-Castresana		Postacchini F	55-190-D-10	Winkelmann W	55-210-E-10
Bachiller F	55-160-C-10	Postel JM	55-160-B-10	Wittner B	55-200-D-10
Goutailler D	55-160-B-10			Zambonin G	55-180-D-10

The shoulder: anterior approaches

L Neumann
IA De Almeida Filho

Abstract. – Many surgical procedures at the shoulder require an anterior approach. As important anatomical structures are close by, an intimate knowledge of the anatomy of the region is absolutely necessary to avoid complications. To obtain a cosmetically acceptable scar, the use of skin tension lines as a guide to the incision is recommended. Pre-operative planning is necessary to select the most appropriate approach for a procedure so as to allow adequate access.

The standard deltopectoral approach is an anatomically attractive way of exposing the anterior aspect of the shoulder, particularly for surgical treatment of shoulder instability.

The extended deltopectoral approach is more suitable for joint replacement surgery of the shoulder and for internal fixation of fractures. For more extensive exposure and particularly to gain access to the superior and posterior part of the rotator cuff and improve access to the glenoid, the modified extensile approach is recommended.

For rotator cuff surgery, limited approach fracture fixation and acromioplasties, the anterolateral approach via a deltoid split is usually sufficient.

It is useful to be able to expose the acromioclavicular joint and the coracoid process via specific approaches.

Keywords: shoulder, surgical approach, anterior approach, extended deltopectoral approach.

Introduction

The majority of pathologies requiring surgical treatment in the shoulder joint complex are accessible from an anterior or anterolateral approach. Therefore those who carry out shoulder surgery need to be familiar with the anatomy of this region, so that the appropriate incision for each individual patient can be chosen. The incision must allow adequate exposure, but also respect the anatomy of the region and the position of the scar must be considered from a cosmetic point of view. Large and important neurovascular structures are located very close to the shoulder joint complex, particularly the axillary and the musculocutaneous nerves. The brachial plexus is also close, and severe complications can arise if any of these structures are injured. Furthermore, the shoulder anatomy is complex and if the surgeon causes unnecessary tissue damage

Lars Neumann, FRCS(Ed), Consultant Orthopaedic Surgeon.
Ildeu Afonso De Almeida Filho, Shoulder Fellow to Prof. WA Wallace and Mr. L Neumann.
The Nottingham Shoulder and Elbow Unit, Nottingham City Hospital, Nottingham NG5 1PB, United Kingdom.

during his approach, complications from adhesions, scarring or fibrosis, can cause stiffness and pain. A disappointing outcome of an otherwise well indicated procedure can be the result. The biomechanics of the shoulder joint complex are complicated, and normal function depends on all of its components - joints, muscles, tendons and neurovascular structures - being in an optimal state.

The shoulder region is notorious for producing very unsightly scars, both hypertrophic, keloid and atrophic, widened ones [17]. The surgeon should therefore plan his incision in such a way as to allow for the scar to heal as well as possible. Skin tension lines [4] are recommended as guidelines for the direction of the incision, and it is worthwhile placing the incision in an area where it can be concealed by the patient's clothes, underwear straps, etc. It is usually possible to achieve this by considering the surgical approach carefully and by using intracuticular stitches, thus avoiding stitch marks. We often use a "bra-strap" incision. The position of the patient's underwear straps are outlined with a marker pen pre-operatively, thereby ensuring the incision is placed where it may be easily concealed.

Approaches

THE STANDARD DELTOPECTORAL APPROACH

▪ Introduction

This approach is probably the most commonly used for the shoulder. It is performed for procedures such as anterior stabilisation of shoulder instability and to access pathologies around the coracoid process, the biceps tendon and the subscapularis muscle and tendon. Fractures of the anterior glenoid, coracoid process and some proximal humeral fractures can be also approached this way.

▪ Approach

We prefer not to use a direct axillary approach as we find this access less satisfactory, although this approach is definitely preferable cosmetically. A relatively distal skin incision is made, starting about 2 to 3 cm distal to the tip of the coracoid and following the tension lines towards the axilla for a distance of about 5 to 6 cm. This incision is cosmetically acceptable to most patients, as with the arm adducted the scar will be barely visible (fig 1).

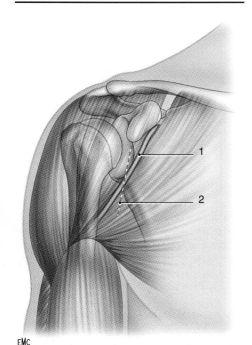

1 *Skin incision for the standard deltopectoral approach. 1. Cephalic vein; 2. line of incision.*

To allow adequate mobilisation and access, it is necessary to undermine the skin surrounding the incision and dissect the subcuticular tissue from the fascia of the deltoid and the pectoralis major for some distance - usually about 3 cm. Once this has been done the landmark of the deltopectoral interval, the cephalic vein, must be identified. It is usually easily found, as it is situated in the fat strip separating the deltoid and the pectoralis major muscles. However, in muscular individuals with little fat, the edges of the two muscles are often almost merged, and it can be very difficult to identify the groove. There are some useful guidelines for locating its position. Proximally, the interval between the muscles will be 1 to 2 cm medial to the tip of the coracoid. Distally it is identified with more ease, as the muscles are usually more clearly separated from each other at this level and the vein is more superficial in the fat tissue. It is important to enter through the interval and not to carry out a split of the medial part of the deltoid muscle. This will result in a division of the terminal branches of the axillary nerve, leading to loss of some function of this important muscle.

Once the cephalic vein has been identified, it can be retracted medially or laterally as the surgeon prefers. It is usually easier to retract it laterally, as there are hardly ever any veins from the pectoralis major draining into the cephalic vein. All that is needed is dissection along the lateral border of the pectoralis major muscle to mobilise the vein and identify the clavipectoral fascia. There are usually several vessels draining the deltoid muscles into the cephalic vein [19]. These veins can be identified with relative ease by careful dissection, and cauterised, allowing the vein to be retracted medially should this be preferred. We routinely retract

the vein medially, as dissection is simple and the vein is better protected. The vein should only be ligated if it is damaged during the procedure. We prefer to sacrifice the small veins from the deltoid in exchange for a preserved cephalic vein. In more extensive anterior approaches, the vein usually has to be retracted medially as its proximal path is directed under the pectoralis major muscle, a few centimetres distal to the clavicle. It is quite easy to damage it if it undergoes stretching when pulled laterally with the deltoid.

Once the interval has been opened, the white clavipectoral fascia becomes visible. At this stage, it is a great help to introduce a narrow Hohmann's retractor over the top of the coracoid process. The distally placed skin incision with the undermined subcuticular tissue will be moved proximally, allowing good access to the upper part of the subcapularis muscle. The clavipectoral fascia is now split, allowing the lateral margin of the conjoined tendon to be identified.

The conjoined tendon consists of the coracobrachialis and the short head of the biceps muscles. The lateral margin of this tendon is made up of muscle fibres and is not tendinous. Care should therefore be taken not to start the dissection along the very clearly visible tendon tissue, which is some distance from the true lateral margin of the tendon. Once this margin has been clearly defined it is easy, after opening the fascia, to release the tendon by blunt dissection from the underlying bursa. The surgeon can be assured of the proximity of the brachial plexus by placing a finger underneath the conjoined tendon. The plexus can usually be palpated 2 to 3 cm medially. Particular attention should be paid to protecting the musculocutaneous nerve, which enters the deep surface of the conjoined tendon at very variable distances from the tip of the coracoid process. We have seen musculocutaneous nerves enter the conjoined tendon less than 2 cm from the tip of the coracoid, and recommend that the nerve be always identified if mobilisation of the conjoined tendon and the coracoid tip is required.

If a coracoid osteotomy is not carried out, the anterior part of the coraco-acromial ligament can be released close to its insertion on the coracoid tip. This gives easier access to the top of the shoulder and, in particular, to the rotator interval. A similar release can be done at the lateral part of the conjoined tendon with an incision of about 5 to 8 mm into the tendon at a level of 5 mm distal to the coracoid tip *(fig 2A)*. This release is easy to repair during closure, and greatly improves access.

It is important to have good self-retaining retractors available, to retract the deltoid to one side and the conjoined tendons to the other. Several excellent retractors are available. We prefer the Kölbel ratchet type retractor with interchangeable blades for

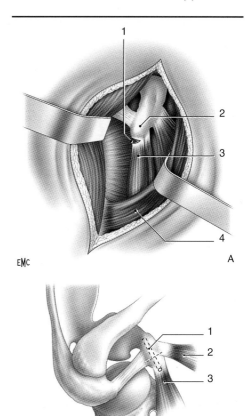

2 *A. Release of the lateral part of the conjoined tendon. 1. Release of conjoined tendon; 2. tip of coracoid process; 3. conjoined tendon. 4. pectoralis major.*
B. Drillhole and line of osteotomy of the coracoid process. 1. Coracoid process with drill hole and line of osteotomy; 2. pectoralis minor muscle; 3. conjoined tendon.

different tissue thicknesses, as it is extremely flexible and allows excellent exposure.

If the surgeon needs to approach the anterior aspect of the scapular neck, if he is carrying out surgery on patients with a medialised glenoid joint surface or very deformed joint, or if he wants to reconstruct anterior glenoid defects with a Bristow-Latarjet type procedure [7, 8], it is useful to carry out a coracoid osteotomy which allows for a more extensive exposure. The coracoid process has a very complex shape, curved in two planes, and the surgeon must be certain he has identified the exact orientation of the process by palpating its upper and deep surfaces. If the process has to be reattached later, it can be of help to pre-drill it before carrying out the osteotomy. The drill is introduced into the bone under careful guidance with a finger along the upper surface of the process. The hole is in the correct position if it is started right at the tip of the coracoid and if a bone depth of at least 30-35 mm is achieved. After predrilling, pre-tapping (we use a half-threaded 4 mm cancellous AO screw) and depth gauging the drill hole, the coracoid tip is osteotomised about 1 to 1.5 cm from its tip using an oscillating saw *(fig 2B)*. (If a coracoid transfer procedure is carried out, a slightly larger part of the coracoid should be detached). In our experience an osteotome is not ideal for this procedure as it tends to fracture the cortex of the coracoid process as it exits on the deep surface.

During reattachment of the coracoid process, complications can occur such as a fracture of the detached tip. Non-unions can be seen if good apposition has not been achieved.

In some cases it is not necessary to carry out further mobilisation of the conjoined tendon, as the osteotomy of the coracoid tip allows the tendon to be deflected medially about 2 cm. If a formal mobilisation is necessary, for instance if the surgeon wants to carry out a Bristow-Latarjet procedure, he then has to identify the musculocutaneous nerve by very careful dissection on the deep surface of the conjoined tendon. The nerve is of a relatively heavy calibre but cannot always be palpated directly so care must be taken. The nerve is then released from the conjoined tendon, as far down as necessary, to allow the tendon to be mobilised as required for the procedure in question. If inadequate release is performed, stretching of the nerve can result, leading to neuropraxia or even permanent nerve injury.

Once the retractor has been introduced between the conjoined tendon and the deltoid, the surgeon can identify the musculotendinous junction of the subscapularis muscle. This is done with the arm in external rotation, and the long head of the biceps tendon is used as a landmark to identify the lateral margin of the lesser tuberosity, in particular in cases where the anatomy is not straightforward, such as in open reduction of posterior dislocations. Another important landmark in this region is the rotator interval (between the subscapularis and supraspinatus) which is usually easy to palpate close and deep to the coraco-acromial ligament where the thick tendinous superior edge of the subscapularis can be identified. The inferior boundary of the subscapularis is marked by two small vessels, branches of the anterior circumflex artery, which are almost always present about 5 mm from the lower margin of the tendon. These vessels are useful landmarks but often have to be coagulated during the mobilisation of the subscapularis *(fig 3)*.

It has been shown that it is safe to split the subscapularis up to 6 cm medial to its insertion, without putting the subscapular nerve at risk [5]. This is anatomically an attractive way of approaching the joint capsule and requires less protection during post-operative rehabilitation than division of the muscle. The split is usually carried out at the junction of the upper two-thirds and the lower one-third of the muscle by blunt dissection with scissors *(fig 3)*. Once the white joint capsule is visible, a two-point retractor (Jackson Burrows) can be inserted and a capsulotomy can be carried out. Before the capsulotomy is performed, a retractor should always be passed along the antero-inferior joint capsule, retracting the

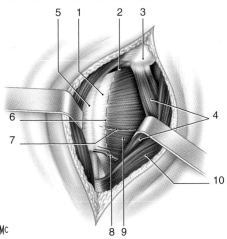

3 *Landmarks for subscapularis division or subscapularis split. 1. Subscapularis tendon; 2. rotator interval; 3. coracoid process; 4. conjoined tendon; 5. long head of biceps tendon; 6. suggested tenotomy line; 7. suggested level for subscapularis split; 8. vessels on subscapularis surface marking lower limit of tenotomy; 9. subscapularis muscle; 10. pectoralis major muscle.*

inferior part of the subscapularis and thus protecting the axillary nerve which is very close.

We usually prefer to divide the subscapularis vertically, just lateral to its musculotendinous junction, as this gives a better exposure, particularly of the inferior aspect of the glenoid rim, and it allows for suture anchors to be optimally positioned in Bankart repairs. Before the division is carried out the subscapularis muscle must always be secured with two stay sutures. This allows the surgeon to retain control of the muscle during the procedure and facilitates subsequent repair. When the tendon is divided within its tendinous part, the subsequent repair is very strong and allows early mobilisation. Dividing the subscapularis more medially in the muscle tissue denervates the part of the muscle lateral to the division, and the sutures used for the repair are in risk of pulling out of the weak muscle tissue, if put under load. The division should include all the upper, thick tendinous parts of the subscapularis, extending as far down as the two aforementioned vessels. In addition, leaving the lower fibres of the muscle intact provides protection of the axillary nerve. The nerve should also be protected by a retractor, as described above, as soon as the lower aspect of the joint capsule has been exposed - axillary nerve lesions are serious complications and must be avoided. The level of the shoulder joint capsule, deep to the subscapularis muscle, as well as the thickness of the muscle, can usually be gauged inferiorly in the division by blunt dissection through the muscle at the musculotendineous junction as, at this level, the muscle separates easily from the capsule. If dissection is carried out with the capsule under tension, i.e. with the arm in external rotation, there is less risk of damaging the capsule. The subscapularis tendon is carefully divided either by diathermy or

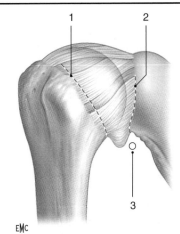

4 *Lines of capsulotomies for medial or lateral approaches to the joint. 1. Suggested line of capsulotomy for Neer's capsular shift; 2. suggested line of capsulotomy for Bankart repair; 3. axillary nerve.*

using a scalpel. When the division reaches the capsule, the tissue quite evidently changes from tendon fibres into the smooth texture of the capsule. Once the tendon has been divided from superior to inferior, it can be released from the capsule using blunt dissection with, for example, a periosteal elevator, while maintaining external rotation and tension of the joint capsule.

Depending on which surgical procedure is to be carried out in the joint, the surgeon will have to decide where to perform the capsulotomy: 1) along the glenoid rim, which is indicated for procedures such as Bankart repairs [2, 3, 15] and for modified capsular shifts [1], or 2) a lateral capsulotomy for a Neer's capsular shift [13] or for other procedures in joints without a Bankart lesion *(fig 4)*.

■ *Closure*

The closure should be carried out in such a way that anatomy is restored as closely as possible to normal, and which allows early mobilisation. The shoulder will scar up very easily if immobilised postoperatively for a prolonged period, and an inferior outcome will result. The cosmetic aspect must also be borne in mind.

The capsule is closed with No. 1 Vicryl® mattress sutures, if a lateral capsular shift or a simple arthrotomy has been carried out. If a medial arthrotomy for a medial capsular shift or a Bankart repair has been the procedure, the capsulotomy will be closed when the Bankart lesion is repaired. The surgeon has to remember that often the upper part of the capsule is very thin, or has defects where the joint communicates with the subcoracoid and subscapular bursa, and care has to be taken when repairing any such defects. By doing so, it is possible to overtighten the joint, so once completed, the repair of the capsule should be tested to ensure that an adequate range of shoulder movement is possible.

If the subscapularis has been split, this only needs to be approximated with one or two interrupted Vicryl® No. 1 sutures. If the subscapularis has been divided the repair is carried out using Vicryl® No. 1 mattress sutures; usually a total of 4 or 5 is necessary. The repair should be end to end and no overlap or shortening should be attempted. By doing so, there is a high risk of distorting the muscle balance of the shoulder and creating a stiff joint, limiting external rotation in particular. The upper, thick tendinous part of the subscapularis should always be identified and carefully closed. If the rotator interval is widened, it may be indicated to close it with interrupted Vicryl® sutures as part of the procedure.

If a coracoid osteotomy has been carried out, the musculocutaneous nerve is checked, and the tip of the coracoid is reattached with a screw. The way the osteotomy has been carried out allows for an anatomical reattachment. Care must be taken not to overtighten the screw and cause a fracture of the coracoid tip. This is difficult to repair and this complication can lead to non-union and painful, lasting fragmentation of the coracoid tip.

If the conjoined tendon has been released, it is repaired with one Vicryl® No. 1 mattress suture.

The deltopectoral interval is closed with one or two loosely applied 2-0 Vicryl® sutures. This prevents a lasting widened interval and, in patients with little sub-cuticular fat, an unsightly defect.

The subcuticular tissue is closed with interrupted 2-0 Vicryl® sutures.

We prefer to use No. 2 Prolene® sutures intracuticularly as stitch marks are avoided. Even if the scar should become widened or keloid, it will at least be linear, and if corrective surgery is later required, less skin will have to be excised to remove the scar. The skin suture is further supported with Steristrips®.

THE EXTENDED DELTOPECTORAL APPROACH

■ *Introduction*

Neer, Watson and Stanton [12] described this approach, and it is probably the most commonly used for indications such as glenohumeral arthroplasty and reconstruction of the upper humerus following fractures. We use this approach with some slight modification for hemiarthroplasty and for fixation of fractures in particular.

■ *Approach*

The incision is 15 to 17 cm long, starting just above the tip of the coracoid, and follows the medial margin of the deltoid towards its insertion on the humerus. It is taken laterally and distal to the anterior axillary fold *(fig 5)*.

After mobilisation of the skin and the subcuticular tissues surrounding the skin incision, the deltopectoral groove and the

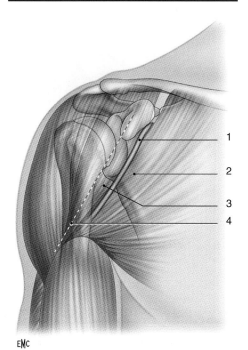

5   *Skin incision for the extended deltopectoral approach. 1. cephalic vein; 2. pectoralis major muscle; 3. deltoid muscle; 4. line of incision.*

cephalic vein are identified, as described for the standard deltopectoral approach.

We prefer to bring the cephalic vein medially, although this requires slightly more dissection. However, once the vein has been mobilised this way, it can be very well protected and is less likely to suffer any damage during the procedure. If the vein is retracted laterally, it will still be possible to access the upper humerus and the sub-acromial area but, in our experience, by doing so, the risk of damaging the vein is greater. The considerations discussed in the previous section also apply to this approach.

After exposure and opening of the clavipectoral fascia, the anterior deltoid muscle can be freed from the underlying bursa. It is usually easier to enter the bursa just anterior to the coraco-acromial ligament, and from this point slide a retractor behind the humeral head, inside the bursa. By doing so, the superficial part of the bursa is left on the deltoid, no formal dissection is necessary and the risk of damaging the axillary nerve on the deep surface of the deltoid is reduced. In this approach, if the deltoid is very tight, release of the anterior part of its distal insertion on the humerus can be performed. It is of the utmost importance that the intended procedure should be performed comfortably through the approach, as forceful pulling and retracting of the anterior deltoid results in a traction injury to the fragile, often thin, deltoid muscle, and leads to a poorly functioning deltoid. The surgeon must therefore be prepared to extend this approach to allow sufficient exposure.

With the arm in external rotation, the long head of the biceps is identified, and the subscapularis is divided close to the lesser

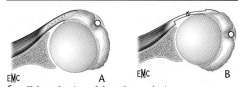

6   *Z-lengthening of the subscapularis.*
A. Z-shaped incision dividing the subscapularis.
B. The joint capsule is sutured to the lateral end of the subscapularis tendon.

tuberosity. In cases with marked contracture and loss of external rotation, it is advisable to dissect the subscapularis tendon off the tuberosity. This facilitates subscapularis lengthening during closure, by reattachment of the tendon more medially on the lesser tuberosity. Alternatively, the tendon may be divided in a Z-shaped manner, which also allows lengthening to take place during closure *(fig 6A)*. The division/detachment should extend from the rotator interval superiorly, and almost to the inferior aspect of the muscle. At this point, the axillary nerve is close and we advise the surgeon to palpate it and then introduce a retractor on the antero-inferior joint capsule. This will retract and protect the inferior fibres of the muscle and the nerve.

The pectoralis major muscle is often tight and contracted and can restrict the important external rotation movement. To improve access, and to provide more movement, it is often useful to divide the upper 1 to 1.5 cm of the tendon near its insertion on the humerus.

The coraco-acromial ligament can be partly released or divided, depending on the need for access. If it is divided we recommend it be repaired afterwards, to reconstruct the coraco-acromial arch.

The coraco-humeral ligament is usually tight and can be palpated easily with the arm in external rotation towards the base of the coracoid process. Releasing this ligament close to the base of the coracoid process is important in patients who have marked loss of external rotation.

The joint capsule is exposed underneath the divided subscapularis muscle when it is reflected medially. If there is an internal rotation contracture present, this approach enables the surgeon to lengthen the anterior soft tissues. He does this by carrying out the capsulotomy at a more medial level than the tenotomy, so the joint is approached via a Z-shaped incision. In some procedures, the capsule can be opened at the level of the tenotomy.

With the arm abducted and externally rotated, the joint can be dislocated. However, this places the axillary nerve at maximum risk and, to prevent accidental surgical nerve injury, it is important that the surgeon identify it by palpation and that a retractor be passed between the joint capsule proximally and the nerve, and remain there during the procedure. It has been suggested that this approach carries an increased risk of temporary neurological complications [9].

■ *Closure*

If a shoulder replacement has been inserted, the closure must be carried out in such a way as to provide adequate soft tissue cover of the implant, and give correct soft tissue balance. The general rule that it is important to close the approach in a way that ensures early mobilisation also applies to this approach.

Depending on the degree of contracture, the joint capsule is either repaired end to end or its lateral stump (which will be of some length if the joint was approached through a Z-shaped division of the subscapularis and joint capsule) is now sutured to the lateral end of the divided sub-scapularis tendon (*fig 6B*). This is carried out with interrupted No. 1 Vicryl® mattress sutures. If the tendon has been dissected off bone, a subscapularis lengthening can be achieved by reattaching the tendon in a more medial position, i.e. close to, or at the margin of, the osteotomy site on the humeral head. The rotator interval should be repaired so that any implant is fully covered by soft tissues. The interval should not be closed all the way to the base of the coracoid, as this will restrict movement of the arm [6]. The supraspinatus and subscapularis are supposed to slide on either side of the coracoid and, by carrying out the closure too far medially, this movement may not be possible.

If the coraco-acromial ligament has been divided, it should be repaired with Vicryl® sutures to restore the coraco-acromial arch. If this structure is not intact an important superior support for the humeral head is lost and superior subluxation, pain and poor function - particularly after a shoulder joint replacement - can result.

The remaining closure is as described for the deltopectoral approach.

THE MODIFIED ANTERIOR EXTENSILE APPROACH

■ *Introduction*

This approach was described by Redfern et al [16] and is our preferred approach for total shoulder joint replacements or for reconstruction procedures around the glenohumeral joint, such as osteotomies following malunions of the proximal humerus, or for hemiarthroplasties associated with rotator cuff reconstruction.

■ *Approach*

The incision is about 12 cm long starting just above the clavicle and extending in a straight line across the tip of the coracoid and down just lateral to the axillary fold but not distal to it (*fig 7*).

These subcuticular tissues are mobilised as described above.

In this approach the cephalic vein must always be retracted medially, otherwise it will have to be divided when the deltoid is reflected laterally after the clavicular osteotomy.

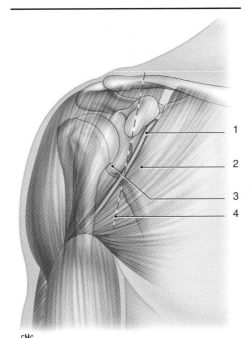

7 *Skin incision for the modified extensile approach. 1. cephalic vein; 2. pectoralis major muscle; 3. deltoid muscle; 4. line of incision.*

To allow for the clavicular osteotomy to be carried out, two artery clips are placed as retractors behind the clavicle, exposing the lateral third of the bone, one at the level of the medial border of the deltoid muscle, the other just medial to the acromioclavicular joint. If the acromioclavicular (AC) joint is not readily palpable, a hypodermic needle can be inserted into the joint to identify the joint line. The surgeon should be familiar with the relatively complex shape of the distal clavicle when he prepares the osteotomy. Using diathermy, a curved osteotomy line is marked along the anterior margin of the clavicle starting just medial to the joint and finishing at the level of the medial border of the insertion of the anterior deltoid. The intention is to osteotomise a thin sliver of bone - no more than 3-4 mm thick and always less than one-third of the width of the clavicle - with the attachment of the anterior deltoid. In some patients, particularly those with rheumatoid arthritis, the clavicle can be very narrow medially and the utmost care should be taken not to make the sliver too thick. The osteotomy line must be curved to avoid stress at the distal margins. We prefer to use an oscillating saw with a thin 12 mm wide saw blade. The blade must also be short to limit the excursion of the oscillations (*fig 8*). The osteotomy must be completed with the saw until the fragment of the anterior clavicle is mobile. No hammering or levering with instruments should be done, as this carries a risk of fracture of the clavicle. Once the osteotomy is completed the anterior deltoid is tacked with a stay suture.

When releasing the soft tissues underneath the osteotomised sliver of the clavicle, the surgeon will usually find a branch of the thoraco-acromial artery, which has to be

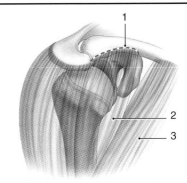

8 *Line of osteotomy of the anterior aspect of the lateral clavicle. 1. Line of osteotomy; 2. deltoid muscle; 3. pectoralis major muscle.*

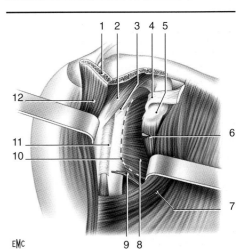

9 *Exposure of the anterior aspect of the humerus after clavicular osteotomy and release of the coraco-acromial ligament. 1. Osteomised fragment of anterolateral clavicle; 2. supraspinatus tendon; 3. rotator interval; 4. coraco-acromial ligament detached from acromion and deflected medially; 5. coracoid process; 6. partial tenotomy of the conjoined tendon. This partial tenotomy is optional, and not routine; 7. pectoralis major muscle; 8. subscapularis muscle; 9. vessels; 10. line of incision for lesser tuberosity osteotomy; 11. long head of biceps tendon; 12. anterior deltoid deflected laterally.*

cauterised. Occasionally the anterior part of the clavicular insertion of the coraco-clavicular ligament is attached to the osteotomised sliver and has to be released. At this stage a Hohmann's retractor can be placed behind the greater tuberosity inside the bursa, to deflect the anterior deltoid laterally and to expose the humeral head (*fig 9*).

As this approach is more anterosuperior than directly anterior, it often requires mobilisation of the coraco-acromial ligament. We detach it at its lateral insertion, as it is easier to re-attach it at this site during closure. The ligament is easily identified once the deltoid is reflected laterally and it can be seen in its full length. It is stripped off the acromion, using blunt dissection and a periosteal elevator. It is then tacked with a stay suture and reflected medially. If the ligament is detached at the coracoid insertion, it will not be possible to carry out an acromioplasty as such an additional procedure would lead to loss of the remaining insertion of the ligament, and the coraco-acromial arch would be impossible to reconstruct.

We prefer to carry out an osteotomy of the lesser tuberosity, rather than a tenotomy, as this allows a very strong repair, which permits immediate intensive rehabilitation. The disadvantage is that subscapularis lengthening around the insertion on the lesser tuberosity is not possible, and if required, release and mobilisation of the muscle have to be carried out at its medial end, along the anterior margin of the glenoid and the deep surface of the subscapularis. The osteotomy line is marked by diathermy about half a centimetre medial to the bicipital groove, extending from the lateral aspect of the rotator interval superiorly, to a level of the inferior fibres of the subscapularis inferiorly. The rotator interval is opened in a line from the proximal exit point of the osteotomy, towards the base of the coracoid, and the lesser tuberosity is osteotomised, using either an osteotome or an oscillating saw. Once the fragment with the sub-scapularis tendon attached to it has been elevated, it is tacked with two stay sutures, facilitating later mobilisation and manipulation.

When the lesser tuberosity has been reflected medially, the joint is opened via the osteotomy and the humeral head can be dislocated by release of the soft tissues inferiorly. This is done from inside the joint with a retractor placed deep to the inferior fibres of the subscapularis, to protect the axillary nerve. Release of the inferior capsule from the bone is almost always necessary. The whole procedure can be carried out with the arm in an adducted position, placing the axillary nerve in far less danger of damage than when the arm is abducted, as it is in the traditional extensile anterior approach.

■ *Closure*

This approach has been developed not only to provide better access during surgery, but also to make very strong tissue repair possible, thus allowing for early and intensive rehabilitation.

The lesser tuberosity and the subscapularis tendon with its insertion on bone are repaired back into the anatomical position from which they were osteotomised. The lesser tuberosity is fixed with two or three double loops of No. 2 Ethibond® sutures which are taken through the subscapularis tendon medially, around the fragment of the lesser tuberosity, and through the bone laterally, crossing the bicipital groove (*fig 10*). The sutures will not cut through the fragment, and the bicipital groove will prevent them from cheese wiring through the bone of the proximal humerus. This reinsertion is resistant to stress and allows immediate mobilisation, including external rotation.

When the lesser tuberosity is repaired back in its anatomical position, the split along the

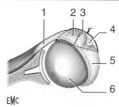

10 *Reattachment of the lesser tuberosity with transosseous sutures. 1. Subscapularis; 2. lesser tuberosity reattached; 3. osteotomy line; 4. long head of biceps tendon; 5. greater tuberosity; 6. humeral head.*

rotator interval should come together anatomically and it only needs to be closed with a couple of No. 1 Vicryl® mattress sutures. However as mentioned in the section on the extended delto-pectoral approach, the medial part of the interval should be left open to preserve mobility of the subscapularis and supraspinatus tendons on either side of the coracoid [6].

The coraco-acromial ligament is repaired back to the soft tissues at the front and under the surface of the acromion, just lateral to the acromioclavicular joint, using Vicryl® sutures. The ligament, which is normally very taught, cannot be repaired in a way that immediately restores tension. However, once healed, the coraco-acromial arc is reconstructed and we have found in revision operations that the ligament is an easily identifiable anatomical structure, which seems to have regained its previous tension.

To reattach the anterior deltoid, three double loops of No. 1 Vicryl® sutures are passed around the osteotomised fragment and round the clavicle as cerclages. It is better to use a blunt tipped needle, which slides on the bone, thereby avoiding catching any soft tissue during the passing of the suture. The most medial cerclage suture is close to the brachial plexus and the subclavian vein and there is a risk of damaging these structures if the technique is not followed strictly. The fragment should easily repair back into an anatomical position. This closure allows immediate mobilisation and no special precautions are needed to protect the deltoid during rehabilitation [10].

Remaining closure is as described for the approaches above.

ANTERO-LATERAL APPROACH (DELTOID SPLIT)

■ *Introduction*

To approach the rotator cuff, to carry out an open sub-acromial decompression or to fix fractures of the greater tuberosity, an approach through the antero-lateral aspect of the deltoid is useful. This can be made either as a simple split, or as a more extensive procedure requiring the release of the deltoid muscle from the anterior acromion.

■ *Approach*

A sagittal incision is performed, starting about 2 to 3 cm posterior to the anterior

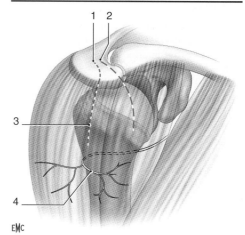

11 *Skin incision and line of deltoid split for the antero-lateral approach. 1. Line of division of soft tissues on acromion; 2. line of incision; 3. line of deltoid split; 4. axillary nerve.*

margin of the acromion and extending from 3 to 4 cm distal to its anterior margin depending on the surgeon's choice of procedure. The incision is just lateral to the AC joint (*fig 11*). At this site the scar will be easily concealed under clothes, and it follows the skin tension lines.

The fat is then released from the fascia of the deltoid and from the soft tissues overlying the acromion.

Between the anterior and lateral parts of the deltoid, there is usually an easily identifiable raphe. This is a useful landmark and by splitting the deltoid at this level, it is possible, depending on what is to be approached in the sub-acromial space, to detach either part of the deltoid anteriorly or laterally or both. If a mini open procedure is carried out, the deltoid is not detached from the acromion, and using blunt dissection, the muscle is split at the appropriate level in the direction of the fibres from its insertion on the acromion and distally. Usually a split of about 3 cm will suffice for a small procedure.

It is very important to remember that on the deep surface of the deltoid, some 5 cm distally to the acromion, the branches of the axillary nerve are located. If the split is extended too far distally and the nerve becomes damaged, any part of the deltoid anterior to the split will be denervated. To prevent the split from propagating during the procedure, it is useful to insert a temporary loose suture, bridging the distal end of the split.

If more extensive procedures, such as cuff repairs, are to be carried out, a release of the deltoid from its insertion on the acromion is often necessary. Our approach varies slightly to that originally described by Neer et al [14]. At the site of the raphe, where the deltoid split starts from the acromion, a retractor is placed through the deltoid split underneath the acromion, thus allowing depression of the humeral head and protection of the cuff during release of the deltoid. Cauterising is usually used to divide the soft tissues on the

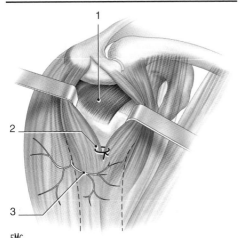

12 *Exposure of the lateral aspect of the humeral head via the deltoid split. 1. Rotator cuff exposed; 2. protective suture; 3. axillary nerve.*

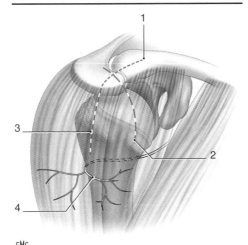

13 *Skin incision and line of division of deep tissues for an approach to the acromioclavicular joint and subacromial space. 1. Line of division of soft tissues on acromion and clavicle; 2. line of skin incision; 3. line of deltoid split; 4. axillary nerve.*

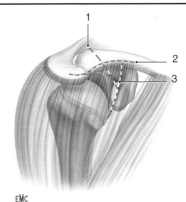

15 *Skin incision and division of deep tissues to approach the acromioclavicular joint and the coracoid process. 1. Line of skin incision; 2. line of division of soft tissues over acromion, acromioclavicular joint and clavicle. 3. line of deltoid split.*

cranial aspect of the acromion down to bone. The direction of this division must ensure the deltoid can be detached with its insertion and fibrous tissue on the cranial aspect of the acromion, leaving the soft tissues covering the acromion in continuity with the deltoid, both medial and lateral to the muscle split *(fig 12)*. This means that even a simple side to side closure of the gap will give the repair good strength immediately.

Using a No. 15 blade, the soft tissues are elevated from the bone anteriorly. We prefer not to use diathermy for this, as we believe that healing of the tissues will be quicker and stronger when the tissues have not been thermally damaged. The acromial end of the coraco-acromial ligament will be exposed when the deltoid medial to the split is mobilised. The ligament is detached from bone, using either a knife or Mayo's scissors, but it is not resected. There are often some bleeding vessels at the insertion and the surgeon should be prepared to cauterise this bleeding. Depending on the procedure undertaken, it may be necessary to perform a similar release of the deltoid insertion laterally, leaving the soft tissues on the acromion in continuity with the deltoid. The deltoid muscle is split in the direction of its fibres using blunt dissection. The precaution described above, to prevent axillary nerve damage, is particularly recommended in the more extensive deltoid splits.

Once the muscle is split and released, the white bursa will be exposed. In cases with inflammation in the subacromial space, the bursa can be very tight and thickened. Once the superficial layer of the bursa has been opened and the inside exposed, the surgeon can pass a finger over the top, front and back of the rotator cuff and tuberosities and free up any adhesions.

If a procedure on the subacromial space has to be carried out in conjunction with an acromioclavicular joint resection, the line of cauterisation of the soft tissues on the cranial aspect of the acromion is swung medially, to cross the AC joint at its centre line *(fig 13)*. The soft tissues including the superior

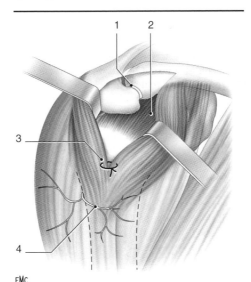

14 *Exposure of the acromioclavicular joint and the acromion. 1. Acromioclavicular joint exposed; 2. rotator cuff; 3. protective suture; 4. axillary nerve.*

acromioclavicular joint capsule and ligament can then be released, as previously described, with the soft tissues over the clavicle and acromion being left in continuity with the deltoid *(fig 14)*.

■ *Closure*

As for the other approaches to the shoulder, a strong repair, allowing early mobilisation, is important. Postoperative detachment of poor deltoid repair causes severe symptoms with pain and weakness with restricted elevation and must be avoided. Similarly, the soft tissues around the AC joint must be carefully repaired so as to stabilise the distal clavicle.

If the incision and the mobilisation of the deltoid muscle have been carried out appropriately, it is sometimes possible to close the deltoid and the soft tissues on the acromion directly side to side with a number of interrupted Vicryl® No. 1 mattress sutures. It is, however, usually

recommended to re-attach the anterior part of the deltoid to the acromion with No. 1 Vicryl® sutures passed through the deltoid insertion and the acromion bone, as this gives a much stronger reattachment. In most cases after acromioplasty, a needle can be passed, with no need for drill holes, from the deep surface of the acromion through bone, without any great force. If the acromioclavicular joint exposure has been carried out in addition to the anterior deltoid split, the soft tissues overlying the joint can be closed side to side with interrupted Vicryl® sutures.

APPROACH TO THE ACROMIOCLAVICULAR JOINT

■ *Introduction*

If the acromioclavicular joint or the distal clavicle is to be approached for excision of the AC joint or fixation of lateral fractures of the clavicle, we always use a sagittal incision. Coronal incisions, either along the clavicle or directly over it, tend to produce some extremely unsightly and widened scars, and if hardware has to be used, for instance for the fixation of a clavicle fracture, there is a risk of wound breakdown, leading to exposure of the metal work.

■ *Approach*

The incision is made sagittally about 1 cm medial to the AC joint and usually does not need to be more than 3 to 4 cm long *(fig 15)*. The supraclavicular nerve is close, and its course should be familiar to the surgeon, as if injured it can produce very painful neuromas [11]. Subcuticular tissue is mobilised from the underlying fascia of the deltoid and trapezium, adjacent to the distal clavicle and the AC joint. A self-retaining retractor is used at this stage.

If the AC joint cannot be palpated with certainty, it is possible to identify it by inserting the tip of a hypodermic needle in the joint space. Once the joint has been found, a longitudinal incision is made along the distal end of the clavicle across the joint and into the soft tissues on the cranial aspect of the acromion *(fig 15)*. Using a knife the soft tissues on either side, including the ligaments and the joint capsule, are released so that two intact sleeves on either side of the incision are in continuity from the clavicle to the acromion. We prefer not to use cauterising for this dissection, as we believe it causes too much tissue damage and that subsequent healing of the repair is hampered.

■ *Closure*

Once the procedure on the AC joint has been carried out, the two tissue flaps that have been mobilised over the joint are closed side to side with interrupted Vicryl® No. 1 sutures. This secures stability of the distal clavicle in relation to the acromion, as the closure will involve the superior acromioclavicular ligament. The fat is closed with 2-0 Vicryl® and the skin with intracuticular Prolene® No. 2.

APPROACH TO THE CORACOID PROCESS

■ *Introduction*

Occasionally the coracoid process has to be exposed, particularly if procedures such as coracoclavicular ligament reconstructions require sutures or implants to be passed around it. Some care needs to be taken to avoid unsightly scar formation and pain.

■ *Approach*

The skin incision is as for the AC joint but extended slightly further distally [18].

Care should be taken not to rely on the clavicle as a landmark, as the anatomy can be grossly distorted, particularly in cases of severe acromioclavicular joint disruption as often the clavicle is displaced posteriorly. The most important landmarks, in particular the anterior margin of the acromion, must be identified with certainty. The approach to the distal end of the clavicle is as described above for the AC joint, but the tissues cranially on the clavicle need to be divided further medially *(fig 15)*. If the clavicle is displaced, it is often necessary to release the soft tissues extensively from the posterior aspect of the distal one-third of the clavicle, as they are responsible for maintaining the clavicle in its posteriorly displaced position.

Once the soft tissue along the clavicle has been split and released, the surgeon carries out a small deltoid split at the level of the coracoid, turning the incision into an L-shape, which allows him to visualise the cranial aspect of the coracoid process *(fig 15)*. The detachment of the deltoid with its insertion on the clavicle, from this level to the medial aspect of the acromion, gives him excellent access to the whole extent of both the coraco-acromial and coracoclavicular ligaments and to the coracoid itself.

■ *Closure*

If a reduction of the clavicle has been performed, this bone has usually been brought so far forward that the deltoid needs to be brought slightly over its cranial aspect and re-inserted onto the trapezius insertion as a double breasted repair. The small deltoid split is closed with interrupted 2-0 Vicryl® and subcuticular tissues and skin, as described above.

References

[1] Altchek DW, Warren RF, Skyhar MJ, Ortiz G. et al. T-plasty modification of the Bankart procedure for multidirectional instability of the anterior and inferior types. *J Bone Joint Surg Am* 1991 ; 73 : 105-112

[2] Bankart AS. Recurrent or habitual dislocation of the shoulder joint. *Br Med J* 1923 ; 2 : 1132-1133

[3] Bankart AS. The pathology and treatment of recurrent dislocation of the shoulder joint. *Br J Surg* 1939 ; 26 : 23-29

[4] Borges AF. Relaxed skin tension lines versus other skin lines. *Plast Reconstr Surg* 1984 ; 73 : 144-150

[5] Duke PF, Frostick SP, Manning P. Subscapularis split: is it safe? *J Bone Joint Surg Br* 1996 ; 78 (suppl 1) : 32

[6] Harriman DT II, Sidles JA, Harris SL, Matsen FA. The role of the rotator interval capsule in passive motion and stability of the shoulder. *J Bone Joint Surg Am* 1992 ; 74 : 53-66

[7] Helfet AJ. Coracoid transplantation for recurring dislocation of the shoulder. *J Bone Joint Surg Br* 1958 ; 40 : 198-202

[8] Latarjet M. À propos du traitement des luxations récidivantes de l'épaule. *Lyon Chir* 1954 ; 49 : 994-997

[9] Lynch NM, Cofield RH, Silbert PL, Hermann RC. Neurologic complications after total shoulder arthroplasty. *J Shoulder Elbow Surg* 1996 ; 5 : 53-61

[10] McMaster J, Duke PF, Neumann L, Kiss J, Wallace WA. The technique and results from clavicular osteotomy as used for shoulder joint arthroplasty. *J Bone Joint Surg Br* 1998 ; 80 (suppl 1) : 106

[11] Metha A, Birch R. Supraclavicular nerve injury: the neglected nerve? *Injury* 1997 ; 28 : 491-492

[12] Neer CS, Watson KC, Stanton FJ. Recent experience in total shoulder replacement. *J Bone Joint Surg Am* 1982 ; 64 : 319-337

[13] Neer CS II, Foster CR. Inferior capsular shift for involuntary inferior and multidirectional instability of the shoulder: a preliminary report. *J Bone Joint Surg Am* 1980 ; 62 : 897-908

[14] Neer CS II. Anterior acromioplasty for the chronic impingement syndrome in the shoulder. *J Bone Joint Surg Am* 1972 ; 54 : 41-50

[15] Perthes G. Uber operationen bei habitueller Schulterluxation. *Dtsch Ztschr Chir* 1906 ; 85 : 199-222

[16] Redfern TR, Wallace WA, Beddow FH. Clavicular osteotomy in shoulder arthroplasty. *Int Orthop* 1989 ; 13 : 61-63

[17] Su CW, Alizadeh K, Boddie A, Lee RC. The problem scar. *Clin Plast Surg* 1998 ; 25 : 451-465

[18] Warren-Smith CD, Ward MW. Operation for acromioclavicular dislocation. *J Bone Joint Surg Br* 1987 ; 69 : 715-718

[19] Watterson PA, Taylor GI, Crock JG. The venous territories of muscles: anatomical study and clinical implications. *Br J Plast Surg* 1988 ; 41 : 569-585

The shoulder: superior and posterior approaches

D Goutallier
JM Postel
P Leguilloux
L Petitclerc

Abstract

Superior approaches: *Superior approaches to the shoulder should respect some anatomical landmarks. The axillary nerve must be protected, but the deltoid muscle, the trapezius muscle and the acromial arch can be reached. Dissection of a muscle by splitting the fibres longitudinally leaves no functional impairment. Osteotomies of the acromion performed parallel to the deltoid fibres heal much better than those carried out perpendicular to it. These anatomical conditions explain the various superior approaches to the shoulder. Vertical approaches through the deltoid fibres are limited to a short distance from the acromion. Extensive surgical procedures are not possible by these approaches. Transacromial approaches with osteotomies parallel to the deltoid fibres are suitable for rotator cuff repair and intra-articular procedures. Approaches through sagittal acromiotomy provide good exposure of the articulation, but they are wider and can be harmful to deltoid function. However, these approaches can be useful for shoulder arthrodesis. Various superior approaches are presented in this chapter with emphasis on Debeyre and Patte's supraspinatus, transacromial, transdeltoid approach.*

Posterior approaches: *The posterior deltoid muscle covers the entire posterior aspect of the shoulder. Surgical procedures needing a posterior access to the shoulder are carried out through the posterior deltoid fibres, as this is the only way to obtain a satisfactory exposure. The osteotomy of the acromion, at the origin of the spine of the scapula, gives a better access to the shoulder, especially the superior part. However, these approaches are quite harmful and it is difficult to rebuild the anatomy. They are almost never used for functional shoulder surgery. The various approaches are presented with emphasis on Dujarrier's subspinal transdeltoid approach.*

Keywords: surgical approaches, superior approach, posterior approach.

Superior approaches

INTRODUCTION

To permit a satisfactory superior approach to the shoulder, it is necessary to reach the middle part of the deltoid muscle, whose integrity must be preserved in as far as possible, and the acromial arch, on which the superior part of the trapezius and the deltoid muscles are inserted. If these structures have been touched, their repair must be perfect. The axillary nerve, which goes around the humerus from back to front, at 4 fingers distance under the lateral edge of the acromion, must be protected at all costs *(fig 1)*.

Daniel Goutallier, M.D., Hôpital Henri Mondor, Creteil, France.
Jean-Marie Postel, M.D., Hôpital Henri Mondor, Creteil, France.
Pierre Leguilloux, M.D., Hôpital Henri Mondor, Creteil, France.
Luc Petitclerc, M.D., Hôpital Enfant-Jésus, Quebec, Canada.

ALL APPROACHES THROUGH THE DELTOID MUSCLE ARE SUBJECT TO CRITICISM

Incisions which are parallel to muscular fibres are limited in length by the acromion above, and by the route of the axillary nerve below. They entail no functional risk, but they allow exposure only of the lateral part of the supraspinatus, the infraspinatus and the coracohumeral ligament. They can be used for limited procedures only: repair of non-retracted distal ruptures of the cuff, excision of tendinous calcification, or even performance of an acromioplasty, if the incision is shifted towards the front.

Incisions which are perpendicular to deltoid fibres are situated above the route of the axillary nerve and can be extended forwards or backwards as much as necessary. No matter how carefully the deltoid muscle is repaired, it leaves a fibrous scar which breaks the contractile continuity of the muscle. Repair after detachment of the deltoid muscle of the acromion should avoid this problem, but reinsertion with transosseous sutures is not without its failures.

APPROACHES THROUGH THE ACROMIAL ARCH

These are of two types: frontal or sagittal.

Approaches by frontal acromiotomy, parallel to the deltoid fibres, are satisfactory, and syntheses after reduction of the acromiotomy are only a little strained by deltoid traction.

■ **Debeyre and Patte's supraspinatus, transacromial, transdeltoid approach** [6]

Setting up the patient

Having the patient in a sitting position is more comfortable for the surgeon. The patient's head is kept in position by a

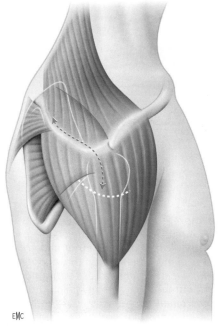

1 *Anatomical difficulties for the superior approaches: the acromial arch and the axillary nerve. Debeyre and Patte's skin incision.*

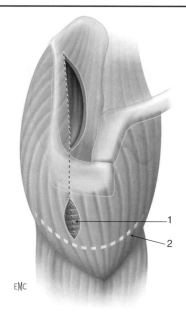

3 *The trapezius muscle incision, with separation of the deltoid muscle fibres and the vertical section of its deep aponeurosis. 1. Deep aponeurosis of the deltoid muscle 2. axillary nerve.*

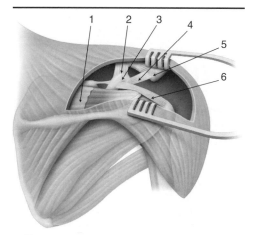

4 *The view given by the Debeyre and Patte's approach. The powerful curved retractor is necessary to improve the exposure. 1. Supraspinatus; 2. coracoclavicualr ligaments; 3. coracoid process; 4. coraco-acrominal ligament; 5. acromion; 6. coracohumeral ligament.*

headrest on the back of the head (a headrest on the face may cause eye compression entailing blindness). The lower limbs are strapped, slightly flexed, to a cushion placed under the knees, and footrests stabilise the patient and prevent him from slipping when the position of the operative table is changed. The forearm of the operated limb rests on a pad with the elbow flexed. Wearing a head light is recommended *(fig 2)*.

Cutaneous incision

The cutaneous incision is located and marked with a dermographic pencil before the sterile fields are applied. These leave the whole upper limb available and sterile (so as to facilitate mobilisation during the operation), as well as the whole shoulder (for complementary posterior or anterior approaches, if necessary). The cutaneous incision starts at the level of the tubercle of the spine of the scapula, parallel to it and

1 cm above it. It bends slightly backward above the acromion to emerge 1 cm in front of the posterior angle of the acromion. It then goes down slightly forward, parallel to the fibres of the deltoid and must end 5 cm from the external edge of the acromion to eliminate all possible aggression to the axillary nerve *(fig 1)*.

Incising the trapezius, acromion and deltoid

The superior part of the trapezius muscle is incised with an electrocautery 1 cm above the spine. This incision cuts the muscular fibres. The fibres of the middle part of the deltoid are split vertically, 1 cm in front of the angle of the acromion. The deep aponeurosis of the deltoid is incised vertically and its deeper face is peeled off the subacromial bursa at the front and back *(fig 3)*.

The acromiotomy is performed with an oscillating saw 1 cm in front of the angle of the acromion and the anterior part of the

acromion is freed from its adherences to the superficial layer of the subacromial bursa. It is tilted around the acromioclavicular joint with a powerful curved orthostatic retractor. Peeling off the cutaneous and subcutaneous front edge of the incision towards the acromioclavicular joint makes tilting the anterior acromion easier. The tongs of the retractor bear upon the deeper face of the posterior and anterior acromion. For the section or resection of the coraco-acromial ligament, it is not necessary to tilt the anterior acromion. The superficial layer of the bursa, which is separated from the deeper face of the deltoid, the inferior face of the acromion and the coraco-acromial ligament, is resected. External rotation of the shoulder allows anterior resection, and internal rotation allows posterior resection *(fig 4)*.

The fat pad found on the superior face of the distal part of the supraspinatus within the subacromial bursa is resected after being peeled off the coraco-acromial ligament and the coracoclavicular ligaments from front to back. The expansion of this fat pad beyond the external edge of the spine of the scapula is also resected; this generally provokes haemorrhaging for which haemostasis is performed with an electrocautery.

Exploring the rotator cuff and the articulation

Exploring the rotator cuff is easy by this approach. It enables the cuff ruptures, however wide, to be repaired and a total shoulder prosthesis to be inserted. When the cuff has no transfixed rupture, the various musculotendinous elements can be explored in turn, by rotating the humerus.

Neutral or slight external rotation reveals the tendon and the distal muscle of the supraspinatus. By increasing the external rotation, with the elbow near the body, the sharp anterior edge of the coracohumeral ligament can be seen and palpated. By adding antepulsion to the arm, the

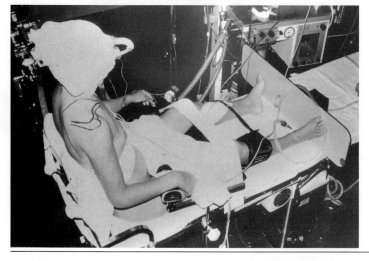

2 *The sitting positon.*

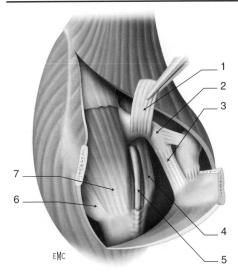

5 *The view given by Debeyre and Patte's approach with slight external rotation of the humerus.*
The arthrotomy is obtained by raising the coracohumeral ligament separated from the supraspinatus and subscapularis tendons. 1. The raised coracohumeral ligament; 2. coracoid process; 3. coraco-acromial liagament; 4. subscapularis tendon; 5. long head of the biceps tendon; 6. infrasupinatus tendon; 7. supraspinatus tendon.

subscapularis, gliding medially under the coracoid, can also be easily seen and palpated. In internal rotation, the tendon and the distal infraspinatus muscle appear. It is easy to locate the separation between the tendon of the supraspinatus and that of the infraspinatus. The confluence between the supraspinatus and the infraspinatus muscle appears clearly on the lateral edge of the spine of the scapula. Starting from this confluence and following the direction of the muscular fibres, it is easy to locate the tendinous fibres belonging to either tendon. Adding lateral elevation to internal rotation allows exposure of the teres minor, with its musculotendinous fibres that differentiate it from the tendon of the infraspinatus. Arthrotomy is performed by raising the coracohumeral ligament. Articular penetration is secured by separating its posterior edge from the tendon of the supraspinatus. The long portion of the biceps can be located. The distal coracohumeral ligament is separated from the transverse humeral ligament and its anterior edge is then separated from the subscapularis by cutting the reflected pulley of the coracohumeral, after locating the edges and allowing them to close exactly (*fig 5*). To enlarge the arthrotomy (so as to insert a prosthesis for instance), the tendon of the supraspinatus is cut 1 cm from its insertion on the greater tuberosity. The humeral head is then separated from the humeral shaft along the capsular insertion with a chisel. After its removal, the view on the glenoid surface and on the superior humeral shaft is excellent. To insert the humeral implant more easily, the superior approach can be enlarged by an osteotomy of the distal part of the clavicle. The osteotomy is performed upwards with an

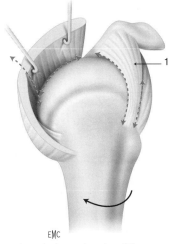

6 *The endo-articular exploration of the supraspinatus and infraspinatus tendons and the incisions for raising the coracohumeral ligament. 1. Coracohumeral ligament.*

oscillating saw. The lateral part of the clavicle is pushed forward with the anterior part of the acromion.

A vertical section of the transverse humeral ligament enables the long head of the biceps to be wrenched forwards and backwards. The arthrotomy is closed by suturing (X stitches with non-resorbable thread) the transverse humeral ligament, the reflected pulley of the coracohumeral ligament, the distal coracohumeral ligament to the intertuberosity ligament, the anterior edge of the coracohumeral ligament to the subscapularis tendon, and the posterior edge of the coracohumeral ligament to the supraspinatus tendon previously sutured with non-resorbable thread, if it has already been opened.

When the superior cuff is ruptured, the tendinous lesions can be assessed by an endo-articular examination.

The upper limb being in adduction and slight external rotation, with the table in a slanted position, the deeper face of the infraspinatus is easily explored visually and with the spatula. It is then possible to detect total or partial ruptures and cleavages of the infraspinatus (with possible detachment of the deeper layer of the cleavage) (*fig 6*).

When the upper limb is put into antepulsion, after raising the coracohumeral ligament if it is still inserted, it is easy to explore the deeper face of the insertion of the subscapularis on the lesser tuberosity thoroughly, both visually and with the spatula (the operative table being in a horizontal position). The long head of the biceps, if it is still there, can be explored easily. Severing the transverse humeral ligament facilitates its mobilisation (the ligament is closed at the end of the operation with non-resorbable thread) (*fig 7*).

Antero-inferior acromioplasty and resection of the coraco-acromial ligament can be performed. Acromioplasty is performed with an oscillating saw on the raised acromion. The edge of the bony section is covered with bone wax (*fig 8*).

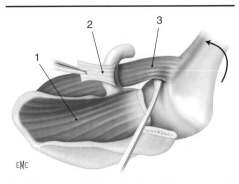

7 *The endo-articular exploration of the subscapularis tendon. 1. Supraspinatus; 2. the raised coracohumeral ligament; 3. subscapularis.*

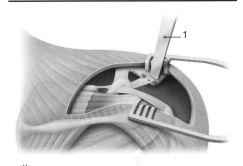

8 *The acromioplasty is performed on the raised anterior part of the osteotomised acromion. 1. Oscillating saw.*

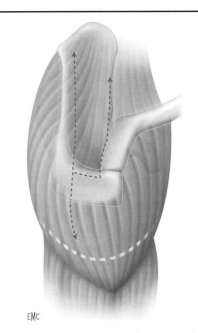

9 *The landmarks of the osteo-tendinous-muscular trapezius flap.*

This approach allows harvesting of an osteo-tendinous-muscular flap of the superior part of the trapezius muscle [5]. This can be used to replace non-reinsertable ruptures of the subscapularis tendon (*fig 9*).

A proximal extension of the supraspinatus, transacromial, transdeltoid approach allows advancement of the supraspinatus muscle and enables the repair of previously non-reparable ruptures of the supraspinatus [3, 6] (*fig 10*).

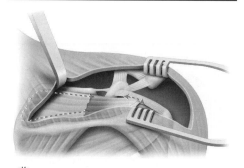

EMC

10 *The medial enlargement of Debeyre and Patte's approach to allow the supraspinatus advancement.*

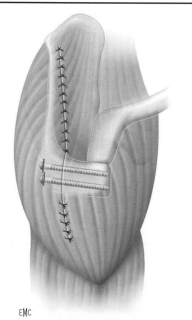

EMC

11 *Closure of Debeyre and Patte's approach.*

Closure of Debeyre and Patte's approach

The anterior part of the acromion is pushed down and reduced to the posterior part of the acromion. The upper limb being raised laterally at an angle of about 40° makes the reduction easier to perform. It is sometimes necessary to run a rugine under the acromion to push back an advanced supraspinatus, for it may become interposed in the trough of the osteotomy. The acromion is kept in place by two parallel screws, preferably titanium, 3.5 mm in diameter, inserted behind the spine of the scapula inside the angle of the acromion and going into the anterior part of the anterior acromion. When the screws are set with washers, compression is excellent and consolidation is obtained in 95% of the cases. Nonunion does not lead to dysfunction of the shoulder.

The trapezius and the deltoid are sutured with non-resorbable X stitches.

Subcutaneous and cutaneous stitching presents no problem (*fig 11*).

APPROACHES WITH ANTEROPOSTERIOR ACROMIOTOMY

These enable the middle part of the deltoid muscle, as well as the lateral part of the acromion, to be pushed outwards and

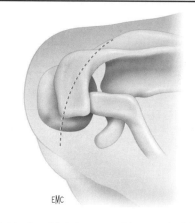

EMC

12 *Mac Laughlin's transacromial approach: skin incision.*

13 *The two possibilities of acromial osteotomy.*

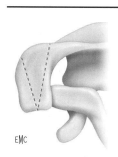

EMC

downwards. They offer a good view of the entire rotator cuff and the glenohumeral joint. Some authors advocate these approaches for inserting a prosthesis, particularly in cases of non-reparable cuff ruptures [1].

■ **The transacromial approach (Mac Laughlin's approach)** [2]

Position

Having the patient in a sitting position is comfortable for the surgeon. The sterile fields leave the upper limb and the shoulder free.

Incision

A sabre incision of the shoulder starts 2 cm beyond and outside the acromioclavicular joint and goes back towards the scapula spine/acromion junction. The cutaneous and subcutaneous lips of the incision are peeled off the underlying muscles and bone over 2 cm (*fig 12*).

Osteotomy of the acromion

The anterior fibres of the deltoid are separated from the acromion over a length of 3 cm and the acromion osteotomy is performed, preferably with an oscillating saw. It starts from the anterior edge, ending either laterally or medially a few millimetres from the posterior angle of the acromion. The lateral part of the acromion and the deltoid inserted onto it are reclined laterally from front to back, to avoid excessive traction on the axillary nerve (*fig 13*).

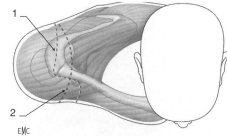

EMC

14 *Widened Mac Laughlin's approach. 1. Muscle and bone incisions; 2. skin incision.*

Closure

Reconstruction of the acromion (and fixing of the middle deltoid) is uncertain. The structure of the acromion (thin and dense) is not favourable to a osteosynthesis which must overcome strong deltoid traction. The reduction of the lateral acromion, mobilised on the proximal acromion, must be kept in place by a strong osteosynthesis to allow early mobilisation of the shoulder. A plate set on the lateral edge of the mobilised acromion and screwed onto the proximal acromion [1] can be replaced by a tension-band wire construct or by more voluminous plates.

■ **Widening Mac Laughlin's approach**

Mac Laughlin's transacromial approach can be widened to enable perfect visualisation not only of the glenohumeral joint, but also of the external part of the spine of the scapula and the margo lateralis scapulae. More aggressive, this approach is mostly used for shoulder arthrodesis [4] (*fig 14*).

Setting up and incision

Having the patient in a sitting position is comfortable for the surgeon. The skin incision starts 5 cm from under the clavicle and 1 cm within the acromioclavicular joint. It goes up towards the clavicle, then towards the acromion to cross its posterior edge 4 cm within its posterior angle, then downward for a length of 3 to 4 cm.

Exposing the deltoid and the acromion; arthrotomy

The two sides of the cutaneous and subcutaneous incisions are peeled off. Dissociating the fibres of the anterior deltoid and anteroposterior acromiotomy and separating the fibres of the posterior deltoid enable the lateral acromion and the deltoid to be pushed outwards. Non-ruptured supraspinatus, infraspinatus and subscapularis tendons are cut from back to front with the capsule, 1 cm from their humeral insertion (*fig 14*).

Pushing back the medial part of their proximal part exposes the coracoid process, the external edge of the spine and the margo lateralis scapula. This enables the bone cuts for the glenohumeral arthrodesis to be performed, and for osteosynthesis to take place (*fig 15*).

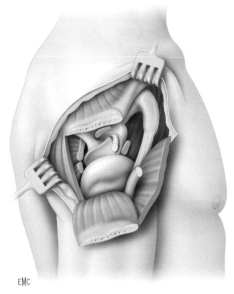

15 *After the incision of the rotator cuff, the articular surfaces, the lateral edge of the spine and the coracoid process are widely exposed.*

Posterior approaches

The posterior part of the deltoid muscle completely covers the posterior part of the shoulder. It is inserted far into the spine of the scapula and on the lower part of the superior third of the humerus. It uncovers the posterior face of the shoulder articulation only when the arm is in a position of lateral elevation.

SUBDELTOID APPROACH [2]

This is the only posterior approach to the shoulder that leaves the posterior deltoid intact. The cutaneous incision follows the postero-inferior edge of the deltoid muscle, from the spine of the scapula towards the humerus. This approach is narrow and it does not allow for any precise intra-articular procedures. It must be used only for posterior drainage arthrotomies.

All posterior approaches that allow intra-articular procedures should go through the posterior deltoid muscle. They must also go through the acromial arch to expose the posterior as well as the superior part of the joint.

■ *The subdeltoid transacromial approach (Kocher's approach)* [2]

This approach enables the superior and posterior aspects of the articulation to be exposed. It is the superior extension of the subdeltoid approach. The acromion separated from the spine can be tilted around the acromioclavicular articulation. This means sectioning the superior trapezius and a vertical section of the posterior deltoid directly below the osteotomy. Too harmful, this approach cannot be used for modern repair surgery of the shoulder.

■ *The subspinal transdeltoid approach (Dujarrier's approach)* [2]

This approach exposes the posterior aspect of the articulation. It goes through the

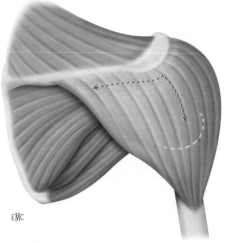

16 *Dujarrier's approach: skin incision.*

posterior deltoid along the spine of the scapula. The insertion of the deltoid onto the spine of the scapula being more fibrous than muscular, satisfactory repair is possible. This approach is used by some to deal with posterior instability of the shoulder, to insert prostheses, particularly those that use glenoid implants with acromial bearing, and to expose the margo lateralis scapulae and the posterior face of the scapula neck.

Setting up

A sitting position as well as lateral decubitus are used. If the patient is in a lateral decubitus position, the chest and the pelvis must be secure, with anterior and posterior rests. A cushion under the thorax releases the fossa axillaris and avoids neurovascular compressions on the upper limb on which the body rests. The head is on a cushion. The table position elevated the head so as to diminish intraoperative bleeding.

Cutaneous incision (fig 16)

The cutaneous incision is located and marked with a dermographic pencil before the sterile fields are applied. These leave the whole upper limb available and sterile (to mobilise it easily during the operation) as well as the whole shoulder (for complementary posterior or anterior approaches if necessary). The incision begins medially, on the tubercle of the trapezius muscle. It runs parallel to the spine of the scapula a little below it. Directly under the posterior angle of the acromion, it runs down a little to the front, for 3 cm. The cutaneous and subcutaneous edges opposite the spiny part of the incision are slightly peeled off the underlying bone and aponeurotic planes.

Separation of the posterior deltoid muscle (fig 17)

The posterior deltoid is separated from the spine either by an 1/2 cm incision under the lower edge of the spine or by detaching it with a thin bone slab using a chisel. The medial part of the deltoid can be left.

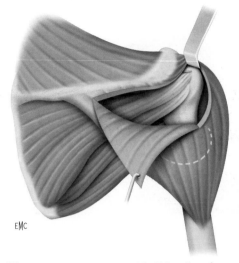

17 *Pulling down the posterior deltoid flap allows for exposure of the inferior part of the supraspinatus, the infraspinatus and the teres minor.*

Starting from the angle of the acromion, the posterior deltoid muscle is separated from its middle part by dissecting the fibres over a length 3 cm.

Exposing the posterosuperior rotator cuff and joint

The inferior deltoid flap is retracted gently downwards. A thread linking the deltoid flap to the underlying cutaneous plane avoids using retractors. The superficial layer of the subacromial bursa is excised. The anterior flexion of the shoulder enables the tendon of the supraspinatus to be seen. The internal rotation of the shoulder enables the tendon of the infraspinatus and the ending of the teres minor to be observed (*fig 17*).

Locating the suprascapular pedicle

It is important to locate the suprascapular pedicle on the lateral edge of the origin of the spine of the scapula. The infraspinatus muscle is detached from the lateral part of the inferior face of the spine with a rugine. It is pushed downward. This gives a good view of the most distal confluence of the supraspinatus and the infraspinatus muscles. The external edge of the spine is located and freed in its superficial part first, then in its deeper part, with a spatula. Right outside it, the neurovascular pedicle is very gently separated from the posterior face of the neck of the scapula with the spatula (*fig 18*).

■ *Arthrotomy*

Arthrotomy can be performed in two different ways.

1) The distal tendons of the infraspinatus and supraspinatus are separated from each other. It is easy to find the separation between the two tendons from the confluence of the supraspinatus and infraspinatus muscles, following the outward direction of the muscular fibres.

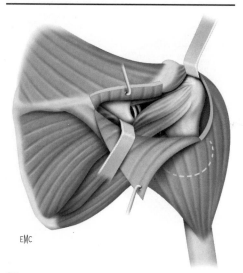

18 *Exposure of the suprascapular pedicle by detachment of the infraspinatus muscle from the lateral part of the spine of the scapula.*

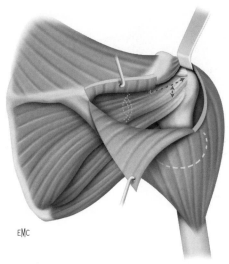

19 *The separation between the infraspinatus and supraspinatus tendons. The vertical partial section of the infraspinatus tendon.*

The separation is begun distally; it is enlarged medially while retaining the possibility of locating the suprascapular pedicle. The tendon of the infraspinatus is then separated from the capsule from top to bottom. The tendon of the supraspinatus is dissected (often with difficulty) from the underlying capsule *(fig 19)*.

The capsule is more conveniently exposed by cutting the infraspinatus vertically at three-quarters of its height, 1 cm from its insertion on the greater tuberosity. The arthrotomy is performed either by a horizontal, vertical or T-incision. Medially, the capsule can be detached from its posterior and superoposterior glenoidal insertion with the scalpel from outside in, taking great care of the position of the suprascapular pedicle *(fig 20)*.

Capsular closure is easily performed with resorbable thread if it has been incised. The tendon of the infraspinatus is sutured with non-resorbable thread. The tendons of the supraspinatus and the infraspinatus are brought edge to edge with non-resorbable thread.

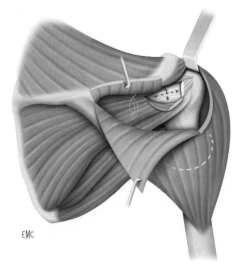

20 *The arthrotomy can be carried out by vertical, horizontal or T incision.*

2) After separating the tendon of the supraspinatus from the tendon of the infraspinatus and locating the inferior edge of the teres minor (while keeping contact with the humerus to avoid injuring the axillary nerve), the infraspinatus and the teres minor are detached from the humerus with a thin 3 mm thick bone slab, using a chisel. The capsula generally comes away with the bone tendinous detachment. A transosseous suture with non-resorbable thread or with a steel thread ensures articular closure.

Closing the approach

The posterior deltoid is stitched up with non-resorbable thread by edge to edge sutures or by transosseous sutures, according to how the incision was made. The middle and posterior parts of the deltoid muscle are brought together with non-resorbable thread.

Postoperative care

For the posterior deltoid to heal, the upper limb rests on an abduction splint that gives a slight lateral elevation with neutral rotation. Passive mobilisation, above the pillow in the plane of the scapula and avoiding internal rotation, is started immediately and carried on for 25 to 30 days. Then, mobilisation becomes progressively active and internal rotation is slowly increased.

References

[1] Baulet E, Chabernaud D, Grammont PM. Résultats de la prothèse inversée de Grammont pour les omarthroses associées à de grandes destructions de la coiffe (16 cas). *Acta Orthop Belg* 1995 ; 61 (suppl 1) : 112-119

[2] Debeyre J, Patte D. Voies d'abord de l'articulation scapulo-humérale. *Encycl Méd Chir* (Éditions Scientifiques et Médicales Elsevier SAS, Paris), Techniques chirurgicales - Orthopédie-traumatologie, 44-250, 1966

[3] Debeyre J, Patte D, Elmelik E. Repair of rupture of the rotator cuff of the shoulder with a note on advancement of the supraspinatus muscle. *J Bone Joint Surg Br* 1965 ; 47 : 36-42

[4] Debeyre J, Patte D, Perrin J. L'arthrodèse de l'épaule. *Encycl Méd Chir* (Éditions Scientifiques et Médicales Elsevier SAS, Paris), Techniques chirurgicales - Orthopédie-traumatologie, 44-260, 1978

[5] Goutallier D, Lavau L, Postel JM. The trapezius flap in non reinsertable tears of the subscapularis. In : Vastamäki M, Jalovaara P eds. Surgery of the shoulder. Amsterdam : Elsevier Science, 1995 : 79-83

[6] Patte D, Goutallier D. Chirurgie de la coiffe des rotateurs. *Encycl Méd Chir* (Éditions Scientifiques et Médicales Elsevier SAS, Paris), Techniques chirurgicales - Orthopédie-traumatologie, 44-285, 1984

Shoulder arthroscopy

F Gómez-Castresana Bachiller
J Tena Arregui
F Peña Gómez

Abstract. – Shoulder arthroscopy is a surgical procedure performed almost as frequently as knee arthroscopy. The development of instruments and equipment (such as power tools and especially laser and radiofrequency probes, both uni- and bipolar) has allowed the performance of multiple techniques in a safe and simple fashion – with good visualisation, the ability to ablate soft tissues and no need for an arthroscopic pump. Similarly, special irrigation solutions such as bidistilled water, glycine or glycerol, previously used with electrosurgery, are no longer necessary, thus avoiding their related complications. Either a beach chair or a lateral decubitus position with soft tissue traction may be used for any arthroscopic technique. The most modern and recent image recording systems allow excellent documentation of interventions as well as exchanges of valuable scientific information within the orthopaedic community. With the development of various arthroscopic techniques, orthopaedic surgeons can progressively address increasingly complex pathology with very similar results to the gold-standard of open techniques. They are able deal with a wide spectrum of pathology, from post-traumatic lesions in the younger population to degenerative conditions in elderly individuals. This chapter will discuss the material required to perform a safe shoulder arthroscopy, as well as the different options for patient positioning and anaesthesia and their potential disadvantages. A detailed description of intra-articular anatomy and some normal anatomial variations, followed by complications during shoulder arthroscopy, will complete this chapter.

Keywords: shoulder, arthroscopy, complications, indications.

Introduction

Ever since Burman [8] first performed glenohumeral joint arthroscopy in a corpse back in 1931, this technique has experienced an exponential progression. The shoulder is one of the most arthroscopically examined and treated joints, second only to the knee. The specific characteristics of the shoulder have favoured the development of both absorbable and non-absorbable bone attachment systems, either with anchors or directly to tissue, as well as several types of suture passers. Various types of knots, both sliding and non-sliding, have been devised to reattach or repair avulsed or torn capsular-ligamentous or tendinous structures. For ablation or thermal retraction of tissue, the development of laser and unipolar (Oratec) and bipolar (ArthroCare,

Fernando Gómez-Castresana Bachiller, M.D., Ph.D., Associate Professor, Department of Orthopaedic Surgery, Universidad Complutense de Madrid, Spain.
Jose Tena Arregui, M.D., Orthopaedic Surgeon, Clínica Santa Elena Madrid, Spain.
Fernando A Peña Gómez, M.D., Orthopaedic Surgeon, Clínica Santa Elena Madrid, Spain.

Vapr) radiofrequency (RF) probes has eliminated the use of distilled water, glycine or glycerol as non-ionic, non-conductive media. If these devices are utilised in a conventional saline setting, cutting and coagulating are simplicity itself when RF probes are used, which makes an arthroscopic pump system to control bleeding an option more than a necessity. Such advances have allowed the improvement of arthroscopic techniques for the repair of a variety of conditions, with a precision as good as that of open surgery (table I); however, the track record for other conditions is poorer. Modern image recording systems (video or printer) facilitate case documentation and allow scientific information to be standardised.

Materials

ARTHROSCOPE

Arthroscopes similar to those used for the knee joint are required, 4.5 mm in diameter and angled at 30°. In some rare instances, a 70° angled arthroscope may be more useful,

compared to the standard 25-30° angled arthroscope. Smaller arthroscopes are not necessary for children. The arthroscope-TV camera transmits images to the monitor display on the arthroscopy tower, where the camera, light source, shaver power system, RF unit, video recorder and printer are also located.

EQUIPMENT

To begin the procedure, the following are required: an arthroscope cannula fitted with a sharp and a blunt trocar, a syringe to drive surgical irrigation into the joint for initial distension, and an 11-gauge blade for skin incision. A spinal needle to guide accessory portal location is often useful, allowing the joint to be punctured from outside and the needle to be seen from inside. Through these accessory portals, variously gauged arthroscopic cannulae may be introduced with a blunt trocar to facilitate placement. To prevent backing up, cannulae may be threaded along their stems, and made in different colours to enhance illumination (fig 1). Some cannulae have a saline outlet to help control flow and pressure inside the joint. The use of cannulae is not essential

Table I. – Possible arthroscopic techniques for shoulder joint conditions.

Glenohumeral joint	Technique
Uni- or multidirectional instabilities	Labrum reattachment with transglenoid suture, suture, or direct fixation with anchors. Retensioning ligaments with sutures or anchors. Capsular thermal shrinkage
SLAP lesions	Debridement, reattachment with anchors and sutures
Stiff shoulder	Capsular release and adhesiolysis
Biceps tendon pathology	Debridement. Tenotomy or tenodesis with anchors
Subscapularis tendon rupture	Reattachment with anchors
Capsular partial rotator cuff tears	Suture
Miscellaneous conditions:	
Fractures and their sequelae	Osteosynthesis. Osseous abrasion, chondral shaving
Synovitis	Excision, thermal ablation
Degenerate arthritis	Debridement, osseous abrasion
Tumours and tumour-like conditions	Excision, debridement, thermal ablation
Chondral injuries	Fixation, shaving, drilling
Infection	Debridement, drainage
Loose bodies or implants	Removal
Inflammatory arthritis and undiagnosed conditions	Debridement, synovial fluid analysis. Biopsy
Subcromial space and acromioclavicular joint	**Technique**
Subcromial impingement	Decompression (osseous and soft tissues)
Rotator cuff tears	Repair: suture, suture with anchors, direct fixation by anchors. Debridement and decompression
Coracoid impingement	Decompression
Acromioclavicular joint pathology	Debridement. Distal clavicle resection (Mumford)
Acromioclavicular instability	Coracoid-clavicular fixation
Calcifications	Excision
Miscellaneous:	
Captured shoulder	Adhesiolysis
Tumours and tumour-like conditions	Excision, debridement. Thermal ablation
Bursitis	Excision
Degenerative arthritis	Debridement. Osseous abrasions
Infection	Debridement, drainage

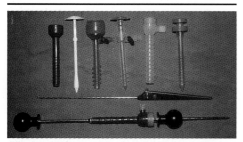

1 *Different models of arthroscopic cannulae and an arthroscopic probe. At the bottom, cannula through a Wissinger rod in a retrograde fashion.*

except for specific surgical procedures, as instruments may be directly introduced through skin portals.

Basic mechanical instruments for arthroscopic shoulder assessment are: the probe, toothed grasping forceps, 3.5 and 5.0 mm basket forceps, and Wissinger switching guide rod [2] or Steinmann pin. The guide rod facilitates positioning of an accessory portal, as a cannula can be passed over it. Once the arthroscope has been withdrawn from its sheath, the rod is pushed through it, and both the capsule and the contralateral peri-articular soft tissues are pierced, resulting in a tent-shaped bulging of the skin. There, at the rod exit point, the skin is incised and the rod pushed farther to be used to guide a cannula into the joint in an outside-in fashion.

Motorised tools such as shaver systems are essential for shoulder arthroscopy, particularly for debridement and adequate visualisation of the subacromial space. Alternatively, a Ho Yag laser – best suited

for arthroscopy [41] – or unipolar (Oratec) and bipolar (ArthroCare, Vapr) RF probes may be used. This type of probe has been extremely effective for soft tissue excision and coagulation, and is less costly than laser.

Each arthroscopic technique requires specific instruments such as: anchorage systems, guides, stitchers, suture retrievers, knot pushers and other sophisticated tools. Some interesting tools designed for passing sutures through the capsule, tendons or ligaments have facilitated the development

of new arthroscopic techniques. Some of the most commonly used instrumentation are the Caspari™ suture punch, several stitchers and suture passers, either monofilament, curved or corkscrew-shaped. We may also find on the market: forceps allowing braided sutures to be directly threaded on the needle at one of the jaws once the tissue has been run through, and other useful instruments capable of shuttling braided suture between both punch jaws while piercing any tissue (Acufex Suture Punch™, ArthroSew™). Such tools, in association with suture retrievers, place suture ends outside the cannula, where they may be tied into knots. Knots are slid into the joint by using knot pushers, thus fixing tissues to bone or closing any tears present. Snyder's Shuttle Relay™ (Concept, Inc.), a nylon-coated steel wire resembling a no. 1-gauge monofilament suture with a central 3 mm eyelet, may be passed through tissues by using a Caspari™ punch or a stitcher. Then, a thick, resilient braided suture is threaded through the eyelet and taken through tissues for definite tying (fig 2). Ultrasonic suture welding (AxyaLoop™, Axya Medical, Inc.) represents a recent, easy-to-use technique that may prove revolutionary for suture knot tying, although no long-term studies to unequivocally determine effectiveness have been conducted so far. Tack-, screw-, screw-washer-, and button-shaped soft tissue direct anchorage systems, both absorbable and non-absorbable (Arthrex, Mitek Products, Bionx, Linvatec), have the advantage of eliminating technically demanding knot tying. The Knotless Suture Anchor™ (Mitek Products) is a novel direct suture anchorage system that has proven very useful for arthroscopic repair of a Bankart lesion for joint instability.

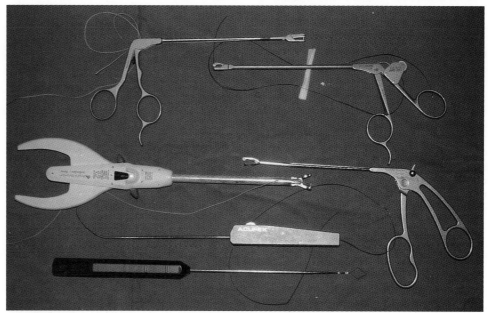

2 *Different models of arthroscopic suture devices. From top to bottom; suture punch by Arthrotek, Caspari™ punch by Linvatec, suture punch by Acufex, Anchor Sew™ by Surgical Dynamics, Stitcher™ by Acufex and Blitz™ suture passer/retriever by Linvatec.*

IRRIGATION

Since the introduction of laser devices and RF probes, which facilitate accurate coagulation of the arthroscopic space to allow a suitable view, the use of an arthroscopic irrigation pump is not considered mandatory. However, the pump may facilitate surgery in selected cases, and therefore it remains an option at the surgeon's discretion. Two 3-litre saline bags mixed with two epinephrine vials (1mg/mL) induce vasoconstriction and thus help to decrease bleeding; they hang from the operating room ceiling at a variable height, allowing satisfactory irrigation similar to that offered by pumps, as a result of hydrostatic pressure. The irrigation system is connected to the arthroscope's sheath or an independent cannula after residual bubbles have been eliminated by purging. This irrigation system may also serve for drainage and aspiration purposes.

Anaesthesia

General anaesthesia is the most commonly used as it offers several advantages: optimal muscle relaxation allowing traction to be applied, a familiar induction routine, and available blood pressure control for prevention of intra-articular bleeding. Arterial hypotension is achieved by using hypnotics, such as propofol (1-2 mg/kg), narcotics such as fentanyl (3-4 mcg/kg), or anaesthetics such as 2% isoflurane. Sodium nitroprusside, a peripheral vasodilator, is used as an effective hypotensive agent in doses of 1-1.5 mcg/kg/min with 0.01% dilution. The interscalene block technique, aided by a nerve stimulator, has fewer side effects and shortens the in-patient hospital stay [30], but its administration requires a well-trained team. A combination of 2% mepivacaine (400 mg), 0.5% bupivacaine (50 mg), and sodium bicarbonate (2 mL), either with or without epinephrine (150 mg) added to the solution, has proven very effective [19].

An anaesthetic block is in itself hypotensive, which facilitates surgery. This technique has some contraindications such as coagulopathy, local infection or a previous history of plexus disease. It is also contraindicated in the presence of chronic obstructive pulmonary disease, contralateral pneumonectomy, pneumothorax, phrenic nerve palsy and ankylosing spondylitis [30]. A combination of both techniques may help in controlling post-operative pain, particularly for patients requiring continuous passive motion (CPM) therapy following arthrolysis [39]. Prior to any planned procedure, shoulder examination under anaesthesia is mandatory to confirm the preoperative diagnosis.

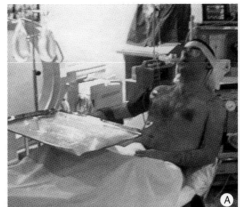 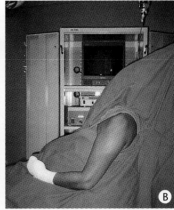

3 *Beach chair position before (A) and after draping (B). Note the eye pads and fixed head position as well as the bolster at the hip level and the flexed hip and knee joints.*

Patient position and preparation

Two positions may be used according to the surgeon's preference. The beach chair position places the patient in a semi-seated position with the upper body minimally elevated at 60°, flexed hips and knees, a sandbag under the ipsilateral hip, head fixed to the table, body near the edge with the shoulder jutting out [38] (*fig 3*). This position allows the shoulder to be freely approached from the anterior, lateral and posterior aspects. Devices that attach to standard operating room tables to facilitate this position are available (Schlein II™, McConnell System™). They provide head fixation while freeing the scapular girdle on the affected side. Special attention must be paid to the head position, which should not be too extended, nor rotated and/or tilted to the contralateral side. There have been reports of injuries to the brachial plexus in patients with incorrect head positions after manipulations during the procedure. Neutral rotation, tilt and flexion must be ensured to avoid neurological complications.

The beach chair position offers the following benefits: rapid patient positioning, lack of traction (avoiding the risk of brachial plexus elongation), a free upper extremity, optimal joint visualisation for all techniques, easy conversion to a position suitable for an open procedure, and no assistant required in front of the patient (in contrast to the lateral position).

In the lateral decubitus position, the upper body is usually externally rotated around 30-40°; arm traction is applied at about 5 kg, while the shoulder is flexed 10° with varying abduction (10-15° for a subacromial exploration, 70° for a glenohumeral examination [16] (*fig 4*). Arm traction is of the cutaneous adhesive type along the forearm, and padding under the wrist must be checked to prevent pressure bearing on the dorsal branch of the radial nerve. Devices are available to achieve traction while providing great protection. Traction force varies according to the patient biotype (5-10 kg) and may be applied along the axis of

the arm or in association with the zenithal force operating on the arm to separate the humeral head from the glenoid fossa by using a supplementary clamp. Devices which can be attached to operating tables to apply traction are available (Arthrex). As the trunk is tilted back, the scapulohumeral joint line is rendered horizontal, which facilitates surgical manoeuvres requiring anteriorly supplied instrumentation, and a potential open procedure conversion as well, by tilting the table into a supine position. Subacromial open surgery is facilitated by widening this space via traction. Special attention must be paid to the padding under the axilla, elbow and knee areas on the weight-bearing side, as well as the padding in the space between both knees and at the paraspinal area resting on a lateral support.

With the surgical site already scrubbed aseptic and isolated by sterile draping, it is highly recommended to use a skin marker to draw the bony contours of the scapular spine, the acromion with its anterior and posterior corners, the acromioclavicular joint, the clavicle, the coracoid tip, and the posterior soft spot as the initial entry point into the glenohumeral joint [39]. This will lower the risk of damaging neurovascular structures, whose anatomy should be thoroughly understood [39]. Using a U-shaped adhesive bag to collect drained saline (3M Co.) is a wise measure which helps to prevent contamination of the surgical field.

The locations of equipment, the assistant and the scrub nurse will depend on the patient's position and on how much space is available in the operating room. The arthroscopic cart with the TV monitor and the previously-described equipment, Mayo stand, irrigation bags, and occasionally a laser unit, are usually located facing the surgeon on the opposite side of the table (*fig 5*). The scrub nurse, instrument table and assistant remain on the surgical side by the surgeon, who watches the TV display, except when anterior portals are used in the lateral decubitus position, where the assistant must stand by the opposite side of the operating table.

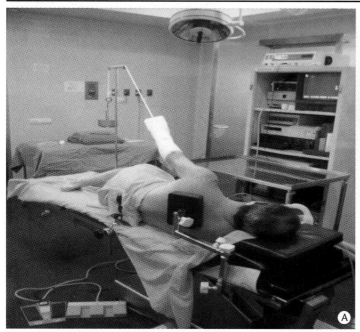

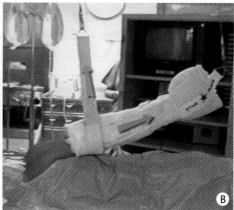

4 *Lateral decubitus position before draping (A). Traction applied to the upper extremity with longitudinal and zenithal components (B).*

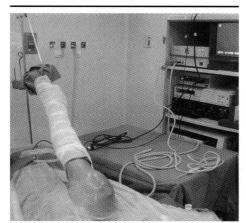

5 *Location of tables and arthroscopic tower prior to surgery with the patient in the lateral decubitus position.*

Arthroscopic examination of the shoulder joint: access portals

GLENOHUMERAL JOINT

The initial entry portal is the posterior one, determined by palpation of the soft spot 2 cm below the acromion and 1 cm medial to the acromial posterior corner [2, 39]. After a minimal skin incision is made, the arthroscope's cannula is introduced; it is fitted with the sharp trocar which is replaced by the blunt trocar before going through the capsule. It is directed towards the coracoid tip by careful palpation with the free hand. The posterior glenoid labrum and the humeral head may then be felt. Distension by previous saline injection, associated humeral abduction by the assistant, and zenithal traction all contribute to widening the joint space. Capsule perforation may be felt as a "pop", and fluid flows back from the joint upon trocar removal, if the joint was previously distended.

With the arthroscope in place within the joint cavity, the biceps is the first, easily identifiable structure to become apparent. No risk of vascular or nerve damage is run, as both the circumflex artery and nerve are located at the quadrangular space 9 cm below. Anterosuperior portal positioning is determined by moving the arthroscope's tip to the space between the biceps and the glenoid fossa in its upper and slightly lateral area, just at the rotator interval between the supraspinatus and subscapular tendons. The arthroscope is then removed and a Wissinger rod or Steinman pin is passed through the cannula, perforating the capsule as well as the deltoid from inside-out and tenting the skin. At this level, the skin is incised and a cannula is retrograded over the rod through a small incision in an outside-in fashion. Alternatively, the portal may be created from the outside by using a spinal needle (allowing the joint to be seen from within), or in lean individuals, it may be guided by the arthroscope's light which becomes visible through the skin upon intra-joint positioning at the portal location. The portal should be positioned lateral to the coracoid process to prevent damage to the musculocutaneous nerve, at the midpoint between the coracoid process and the acromial anterior corner (*fig 6*).

Joint examination must be carried out systematically, and all structures (including the biceps tendon and its glenoid attachment, the entire labrum, and the labrum's capsular attachment) should be both visualised and palpated front to back. Using both portals, the arthroscope's end may be moved into all corners within the joint; a better superior or inferior viewing angle may be achieved by turning it around on some occasions. Alternatively, initial joint examination may be performed from an antero-inferior portal, particularly when surgery does not require two anterior

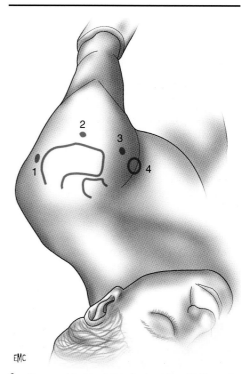

6 *Topographical anatomy of a shoulder with the posterior, lateral and anterior portals marked. 1. Posterior portal; 2. lateral portal; 3. anterior portal; 4. coracoid.*

portals, as is the case with transglenoid or direct labrum reattachment with ligament retensioning or arthrolysis. The antero-inferior portal may be positioned from the inside with the aid of a Wissinger rod passed just over the upper edge of the subscapularis, or from the outside by marking the point with an anteriorly introduced spinal needle. The cannula with the trocar is passed posteriorly, which benefits from a more lateral positioning. Some authors prefer a lower, 5 o'clock position for the right shoulder, with the entry point through the subscapularis to

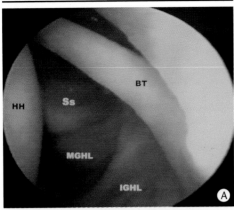

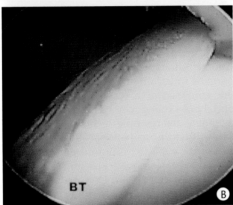

7 A. *Intra-articular view of a left shoulder from the posterior portal. HH = humeral head; BT = biceps tendon; Ss = subscapularis; MGHL = middle glenohumeral ligament; IGHL = inferior glenohumeral ligament.*
B. *Biceps tendon with signs of tenosynovitis.*

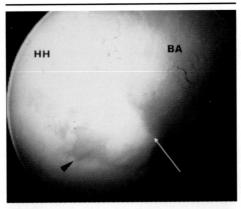

8 *Right shoulder seen from the posterior portal. Humeral head with a Hill-Sachs lesion (arrow head) and the bare area (BA). The thin arrow marks the border between normal cartilage (where the Hill-Sachs lesion is included) and the bare area. HH = humeral head.*

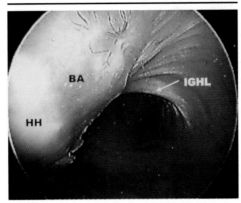

9 *Inferior recess of glenohumeral joint seen from the posterior portal, showing the posterior fold in a hammock shape. BA = bare area; HH = humeral head; IGHL = inferior glenohumeral ligament.*

directly access the glenoid fossa, thus facilitating potential capsular-ligamentous fixation.

Many anatomical variations exist and must be recognised as such to avoid mistaking them for pathological conditions. The biceps tendon may be covered with a synovial membrane and thus escape identification within the anterior area. It must be assessed for tendonitis all the way to the most lateral portion, as it leaves the glenohumeral joint over a portion of tissue that resembles a shelf (horizontal and "holding up" the tendon) – this structure is the superior glenohumeral ligament (fig 7).

Moving laterally, the articular aspect of the rotator cuff tendons may be assessed; the supraspinatus is the most anterior and the most likely to show some pathology and frayed fibres if a partial thickness tear is present. By rotating the scope and backing out slightly, the rest of the humeral head can be evaluated. The bare area over the posterior aspect of the humeral head must not be confused with a Hill-Sachs lesion (fig 8).

Generally speaking, the bare spot is located at the most posterior margin of the articular surface; therefore, it is adjacent to cartilage just anteriorly, whereas a Hill-Sachs lesion is surrounded by articular cartilage in its entire extension. Posteriorly, the capsule looks uniform except in its lower area, where a

fold corresponding to the inferior glenohumeral ligament's posterior fascicle appears. The two fascicles making up this ligament give rise to a hammock-like sling at the inferior recess (fig 9). The labrum may blend into the glenoid fossa, or rather have a meniscus-like appearance with a free margin, which allows positioning the probe's hook between both structures. The presence of the sublabrum foramen, another normal anatomical variation, may be observed from the 1 to 4 o'clock position for a right shoulder. This variation may be easily identified by the presence of articular cartilage under the foramen (as is not the case with a tear), and also by the dramatic decrease in external rotation if an attempt is made to reduce the foramen with either instruments or some type of fixation.

Finally, going back to the most anterior aspect of the glenohumeral joint, the anterior ligaments are examined. Four types of anatomical variations exist for anterior glenohumeral ligaments. In type I, the intra-articular invagination for each glenohumeral ligament (superior, middle and inferior) may be anatomically identified. The middle ligament and the superior ligament come together into a single structure in type II. Type III shows an isolated, cord-like, superiorly attached middle glenohumeral

ligament which gives rise to a large capsular hole together with the humeral glenoid structure. In type IV, the middle and inferior ligaments may not be identified, and only the interval between the superior glenohumeral ligament and the subscapularis upper edge can be seen [39]. As a distinct variation, the Buford complex shows a cord-like middle glenohumeral ligament that is attached to the biceps tendon base; it lacks superior labral tissue, thus resembling a Bankart lesion. Finally, the upper margin of the subscapularis tendon will be seen crossing the joint transversely from medial to lateral and perpendicular to the fibres of the middle glenohumeral ligament. Laterally (although difficult to visualise), we may sometimes find pathology from previous tears.

Other accessory portals may be required for certain arthroscopic techniques. A postero-inferior portal [38], 2 cm below the classic posterior one, is useful for both inferior and posterior capsular thermal shrinkage, anchorage techniques, and posterior capsular re-tensioning. A supraspinatus fossa portal [2, 37] is positioned at the fossa's most lateral area, at the angle between the clavicle, the medial acromion and the scapular spine, and goes through the trapezium, supraspinatus muscle and capsule. Its medial placement within the fossa puts the suprascapularis nerve at risk. The manoeuvre is performed in an outside-in fashion, through a small skin incision and under the guidance of a spinal needle inserted under visual intra-articular control. This portal is useful when a route for joint distension irrigation is set up for the repair of posterior SLAP (Superior Labrum Anterior to Posterior) lesions or posterior capsular lesions, and to pass and tie sutures for posterior capsular re-tensioning [31] (fig 10). Some authors use supraspinatus transtendinous portals to repair type II SLAP lesions, as is the case with Wilmington's portal, positioned 1 cm lateral and anterior to the acromial posterior corner [7].

Relatively common injuries may be identified by means of a systematic arthroscopic approach. Such injuries are Bankart lesions at the anterior labrum, Hill-Sachs lesions at the posterior aspect of the humeral head, complete or partial rotator cuff injuries [11], SLAP lesions with their four variations [7], anterosuperior labral tears and anterior supraspinatus cuff tears or SLAC (Superior Labrum Avulsion Capsule) lesions and reverse Hill-Sachs lesions on the anterior aspect of the humeral head, characteristic of posterior dislocation. Degenerative lesions, and rupture or ablation of the long head of the biceps tendon are all accurately detected. Assessment may be equivocal for multidirectional laxity with no apparent lesion, where only increased mobility of the humeral head is encountered.

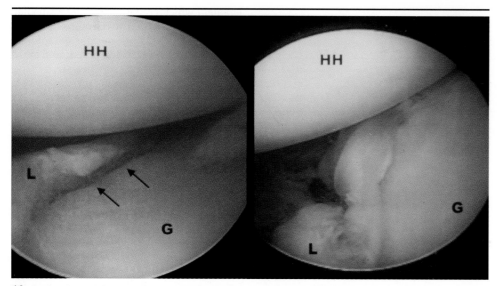

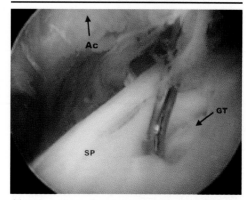

11 *From a posterior portal, view of the subacromial space of a right shoulder with a supraspinatus tear. Ac = acromion; SP = supraspinatus; GT = greater tuberosity.*

10 *Bankart lesion before and after repair with the transglenoid suture technique. The arrows mark the subperiosteal avulsion of the labrum and periosteum from the infero-anterior glenoid. HH = humeral head; L = labrum; G = glenoid.*

A number of functional markers have been described for arthroscopic assessment, including the drive-through sign [7], when the arthroscope may be passed from posterior to anterior and from proximal to distal toward the inferior recess, which suggests ligament laxity. The peel-back sign [7] is defined as the medial retraction of the labrum on the glenoid neck. It is usually associated with SLAP lesions, in which case the biceps tendon becomes vertical and posteriorly angulated when arm abduction and external rotation are attempted.

In addition, direct visualisation of synovial tissue, occasionally aided by a biopsy or fluid analysis and culture, allows diagnosis and assessment of conditions such as adhesive capsulitis, "frozen shoulder", calcifications, and synovitis of the inflammatory, haemophilic, rheumatic or septic type [18, 29]. Other conditions suitable for diagnosis and treatment by arthroscopic techniques include tumour-like conditions, such as synovial chondromatosis [39], peri-articular cyst [21] or osteochondroma development. Pseudotumour conditions such as pigmented villonodular synovitis [28], and a mix of other conditions such as joint trauma injuries [9] or their sequels [39], bone necrosis with joint involvement, or degenerative arthritic disease, may all be both diagnosed and treated [39].

The glenohumeral conditions susceptible to arthroscopic management are: acute or chronic, anterior or posterior trauma-induced instability (TUBS - Trauma Unilateral Bankart Surgery) [25, 33, 36, 37]; posterosuperior instability [7]; multidirec-tional instability (AMBRI - Atraumatic Multidirectional Bilateral Rehabilitation Inferior capsular shift, occasionally) [42]; SLAP lesions with reattachment of the labrum or the long head of the biceps tendon; ligament re-tensioning by direct suture (capsulorrhaphy or plication), by suture onto direct fixation systems or by means of capsular thermal shrinkage using either laser or radiofrequency energy [1, 7, 11, 33, 39]. Resection of a degenerated long head of the biceps tendon [15] or its residual stump following rupture may be attempted. In the younger patient, tenodesis of a partial or complete rupture of the biceps tendon may also be carried out [14]. Post-traumatic stiff shoulder and primary or secondary adhesive capsulitis, "frozen shoulder", are managed by arthroscopic capsular release and adhesiolysis [18]. Synovitis of all sorts, and tumours or pseudo-tumour lesions may be debrided or excised, and tumour beds may be cauterised. Bone abrasion may be carried out for degenerative conditions or in the presence of osteophytes [13] or post-traumatic joint irregularities [39]. Following intra-articular fracture, bony fragments may be stabilised by direct osteosynthesis using wires or micro-screws, or by loose body removal and implants [39].

SUBACROMIAL SPACE AND ACROMIOCLAVICULAR JOINT

In examining these two areas, four access portals are basically used [2, 39]. The posterior portal is used for the glenohumeral joint; the trocar is pulled back to the skin level and the arthroscope is then redirected toward the subacromial space; the posterior aspect of the subacromial bursa is then perforated with a "pop". The coraco-acromial ligament may be felt with the tip of the arthroscope when it is swung from medial to lateral. The anterior portal is positioned immediately anterior to the acromioclavicular joint, and lateral to the coracohumeral ligament, so that the arthroscope does not become stuck, loosing mobility. This portal is opened up by passing a Wissenger's switching rod through the arthroscope's cannula when located in the posterior portal, thus perforating the capsule and the deltoid muscle outwardly. It then raises the skin, and here an incision is made through which the cannula is introduced and passed over the rod. Another alternative to create the anterior portal is to use an outside-in technique with the guidance of a spinal needle. Anterior portal positioning may vary according to the intended arthroscopic technique, as is the case with arthroscopic resection of the distal end of the clavicle (Mumford procedure), in which it is positioned just anterior to the acromioclavicular joint. Exploration may be performed through both these portals or through the lateral portal located 2 to 4 cm below the acromion, immediately behind the acromioclavicular joint's posterior border. A more distal positioning would jeopardise the axillary nerve, running horizontally 5 cm away from the acromial edge. A power shaver is essential for this part of the procedure, as vision may be blocked by a swollen bursa requiring resection. Alternatively, an electric knife, laser device, or radiofrequency probe may also be used; all these tools decrease bleeding by vessel coagulation. The antero-inferior and lateral borders of the acromion and the coracohumeral ligament should all be inspected, as well as the lateral aspect of the bursa, rotator cuff musculotendinous junction, its tuberosity attachment, and the area where supraspinatus impingement may occur. From the anterior portal, the rotator cuff, posterior acromion and supraspinatus-subscapularis interval area covering the biceps tendon may be examined. The fourth portal that may be necessary is made at the suprascapularis fossa running only through the trapezium; this allows examination of the subacromial space and acromioclavicular joint. It may have a role when performing a Mumford procedure or resecting the articular surface of the acromion at the acromioclavicular joint.

By using a probe or grasping forceps, the rotator cuff may be explored to assess tear size and the amount of lateral displacement, factors to be considered if repair is a feasible option *(fig 11)*. The presence and mobility of an os acromiale may be evaluated, as well as the softness of the coracohumeral ligament if calcifications are sought. This also permits assessment of the presence of outgrowths or osteophytes at the

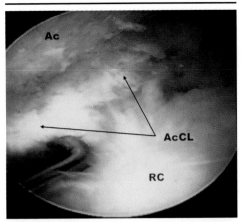

12 *Subacromial space seen from a posterior portal during a decompression by arthroscopic burring. The acromiocoracoid ligament is easily identified after resection of the acromion. Rc = rotator cuff; Ac = acromion; AcCL = acromiocoracoid ligament.*

acromioclavicular joint or anterior acromial edge, including hooked types II and III, and acromions with less than a 30 degree slope from a lateral view. Rotator cuff and subscapular calcifications are identified, and may then be examined using a spinal needle to locate calcified collections, or occasionally with the aid of a C-arm radiographic image intensifier.

■ *Subacromial or acromioclavicular joint conditions susceptible to arthroscopic management*

Subacromial impingement of any etiology may be solved by arthroscopic acromioplasty in association with other arthroscopic surgical procedures such as coracohumeral ligament sectioning and resection of subacromial bursa, calcifications, os acromiale, loose bodies or foreign bodies (fig 12). Partial, total, and massive rotator cuff tears may be managed by direct fixation of tissues to the greater tuberosity using anchors or anchors with suture [20, 24]. Coracoid impingement can be solved by motorised resection of the tip of the coracoid [23]. Different diseases of the acromioclavicular joint may be managed by debridement and the Mumford procedure [32]. Peri-articular calcifications may be debrided using a shaver or with the help of a laser system. Acromioclavicular instabilities may be stabilised by fixation of the clavicle to the coracoid process [39, 43]. Subacromial adhesions (captured shoulder), bursitis, tumours, pseudotumours, loose bodies, and various synovial-based proliferations may all be resected with arthroscopic techniques [29]. Biopsy and culture of tissue or fluid may help in diagnosing many specific conditions [29]. Focal infection within this space may also be drained and debrided [39].

Complications

Some complications inherent to the arthroscopic technique are discussed below; the authors have excluded complications which correspond to specific surgical procedures.

COMPLICATIONS AND SIDE EFFECTS OF ANAESTHESIA

The use of interscalene nerve block has become very popular for arthroscopic shoulder procedures performed on an outpatient basis, which results in financial savings among another advantages [3, 4, 30]. However, complications resulting from faulty technique have been described. Intravascular injection of local anaesthetics may give rise to a toxic reaction potentially evolving into grand mal seizure [30]. This must be prevented by careful technique and by intermittent aspiration with the syringe during the anaesthetic injection. Local anaesthetics may be toxic to nerves, which may result in prolonged paralysis [39]. In this sense, lidocaine, mepivacaine, and bupivacaine are considered the anaesthetics with the lowest potential for complications. Intranervous injection may also result in permanent nerve injury, identified by acute, intense pain and the patient's resistance to continue with the anaesthetic injection, which should be stopped. Hypotensive-bradycardic events during shoulder arthroscopy have been reported in more than 20% of patients when interscalene block is used in the beach chair position [27]. This is the result of vaso-vagal reactions and neurocardiogenic syncope, as induced by Bezol-Jarisch reflex activation [27]. It is reversed by administration of a beta-blocker such as metoprolol. Complete airway obstruction has been reported during a subacromial decompression procedure in a lateral decubitus position, under interscalene block, and with the aid of an irrigation pump [19]. This obstruction was caused by extra-articular soft tissue dissection by the irrigating solution, under high pressure flow from the arthroscopic pump.

A 5 cm increase in neck perimeter may be noted following routine shoulder arthroscopy procedures. In such a situation, immediate tracheal intubation may be necessary, and a life-threatening complication should be suspected if the patient exhibits swallowing difficulties or any other unfamiliar throat-related sensations. Similarly, other complications such as subcutaneous emphysema, pneumomediastinum [19] and pneumothorax [12] have been reported for subacromial decompression, more commonly in patients with chronic obstructive pulmonary disease. Between 13 and 17% of interscalene blocks are not capable of taking the patient through the intervention and must be converted to general anaesthesia. This often results from the development of anxiety or respiratory/swallowing difficulties [3, 4].

The side effects of interscalene block are well known: benign Horner's syndrome in more than 50% of patients from stellate ganglion block, and recurring laryngeal nerve block with hoarseness and a weak voice in less than 10% of patients, which usually resolves within 3-5 hours after surgery [3, 4, 30]. It will also block the phrenic nerve in almost 100% of patients, with a subclinical reduction of pulmonary function by 30% [30]. However, despite a change in the pulmonary function test, these patients rarely complain of dyspnea. The beach chair position facilitates pulmonary function and is thus recommended when interscalene block is used. If the phrenic nerve paralysis affects pulmonary function on the surgical side when the lateral decubitus position is used, then the contralateral lung cannot adequately make up for loss of function, as it is being compressed against the operating table. A positive-pressure ventilation unit should be available and the patient intubated should decompensation develop.

Epidural block may be achieved by epidural, subarachnoid or subdural injection. This does not present any difficulties or require unusual precautions for the surgical intervention [3, 4, 30]. The complications of general anaesthesia are common to all surgical procedures, and arthroscopic techniques are no exception. A study comparing general anaesthesia to interscalene block considered the latter a good option with minimal morbidity, as recommended by Mayfield, who also points out its lower cost. However, in another study, general anaesthesia proved effective in reducing costs and was safely used on an outpatient basis [26].

COMPLICATIONS FROM IRRIGATING SOLUTIONS

Since the introduction of laser and RF probes that may be operated in a conventional physiologic saline environment, there is no need to use special, non-ionic solutions such as sterile water, 1.5% glycine or isosmolar glycerol. Sterile water and to a lesser extent glycine, because of its hyposmolarity, may damage joint cells. The leakage of glycine into the general circulation may cause visual disorders and blindness [6], and in extreme cases brain oedema. Glycerol has proven an appropriate medium when the above-mentioned probes are not available and electrosurgery has to be used. Occasionally (and more frequently during the procedures performed early on), the arthroscopic technique may have to be aborted or converted to an open technique because of significant oedema during the intervention. This situation is more common when a high pressure pump is used. The chance of creating a compartment syndrome and vascular compromise should convince the surgeon to stop the intervention. In most instances, the oedema will resolve within the following hours, although a very large and hard shoulder may be noted by the end of the procedure.

INJURY TO INTRA- AND PERI-ARTICULAR STRUCTURES

Instruments, particularly of the motorised type, which are being handled within a relatively small joint may cause iatrogenic injuries on the articular surfaces. Exposed bony areas, such as the posterior bare area of the humeral head, may be inadvertently pierced upon introduction of the arthroscopic cannula, particularly in tighter shoulders such as those suffering from joint stiffness. Excessive acromial resection during subacromial decompression may lead to posterior fracture due to the resulting weakness in this area. A sound preoperative approach will prevent this complication. Excessive soft tissue resection over the anterior edge of the acromion may result in a release of the deltoid insertion with significant functional loss as a consequence. Other inner structures such as the labrum or the biceps tendon may become injured, particularly when the anatomy is not properly understood and the normal but infrequent anatomical variations are mistaken for lesions. The rotator cuff may become injured when transtendinous portals are used, and when power tools or instruments designed for suture and anchor placement are handled improperly. Particular care must be taken when operating electric knife terminals. Because of the power they require for coagulation and cutting purposes, they may cause burns. Laser or RF probes, particularly if capsular thermal shrinkage is performed using inappropriate power or for an excessive length of time, may lead to disastrous capsular ablation and neuritis of adjacent nerves, most frequently the axillary nerve. Remnants of a broken tool or loosened anchorage systems [22] may result in intra-articular damage when left behind in the joint. Synovial reactions to the presence of such objects or to bio-absorbable materials may also be a source of damage [5].

NERVE INJURY

Injury to the brachial plexus has been reported, as well as to the following nerves: musculocutaneous, circumflex, supras-capular, ulnar, median, cutaneous of the forearm, dorsal digital of the thumb, hypoglossal and lateral femoral cutaneous [40]. The aetiology of such lesions is often difficult to determine. Patient and arm positioning and movement, traction

used during the surgical procedure, joint distension and irrigation fluid leakage, and arthroscopic portal location may all be contributing factors [40]. Care is essential to prevent this type of injury. Bony protuberances should be padded, particularly at the wrist to avoid compressing the sensitive branch of the digital dorsal nerve of the thumb, at the contralateral iliac crest to avoid compression of the femoral cutaneous nerve, and at the tibial plateau region to prevent compression of the peroneal nerve. The lateral decubitus position may cause compression of the contralateral brachial plexus by the humeral head. A roll or a one litre serum bag should be placed under the weight-bearing axilla resting on the table. The arm should be positioned anterior to the thorax, which is facilitated by tilting the trunk backwards [17]. Traction in excess of 7 kg should not be used on the limb axis, or in excess of 5 kg when perpendicular to the arm. Excessive traction results in abnormal somatosensory potentials at the musculocutaneous, median, ulnar, and radial nerves, the former being most susceptible [35]. When perpendicular to the arm, traction may compromise the median and ulnar nerves, so adequate padding should be provided at the point where the force is applied [40]. The beach chair position requires no traction whatsoever, and thus avoids such complications [35]. When in this position, the head stance must be monitored to prevent inadvertent traction on the brachial plexus. Extreme arm extension or abduction positions must be avoided. To reduce tension on the plexus, 30° of forward elevation are recommended. The lowest intra-articular pressure is obtained with 60° of arm abduction and the highest with arm rotation, particularly before drainage portals are set up. Capsular distension and irrigation fluid leakage may result in neurological lesions [36]. Haemorrhage control using RF or laser probes allows lower intra-articular pressures while having a bloodless field, thus avoiding the high pressure flow required for control of bleeding by arthroscopic infusion pumps. Shortening procedure time by diligent practice will prevent excessive leakage and oedema.

Selection of the arthroscopic portals is essential to avoid nerve injury [2, 40]. The posterior portal is at least 9 cm away from the circumflex nerve, and thus no risk of nerve injury should be present. The inferior branch of the suprascapular nerve may be injured at an area medial to the posterior entry point, or when transglenoid

perforation techniques are used for glenohumeral instability. The anterior portal should be positioned lateral to and above the tip of the coracoid process to avoid damage to the musculocutaneous nerve. When an antero-inferior glenohumeral portal is used below the edge of the subscapularis muscle, no distally-directed angulations should be carried out for fear of injuring the brachial plexus. The superior portal at the supraspinatus fossa should be placed as lateral as possible to prevent damage to the suprascapular nerve, at 3 cm in a medial direction. Some techniques such as capsular thermal shrinkage and antero-inferior capsule retensioning may put the axillary nerve, contiguous to the capsule at this level, at risk for either thermal or mechanical damage [1, 16]. Abduction will further approximate the axillary nerve to the capsule, thereby increasing the chance for complications. The possibility that a Charcot's shoulder may develop from denervation brought about by temperature-based techniques cannot be ruled out. Intra-operative monitoring by recording somatosensory evoked potentials may prevent these neurological lesions from developing [13, 35], and checking the neurological status after surgery is always recommended. Reflex sympathetic dystrophy reported as a neurological complication is not specific to arthroscopic techniques.

VASCULAR INJURIES

Vascular injuries are uncommon and develop mostly on the cephalic vein upon establishment of the anterior portal, giving rise to usually irrelevant bleeding and echymosis [10]. Potential vascular injury may develop from an insult to suprascapular vessels when the superior portal is opened, or upon creation of an anterior subacromial portal due to injury to branches from the thoraco-acromial artery located on the medial side of the coracohumeral ligament. Post-operative vascular assessment is mandatory.

INFECTION

Infection rarely develops when arthroscopic techniques are used, as they are minimally aggressive and include continuous washing during the intervention. A superficial infection of a portal site may occur, which resolves with a superficial wash out and a brief course of oral antibiotics. In such a situation, the portal site should never be closed. Some surgeons prefer to leave the most posterior portal open, with no formal closure by sutures or tapes, to guarantee adequate drainage evacuation from the joint.

References

[1] Abrams JS. Thermal capsulorrhaphy for instability of the shoulder: concerns and applications of the heat probe. *Instr Course Lect* 2001 ; 50 : 29-36

[2] Andrews JR, Heckman MM. Basic techniques for shoulder arthroscopy. In : McGinty JB ed. Operative arthroscopy. New York : Raven Press, 1991 : 477-483

[3] Arciero RA, Taylor DC, Harrison SA, Snyder RJ, Leahy KE, Uhorchak JN. Interscalene anesthesia for shoulder arthroscopy in a community-sized military hospital. *Arthroscopy* 1996 ; 12 : 715-719

[4] Brown AR, Weiss R, Greenberg C, Flatow EL, Bigliani LU. Interscalene block for shoulder arthroscopy: comparison with general anesthesia. *Arthroscopy* 1993 ; 9 : 295-300

[5] Burkart A, Imhoff AB, Roscher E. Foreign-body reaction to bioabsorbable suture device. *Arthroscopy* 2000 ; 16 : 91-95

[6] Burkhart SS, Barnett CR, Snyder SJ. Transient postoperative blindness as a possible effect of glycine toxicity. *Arthroscopy* 1990 ; 6 : 112-114

[7] Burkhart SS, Morgan C. SLAP lesions in the overhead athlete. *Orthop Clin North Am* 2001 ; 32 : 431-441

[8] Burman MS. Arthroscopy or the direct visualization of the joints. An experimental cadaver study. *Clin Orthop* 2001 ; 390 : 5-9

[9] Cameron SE. Arthroscopic reduction and internal fixation of an anterior glenoid fracture. *Arthroscopy* 1998 ; 14 : 743-746

[10] Caspari RB. Complications of shoulder arthroscopy. In : Spague NF 3rd ed. Complications in arthroscopy. New York : Raven Press, 1989 : 179-197

[11] Conway JE. Arthroscopic repair of partial-thickness rotator cuff tears and SLAP lesions in professional baseball players. *Orthop Clin North Am* 2001 ; 32 : 443-456

[12] Dietzel DP, Ciullo JV. Spontaneous pneumothorax after shoulder arthroscopy: a report of four cases. *Arthroscopy* 1996 ; 12 : 99-102

[13] Gartsman GM, Hammerman SM. Arthroscopic biceps tenodesis: operative technique. *Arthroscopy* 2000 ; 16 : 550-552

[14] Gartsman GM, Hasan SS. What's new in shoulder surgery? *J Bone Joint Surg Am* 2001 ; 83 : 145-151

[15] Gill TJ, McIrvin E, Mair SD, Hawkins RJ. Results of biceps tenotomy for treatment of pathology of the long head of the biceps brachii. *J Shoulder Elbow Surg* 2001 ; 10 : 247-249

[16] Greis PE, Burks RT, Schickendantz MS, Sandmeier R. Axillary nerve injury after thermal capsular shrinkage of the shoulder. *J Shoulder Elbow Surg* 2001 ; 10 : 231-235

[17] Gross RM, Fitzgibbons TC. Shoulder arthroscopy: a modified approach. *Arthroscopy* 1985 ; 1 : 156-159

[18] Harryman DT 2nd. Arthroscopic management of shoulder stiffness. *Oper Tech Sports Med* 1997 ; 5 : 264-274

[19] Hutchinson MR, Veenstra MA. Arthroscopic decompression of shoulder impingement secondary to os acromiale. *Arthroscopy* 1993 ; 9 : 28-32

[20] Hynson JM, Tung A, Guevara JE, Katz JA, Glick JM, Shapiro WA. Complete airway obstruction during arthroscopic shoulder surgery. *Anesth Analg* 1993 ; 76 : 875-878

[21] Iannnotti JP, Ramsey ML. Arthroscopic decompression of a ganglion cyst causing suprascapular nerve compression. *Arthroscopy* 1996 ; 12 : 739-745

[22] Kaar TK, Schenck RC, Wirth MA, Rockwood CA. Complications of metallic suture anchors in shoulder surgery: a report of 8 cases. *Arthroscopy* 2001 ; 17 : 31-37

[23] Karnaugh RD, Sperling JW, Warren RF. Arthroscopic treatment of coracoid impingement. *Arthroscopy* 2001 ; 17 : 784-787

[24] Kempf JF, Bonnomet F. Rotator cuff tears: the arthroscopic techniques. *Encycl Méd Chir* (Éditions Scientifiques et Médicales Elsevier SAS, Paris), Surgical Techniques in Orthopaedics and Traumatology, 55-190-E-10, 2000 : 1-5

[25] Larrain MV, Botto GJ, Montenegro HJ, Mauas DM. Arthroscopic repair of acute traumatic anterior shoulder dislocation in young athletes. *Arthroscopy* 2001 ; 17 : 373-377

[26] Lewis RA, Buss DD. Outpatient shoulder surgery. A prospective analysis of a perioperative protocol. *Clin Orthop* 2001 ; 390 : 138-141

[27] Liguori GA, Khan RL, Gordon J, Gordon MA, Urban MK. The use of metoprolol and glycopyrrolate to prevent hypotensive/bradycardic events during shoulder arthroscopy in the sitting position under interscalene block. *Anesth Analg* 1998 ; 87 : 1320-1325

[28] Mahieu X, Chaouat G, Blin JL, Frank A, Hardy P. Arthroscopic treatment of pigmented villonodular synovitis of the shoulder. *Arthroscopy* 2001 ; 17 : 81-87

[29] Matthews LS, Wolock BS, Martin DF. Arthroscopic management of inflammatory arthritis and synovitis of the shoulder. In : McGinty JB ed. Operative arthroscopy. New York : Raven Press, 1991 : 573-581

[30] Mayfield JB, Carter C, Wang C, Warner JJ. Arthroscopic shoulder reconstruction. Fast-track recovery and outpatient treatment. *Clin Orthop* 2001 ; 390 : 10-15

[31] McIntyre LF. Arthroscopic capsulorrhaphy for multidirectional instability. *Oper Tech Sports Med* 1997 ; 5 : 233-237

[32] Miller MD, Flatow EF. Arthroscopic debridement of the acromioclavicular joint and distal clavicle resection. *Oper Tech Sports Med* 1997 ; 5 : 192-203

[33] Minola R, Zambonin G. Recurrent anterior instability: the arthroscopic techniques. *Encycl Méd Chir* (Éditions Scientifiques et Médicales Elsevier SAS, Paris), Surgical Techniques in Orthopaedics and Traumatology, 55-180-D-10, 2001 : 1-6

[34] Mormino MA, Gross RM, McCarthy JA. Captured shoulder: a complication of rotator cuff surgery. *Arthroscopy* 1996 ; 12 : 457-461

[35] Pitman MI, Nainzadeh N, Ergas E, Springer S. The use of somatosensory evoked potentials for detection of neurapraxia during shoulder arthroscopy. *Arthroscopy* 1988 ; 4 : 250-255

[36] Romeo AA, Cohen BS, Carreira DS. Traumatic anterior shoulder instability. *Orthop Clin North Am* 2001 ; 32 : 399-409

[37] Savoie FH 3rd, Field LD. Arthroscopic management of posterior shoulder instability. *Oper Tech Sports Med* 1997 ; 5 : 226-232

[38] Skyhar MJ, Altchek DW, Warren RF, Wickiewicz TL, O'Brien SJ. Shoulder arthroscopy with the patient in the beachchair position. *Arthroscopy* 1988 : 4 : 256-259

[39] Snyder SJ. Shoulder arthroscopy. New York : McGraw-Hill 1994

[40] Stanish WD, Peterson DC. Shoulder arthroscopy nerve injury: pitfalls and prevention. *Arthroscopy* 1995 ; 11 : 458-466

[41] Vangsness CT, Smith CH. Arthroscopic shoulder surgery with three different laser systems: evaluation of laser applications. *Arthroscopy* 1995 ; 11 : 696-700

[42] Wichmam MT, Snyder SJ. Arthroscopic capsular plication for multidirectional instability of the shoulder. *Oper Tech Sports Med* 1997 ; 5 : 238-243

[43] Wolf EM, Pennington WT. Arthroscopic reconstruction for acromioclavicular joint dislocation. *Arthroscopy* 2001 ; 17 : 558-563

Fractures of the clavicle

P Wiger
J Karlsson

Abstract. – *Fractures of the clavicle account for 5% of all fractures. Males are more frequently affected. For both genders, the incidence of clavicular fractures decreases with increasing age. The middle third of the clavicle is the weak point of the bone, in particular with regard to axial loading. The majority of patients have sustained a direct blow to the shoulder.*
Most clavicle fractures heal with conservative treatment. Distal fractures are usually the result of a high-energy injury and a direct blow to the shoulder. Without surgery, the risk factors for nonunion include the degree of high-energy trauma, fracture comminution, the degree of fracture fragment displacement, and the anatomical location of the fracture. Function is reduced, with decreased strength in elevation and abduction as well as local pain over the clavicle, which can also involve symptoms from underlying structures such as the brachial plexus or vascular structures. The purpose of treating clavicle nonunion is to reduce shoulder deformity, dysfunction, neurovascular symptoms and pain. The recommended treatment is removal of the hypertrophic nonunion/callus and restoration of the length of the clavicle, using harvested iliac graft and rigid plate and screw fixation.

Keywords: shoulder, clavicle, fracture, classification, nonunion, malunion, osteosynthesis.

Introduction

Fractures of the clavicle account for up to 44% of all shoulder girdle injuries [26]. Only fractures through the proximal humerus are more common in the shoulder region in adults. It has been estimated that 1 out of every 20 fractures involves the clavicle. It has long been thought that this fracture has an inherent reparative capacity [26]. In childhood, the clavicle is the most commonly fractured bone [3]. It heals readily in the majority of patients with remodelling of the deformity [1].

Anatomy

The clavicle is named for its S-shaped curvature, resembling the musical symbol clavicula [17]. The medial curvature provides space for the neurovascular structures through the costo-clavicular interval. The clavicle is made up of very dense bone without a well-defined medullary canal. In cross section, the clavicle changes gradually from a flat lateral aspect, to a more tubular mid-portion and then expands to a flatter medial part. The flat outer third is most compatible with pull from muscles and ligaments, whereas the tubular medial third is more compatible with axial pressure. The junction between the two cross sections varies in its precise location with the middle third of the clavicle. This junction is a weak spot, particularly with regard to axial loading. This may be one reason why fractures occur most commonly in the middle third. The clavicle is the only bony structure connecting the trunk to the shoulder girdle and the arm. The scapula and clavicle are bound securely by both the acromioclavicular and the coracoclavicular ligaments on the lateral side of the clavicle (*fig 1*).

Function of the clavicle

The clavicle supports mobility of the shoulder, overhead activity and actions requiring power and stability. It plays an important functional role in the shoulder girdle; therefore, every effort should be made to preserve or restore its normal length and alignment [11].

Classification of clavicular fractures

There are three main classifications, according to Allman [1], Rockwood [25] and Neer [20].

Allman classified clavicular fractures into three groups, based on a strict anatomical localisation.

– Group I - Fractures of the middle third.

– Group II - Fractures of the distal third.

– Group III - Fractures of the medial third.

Rockwood's classification includes both lateral and medial fractures [25]. It takes into consideration the ligamentous dependency of the bony structures of the clavicle.

– Group I - Fractures of the middle third.

– Group II - Fractures of the distal third.

– Type I - Minimal displacement (interligamentous).

– Type II - Displacement secondary to a fracture medial to the coracoclavicular ligaments.

– Conoid and trapezoid ligaments attached.

– Conoid torn, trapezoid ligaments attached.

Per Wiger, M.D., Ph.D.
Jón Karlsson, M.D., Ph.D.
Department of Orthopaedics, Sahlgrenska University Hospital, Östra, 41685 Göteborg, Sweden.

All references to this article must include: Wiger P and Karlsson J. Fractures of the clavicle. Editions Scientifiques et Médicales Elsevier SAS (Paris). All rights reserved. Surgical Techniques in Orthopaedics and Traumatology, 55-160-D-10, 2002, 5 p.

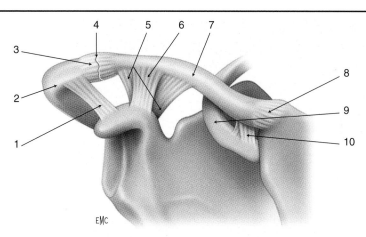

1 *Anatomy and ligaments of the clavicle. 1. Corocoacromial ligament; 2. acromion; 3. superior acromioclavicular ligament; 4. acromioclavicular joint; 5. trapezoid ligament; 6. conoid ligament; 7. clavicle; 8. sternoclavicular joint; 9. first rib; 10. costoclavicular ligament.*

– Type III - Articular surface fractures.

– Type IV - Ligaments intact to periosteum (children) with displacement of the proximal fragment. The fragment ruptures through the thin periosteum, and may be displaced upward by muscular forces.

– Type V - Comminuted; the ligaments are not attached proximally or distally, but are attached to an inferior, comminuted fragment.

– Group III - Fracture of the proximal third.

– Type I - Minimal displacement.

– Type II - Significant displacement (ligaments ruptured).

– Type III - Intra-articular.

– Type IV - Epiphyseal separation (children and young adults).

– Type V - Comminuted.

In Neer's classification, fractures distal to the proximal limit of the trapezoid ligament are defined as distal clavicular fractures.

– Type I is a fracture in which both the trapezoid and conoid ligaments remain intact and are attached to the medial fragments. This provides a stable situation.

– In Type II, the conoid ligament is ruptured and does not maintain reduction of the medial fragment. The wide displacement of the medial fragments increases the risk of nonunion [19].

– The fracture is classified as Type III if the lateral fracture is associated with an acromioclavicular joint dislocation.

Neer's classification is an easy and commonly used classification.

Incidence and mechanisms of injury

The incidence of clavicle fracture decreases with increasing age for both genders. The fracture rarely results from direct injury to

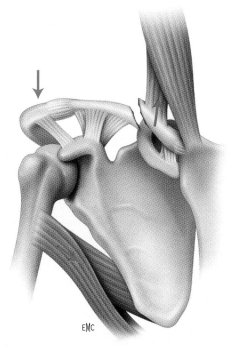

2 *Displacement of the clavicle. The distal part of the clavicle is pulled medially by the pectoralis major and downward by the weight of the arm. The proximal fragment is pulled upward by the sternocleidomastoid muscle.*

the clavicle. Distal clavicle fractures tend to result from a high-energy injury and a direct blow to the shoulder [9].

Clinical presentation

The clinical presentation shows a proximal fragment of the clavicle displaced upward and backward, which may tent the skin. The involved arm droops forward and downward *(fig 2)*. Haemorrhage produces acute swelling of the soft tissues and this may obscure the deformity.

Conservative treatment

The percentage of clavicle fractures (of all types and groups) treated non-operatively and which fail to heal has been reported to

be between 0.1% [18] and 2.2% [6, 7]. Most authors advocate non-surgical treatment of most clavicle fracture types. For ordinary closed fractures, very few studies have compared treatment with a figure-of-eight bandage to treatment using a simple sling [2, 16, 28]. To our knowledge, no study has reported a better result with either treatment. Both the figure-of-eight bandage and the simple sling reduce the pain of the fracture but do not induce callus formation. A sling is normally enough to simply support the arm, but is not intended to reduce the fracture. The more complicated figure-of-eight bandage is more restricting for the patient and there is no documentation to indicate that it leads to better healing.

Surgical technique

Due to the difficulty of surgical treatment, the risk for severe complications with surgery, and a high incidence of healing after non-surgical treatment, surgical treatment is reserved for those rare cases where the risk of skin penetration is acute or for cases of nonunion or malunion. The purpose of treating clavicular nonunion is to reduce shoulder deformity, dysfunction, neurovascular symptoms and pain. Many authors recommend removal of the hypertrophic nonunion/callus, restoration of the length of the clavicle, the use of iliac graft and fixation by a rigid plate and screws [5, 6, 10, 11, 12, 15, 22, 23, 24, 27, 29, 30, 31].

The patient is positioned in the beach chair position *(fig 3)*. The shoulder region and the iliac crest on the same side are draped. A midline incision over the clavicle is to be preferred. The bone is subcutaneous along its entire length and the only structure which crosses the incision is the supraclavicular nerve. The hypertrophic nonunion/callus should be dissected and removed. The desired alignment and length of the clavicle are estimated and restored. Stripping of the periosteum should be avoided to prevent devascularisation of the clavicle. The fragments are stabilised using a 3.5-mm DC plate, usually with at least seven holes *(fig 4, 5, 6, 7)*. The plate is applied to the superior surface of the bone.

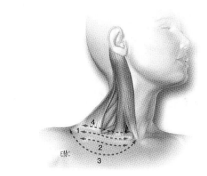

3 *Approaches to the clavicle.*

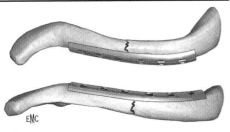

4   *Plate in the anteroinferior or inferior position.*

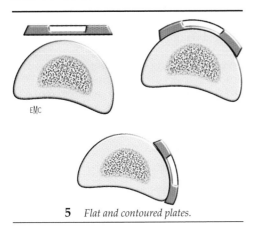

5   *Flat and contoured plates.*

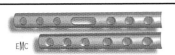

6   *Autocompressive plates.*

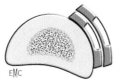

7   *Use of two superimposed contoured plates.*

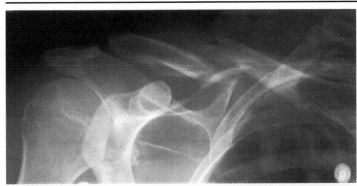

8   *Comminuted fracture caused by high-energy trauma.*

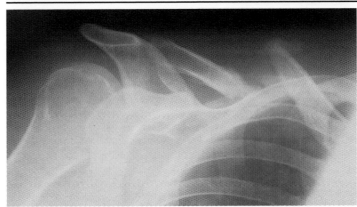

9   *Nonunion of the clavicle fracture presented in figure 8, eight months after trauma.*

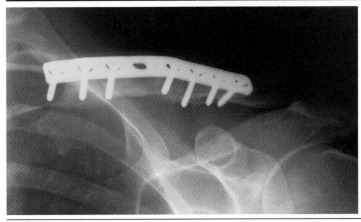

10   *Nonunion of the clavicle fracture one year after surgery. The length of the clavicle was restored, iliac graft was used and fixation was by rigid plate and screws. Callus formation is seen.*

The contours of the clavicle require bending and contouring of the plate. Stable fixation is maintained if three screws are placed in each major fragment *(fig 8, 9, 10)*. A protective instrument is used below the clavicle to avoid injury to the subclavian vein and penetration into the thorax [4, 8]. Iliac crest cancellous bone graft is placed between the fragments to stimulate healing *(fig 11, 12)*.

For an acute two-fragment clavicular fracture with wide dislocation, the McKeever technique or its variations [14] with medullary pin fixation is often used *(fig 13, 14)*. A transverse incision is made over the fracture. A canal is made in the centre of the medial fragment with a Steinmann pin without stripping the periosteum. In the same way, the pin is passed laterally into the centre of the lateral fragment and emerges close to the conoid tubercle of the clavicle. The pin is bent at its extremities to prevent its migration.

A 3.2 mm Steinmann pin which is threaded along half of its length is inserted from the lateral fragment. The fracture is reduced and

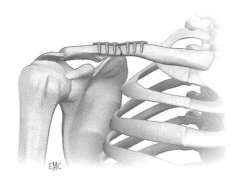

11   *Plate screwed with 6 cortical screws, on both sides of the fracture site.*

the pin is drilled into the medial fragment. The threaded part must not cross the fracture *(fig 15, 16)*.

COMPLICATIONS

Intraoperative complications when using plates or pins are rare despite the important

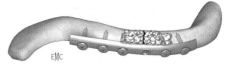

12   *Corticospongious graft and plate fixation with screws.*

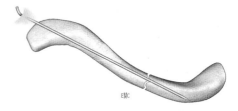

13   *Percutaneous pinning of the clavicle.*

anatomical structures beneath the clavicle. Reported complications are tearing of the subclavian vein, pneumothorax, air embolism and brachial plexus palsy. If

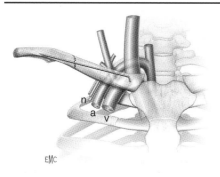

14 *Closed pin fixation from inside out, without "to and fro": n: nerves, a: artery; v: vein.*

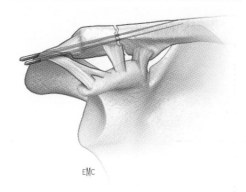

16 *Pin fixation of a fracture of the distal fourth of the clavicle.*

unthreaded pins are used, the risk of pin loosening is high. Many authors find hypertrophic scar formation to be one of the potential complications of surgical treatment [13]. Some patients are unhappy with a prominent callus after conservatively-treated clavicular fracture. It is important to inform these patients of the risk of hypertrophic scar formation after surgery.

Indications for surgery

Indications can be either absolute or relative. The only absolute indications for surgical treatment are an open fracture or an acute vascular complication after the fracture. Relative indications must take into account and evaluate the patient's shoulder deformity, dysfunction, neurovascular symptoms and pain. A sharp fragment or a vertical inferior third fragment presenting a hazard of skin penetration are relative indications for surgical treatment.

The interest in clavicular nonunion or malunion is relatively new. Primary surgical treatment of fractures of the clavicle has been associated with a risk of nonunion on the order of 3.7% according to Rowe [26] and 4.6% according to Neer [18]. In conservative treatment, the risk factors for nonunion include the degree of high-energy trauma, comminution, the degree of fragment displacement and the anatomical region of the fracture [5, 12, 22, 24, 25, 27, 29]. In 1986 a FDA (Food and Drug Administration, USA) panel defined nonunion as "established" when a minimum of 9 months had elapsed since injury and the fracture had shown no progressive signs of healing for 3 months.

The finding that nonunion is more common in mid-clavicle fractures than in distal fractures has been ascribed to the fact that the mid-clavicle fractures are more common [5, 12, 29, 30]. By definition, a malunion is healing with the fragments in a non-anatomical position which impairs function in several ways.

Patients with a nonunited clavicle fracture usually have cosmetic complaints about deformity, with adduction, shortening and protraction of the shoulder girdle. Function is reduced with less strength in elevation and abduction, as well as local pain over the clavicle, which can also involve symptoms from underlying structures such as the brachial plexus or blood vessels [25]. Problems after nonunion include thoracic outlet syndrome, subclavian artery or vein compression, thrombosis and brachial plexus palsy [13, 14, 20].

Post-operative rehabilitation

Postoperatively, the patient uses a sling for comfort during wound healing, i.e. the initial 14 days. Passive shoulder pendulum and flexion exercises of the elbow are permitted. Full overhead activities and exercises with resistance should be avoided for at least two months, until callus formation is visible on the control radiographs. Reliable fracture union usually occurs four months after surgery, and the patient can return to most occupational duties. Hardware may cause skin problems. After consolidation of the fracture, which usually occurs after 12-18 months, the plate can be safely removed.

Conclusion

For acute clavicular fractures, to our knowledge, no study has presented a better result with open reduction and internal fixation than with consevative treatment. The percentage of non-surgically treated clavicular fractures, of all types and groups, which fail to heal has been reported to be between 0.1% and 2.2%. Absolute acute indications for surgical treatment are skin penetration or vascular complications after fracture. Primary surgical treatment of fractures of the clavicle has been associated with an increased risk of nonunion, formation of a "bump", and a visible or sometimes unaesthetic scar, particularly in women.

Secondary surgical treatment is indicated for nonunion or malunion if the patient has severe symptoms, such as pain or decreased strength, or in the case of cosmetic complaints about deformity.

Fixation with a plate, screws and iliac crest cancellous bone graft placed between the fragments can restore the length of the clavicle and supports callus formation. Before this kind of surgery is undertaken, the patient should be well informed about the risks.

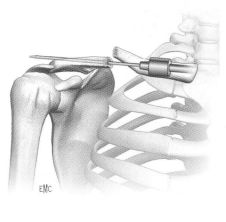

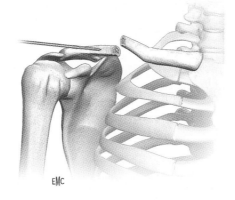

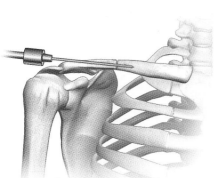

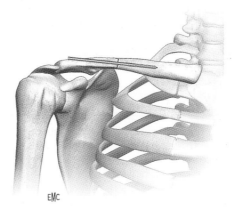

15 *Pin fixation by the "to and fro" technique.*

References

[1] Allman FL. Fractures and ligamentous injuries of the clavicle and its articulation. *J Bone Joint Surg Am* 1967 ; 49 : 774-784

[2] Anderson K, Jensen PO, Lauritzen J. Treatment of clavicular fractures: figure-of-eight bandage vs. a simple sling. *Acta Orthop Scand* 1987 ; 57 : 71-74

[3] Dameron TB Jr, Rockwood CA Jr. Fractures of the shaft of the clavicle. In : Rockwood CA Jr, Wilkins KE, King RE eds. Fractures in children. Philadelphia : JB Lippincott, 1984 : 608-624

[4] DellaSanta D, Narakas A, Bonnard C. Late lesions of the brachial plexus after fracture of the clavicle. *Ann Hand Surg* 1991 ; 10 : 531-540

[5] Edvardsen P, Odegard O. Treatment of posttraumatic clavicular pseudoarthrosis. *Acta Orthop Scand* 1977 ; 48 : 456-457

[6] Eskola A, Vainionpaa S, Myllyen P. Surgery for ununited clavicular fracture. *Acta Orthop Scand* 1986 ; 57 : 366-367

[7] Eskola A, Vainionpaa S, Myllynen P, Patiala H, Rokkanen P. Outcome of clavicular fracture in 89 patients. *Arch Orthop Trauma Surg* 1986 ; 105 : 337-338

[8] Guilfoil PH, Christiansen T. An unusual vascular complication of fractured clavicle. *JAMA* 1967 ; 200 : 72-73

[9] Heppenstall RB. Fractures and dislocations of the distal clavicle. *Orthop Clin North Am* 1975 ; 6 : 447-486

[10] Jablon M, Sutker A, Post M. Irreducible fractures of the middle third of the clavicle. *J Bone Joint Surg Am* 1979 ; 61 : 296-298

[11] Jupiter JB, Leffert RD. Nonunion of the clavicle. *J Bone Joint Surg Am* 1987 ; 67 : 753-760

[12] Kabaharjve E, Joukainen J, Peltonen J. Treatment of pseudoarthrosis of the clavicle. *Injury* 1982 ; 13 : 400-403

[13] Khan MA, Lucas HK. Plating of fractures of the middle third of the clavicle. *Injury* 1978 ; 9 : 263-267

[14] Lengua F, Nuss JM, Lechner R, Baruthio J, Veillon F. Traitement des fractures de la clavicule par embrochage à foyer fermé de dedans en dehors sans va-et-vient. *Rev Chir Orthop* 198787 : 377-380

[15] Manske DJ, Szabo RM. The operative treatment of mid shaft clavicular non-unions. *J Bone Joint Surg Am* 1985 ; 67 : 1367-1371

[16] McCandless DN, Mowbray M. Treatment of displaced fractures of the clavicle. Sling vs. figure-of-eight bandage. *Practitioner* 1979 ; 223 : 266-267

[17] Moseley HF. The clavicle : its anatomy and function. *Clin Orthop* 1968 ; 58 : 17-27

[18] Neer CS2nd. Nonunion of the clavicle. *JAMA* 1960 ; 172 : 1006-1011

[19] Neer CS2nd. Fractures of the distal third of the clavicle. *Clin Orthop* 1968 ; 58 : 43-50

[20] Neer CS2nd. Fractures of the clavicle. In : Rockwood CA Jr, Green DP eds. Fractures in adults. Philadelphia : JB Lippincott, 1984 : 707-713

[21] Nordqvist A, Redlund-Johnell I, VonScheele A, Petersson CJ. Shortening of clavicle after fracture. Incidence and clinical significance: a 5-year follow-up of 85 patients. *Acta Orthop Scand* 1997 ; 68 : 349-351

[22] Olsen B, Vaesel M, Sojbjerg J. Treatment of midshaft clavicular nonunion with plate fixation and autologous bone grafting. *J Shoulder Elbow Surg* 1995 ; 4 : 337-344

[23] O'Rourke IC, Middleton RW. The place and efficacy of operative management of fractured clavicle. *Injury* 1975 ; 6 : 236-240

[24] Pyper JB. Nonunion of fractures of the clavicle. *Injury* 1978 ; 9 : 268-270

[25] Rockwood CA Jr, Matsen FA3rd. The shoulder. Philadelphia : WB Saunders, 1990

[26] Rowe CR. An atlas of anatomy and treatment of midclavicular fractures. *Clin Orthop* 1968 ; 58 : 29-42

[27] Simpson LA, Kellam J. Surgical management of fractures of the clavicle, scapula, and proximal humerus. *Orthop Update Series* 1985 ; 4 : 1-8

[28] Stanley D, Norris SH. Recovery following fractures of the clavicle treated conservatively. *Injury* 1988 ; 19 : 162-164

[29] Thompson AG, Batten RL. The application of rigid internal fixation to the treatment of nonunion and delayed union using AO technique. *Injury* 1977 ; 8 : 88-98

[30] Tregonning G, Macnab I. Post-traumatic pseudoarthrosis of the clavicle. *J Bone Joint Surg Br* 1976 ; 58 : 264

[31] Wilkins RM, Johnston RM. Ununited fractures of the clavicle. *J Bone Joint Surg Am* 1983 ; 65 : 773-778

Acromioclavicular dislocations

J Eulert
TD Böhm

Abstract. – Acute dislocations of the acromioclavicular joint (Rockwood type IV, V, VI and some type III injuries) usually require primary surgical reconstruction. For these conditions, we use a combined acromioclavicular and coracoclavicular fixation. After a bra-strap skin-incision and exposure of the acromioclavicular joint, the deltotrapezius muscle fascia and the coracoclavicular ligaments, the acromioclavicular joint is reduced and held with a single unthreaded 2 mm Kirschner-wire. For coracoclavicular fixation, a 2 mm polydioxanon-sulphate (PDS) cord is used in a figure of eight loop through an drill hole in the clavicle and around the base of the coracoid. In addition, a reconstruction of the acromioclavicular and coracoclavicular ligaments is performed.

In chronic symptomatic acromioclavicular dislocations, we recommend a modified Weaver-Dunn procedure. After a bra-strap skin-incision and exposure of the acromioclavicular joint, the deltotrapezius muscle fascia and the coracoclavicular ligaments, the distal 1.5 cm of the clavicle is resected. The acromial end of the coracoacromial ligament is detached with a bony sliver and fixed into the medullary canal of the distal clavicle with non-absorbable sutures. For coracoclavicular fixation, a 2 mm polydioxanon-sulphate cord is used in a figure of eight loop through a drill hole in the clavicle and around the base of the coracoid.

Keywords: shoulder, acromioclavicular dislocation, reconstruction.

Introduction

Injuries to the acomioclavicular (AC) joint usually are the result of a force applied downwards on the acromion such as in a fall directly on the adducted shoulder. After clinical assessment, specific radiographs of the AC joint are necessary to determine the degree and the direction of the dislocation. Anteroposterior, axillary and stress films give sufficient information to classify the injury into 6 types according to Rockwood [13] (fig 1).

Treatment

ACUTE ACROMIOCLAVICULAR DISLOCATIONS

Type I and II dislocations usually do not require primary surgical intervention [1, 2, 6, 7, 8, 13]. Conservative treatment includes immobilisation in a sling for 10 to 14 days, ice application, analgesics, and within the limits of comfort, an early and gradual

Jochen Eulert, M.D., Professor and Chairman.
T. Dirk Böhm, M.D.
Department of Orthopaedics, Brettreichstrasse II, University of Würzburg, 97074 Würzburg, Germany.

rehabilitation. Most type III dislocations are also treated conservatively, except for type III dislocations in young athletes (especially those involved in overhead sports), in heavy manual or overhead workers, and in very thin persons with a very prominent lateral clavicle [1, 7]. We recommend surgical treatment for type IV, V and VI dislocations. In our opinion, successful treatment should fulfill the following requirements : exposure and debridement of the AC joint, repair of the AC and coracoclavicular (CC) ligaments, reduction and stable fixation of the AC joint. Several surgical procedures, either with reposition and fixation across the AC joint [2, 12], or with reposition and fixation between the clavicle and the coracoid [3], fulfil these requirements. Excision of the distal clavicle [10] and dynamic muscle transfers should not be used in acute cases. In the Phemister procedure [12], two threaded pins are inserted from the lateral acromion, crossing each other at the centre of the articular facet of the acromion to stabilise the AC joint. In addition, the CC ligaments, the AC joint capsule and the AC ligaments are reconstructed [12]. Bosworth uses a specially designed screw, which is placed through a drill hole in the clavicle into the base of the coracoid. The CC ligaments, the superior AC ligament and the deltotrapezius

muscle fascia are reconstructed after insertion of this screw [3]. We use a combined procedure with AC fixation, CC augmentation and repair of the AC and CC ligaments.

■ Surgical procedure

The patient is set up in a beach-chair position, the arm free and the head fixed in a neutral position on the table. A 7-9 cm shoulder strap incision is made in Langer's lines starting 2-3 cm posterior to the clavicle and 1 cm medial to the AC joint, extending down to the tip of the coracoid (fig 2).

The incision is undermined and the AC joint, the anterior deltoid with the deltotrapezius muscle fascia, and the lateral third of the clavicle are exposed. Usually, the deltotrapezius muscle fascia is already detached from the distal clavicle; if not, the interval must be divided by splitting the periostium of the distal 5-6 cm of the clavicle horizontally. The AC joint is explored and if possible the intra-articular disk is preserved or reconstructed. However, if it is too badly damaged, it must be excised and the joint debrided. The clavicle can now be lifted upwards with a bone-clamp and the torn CC ligaments and the base of the coracoid can be visualised after a blunt vertical deltoid split. The torn ends of CC ligaments

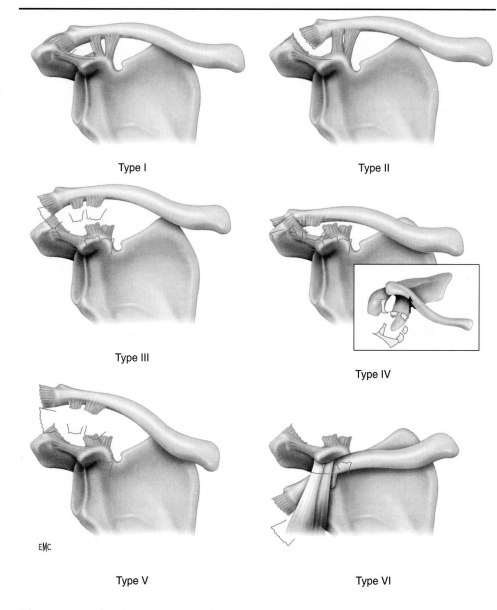

Type I

Type II

Type III

Type IV

Type V

Type VI

1 *Rockwood classification of acromioclavicular injuries.*
Type I: neither acromioclavicular nor coracoclavicular ligaments are disrupted.
Type II: acromioclavicular ligament is disrupted, and coracoclavicular ligaments are intact.
Type III: both ligaments are disrupted.
Type IV: ligaments are disrupted and the distal end of the clavicle is displaced posteriorly into or through trapezius muscle.
Type V: ligaments and muscle attachments are disrupted, and major separation (100-300% of the normal shoulder) between clavicle and scapula has occurred.
Type VI: ligaments are disrupted, and the distal clavicle is dislocated inferior to coracoid process and posterior to biceps and coracobrachialis tendons.

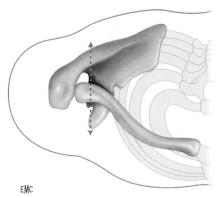

2 *Shoulder strap skin incision following Langer's lines.*

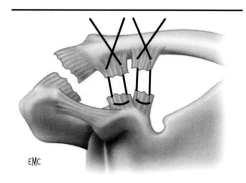

3 *Exposure of the AC joint, coracoid, CC ligaments and re-approximation of the CC ligaments.*

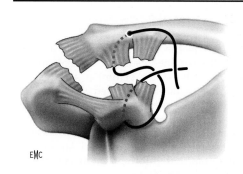

4 *Coracoclavicular augmentation with a 2 mm PDS cord through a drill hole in the clavicle and around the base of the coracoid.*

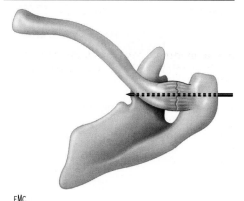

5 *AC joint stabilisation with a smooth 2 mm central Kirschner-wire.*

are freed and tagged with PDS sutures, which are not tied at this time *(fig 3)*.

A vertical 3.2 mm drill hole is then placed in the clavicle directly above the base of the coracoid. A lubricated and stretched (to avoid lengthening) 2 mm PDS cord is passed through this hole. Using a curved clamp, its inferior end is passed from medial to lateral around the base of the coracoid to make a figure of eight circle with the cord. With a trial reduction, the correct anatomical position is checked, but none of the sutures are tied at this time *(fig 4)*.

A smooth 2 mm Kirschner-wire with two pointed ends is placed in the centre of the acromial part of the AC joint and drilled laterally through the acromion until it perforates the skin. If this is technically not possible, the wire must be drilled from the lateral acromion through the centre of the AC joint. After manual anatomical reduction, creating a normal AC joint space, the wire is drilled into the distal clavicle until it perforates the cortex *(fig 5)*.

The lateral end of the wire is bent 90° and cut off. Now the coracoclavicular PDS cord and the sutures of the CC ligaments are tied up. Then, the remnants of the AC ligaments and the capsule are reconstructed, the deltotrapezius muscle fascia is repaired back to the clavicle and, if possible, imbricated. The skin is closed by intracutaneous suture.

■ *Postoperative care*

The arm is kept in a sling for 2 weeks, with physiotherapy starting after removal of the drain. Abduction and anteversion is limited to 90° until removal of the Kirschner-wire after 6-8 weeks. To prevent heterotopic ossification, indomethacin (2 x 50 mg daily) is given for 2 weeks, and no heavy lifting, pulling or pushing is allowed for 3 months.

■ *Special circumstances or variations of the technical procedure*

If there is a fracture of the coracoid in addition to the AC dislocation, the CC fixation must be abandoned, and only an AC fixation and reconstruction of the ligaments and deltotrapezius muscle fascia is performed. Associated fractures of the lateral clavicle or the acromion usually need appropriate fixation of this fracture in addition to the AC fixation. If the AC joint shows significant arthritis, we use the modified Weaver-Dunn procedure as described for chronic AC dislocations.

■ *Complications and results*

Besides general complications such as wound infection, osteomyelitis or nerve injury, the following procedure-associated complications are reported: soft-tissue ossification, migration of the wire, AC arthritis, bone erosion by the wire, metal failure, loss of purchase of the fixation, and fractures through implant holes [8, 13]. AC fixation procedures have good or excellent results in 66% (Bargren JH, Erlanger S, Dick HM. Biomechanics and comparison of two operative methods of treatment of complete acromioclavicular separation. *Clin Orthop* 1978; 130: 267-272), 89% [6], 97% [7] and 98% [17]. CC fixation procedures have good or excellent results in 77% [1], 86% [9], 89% [6] and 94% (Bargren et al, 1978). No results of the presented method with AC and CC fixation combined with a repair of the AC and CC ligaments have been published so far. Similar methods with a combined AC and CC fixation have reported good and excellent results in 85% [11] and 89% [5].

CHRONIC ACROMIOCLAVICULAR DISLOCATIONS

In chronic symptomatic AC dislocations, we use a modified Weaver-Dunn procedure [14, 15] with an additional coracoclavicular PDS augmentation.

■ *Surgical procedure*

The patient's set up and the surgical approach are identical to those described for acute repair of AC dislocations (*fig 2*). After exposure of the AC joint, the coracoacromial and CC ligaments, the deltotrapezius muscle fascia and the base of the coracoid (*fig 3*), the distal 1-1.5 cm of the clavicle are excised (*fig 6*).

The medullary canal of the distal clavicle is then curetted, and two 2 mm drill holes are

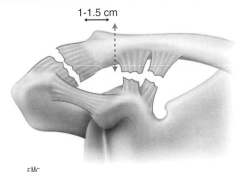

1-1.5 cm

6 *Resection of 1-1.5 cm of the distal clavicle.*

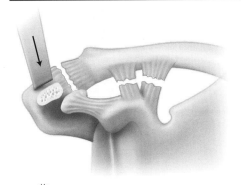

7 *Detachment of the acromioclavicular ligament with a bony sliver from the acromion process.*

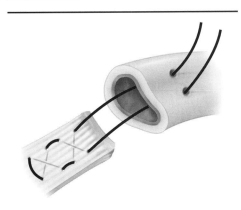

8 *Preparation of the acromioclavicular ligament and the distal clavicle.*

made into the superior cortex leaving a bone-bridge of 1.5 cm to the lateral end of the clavicle. The coracoacromial ligament is detached with a small bony sliver from its acromial insertion using a chisel (*fig 7*).

A heavy No. 2 nonabsorbable suture is woven back and forth through the ligament, so that both ends exit through the acromial end of the ligament. Both suture ends are passed through the drill-holes in the clavicle and a trial reduction is performed to check the achieved correction (*fig 8*).

If the ligament is too long, the excess ligament and the bony sliver are cut away. The preparation of the CC fixation with a 2 mm PDS cord through a drill hole in the clavicle and around the base of the coracoid is performed as described for acute cases without tying them up at that point (*fig 4*).

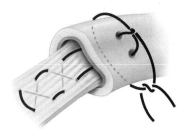

9 *Reduction of the superior migration of the clavicle by pulling the coracoacromial ligament into the clavicle.*

Holding manual correction of the superior migration of the clavicle, the PDS cord is tied in front of the clavicle. The coracoacromial ligament is pulled into the distal clavicle and fixed with two knots, before passing one end of the suture around the clavicle and securing the reduction with 4-6 knots anterior to the clavicle. This avoids a knot bulge on the superior cortex of the clavicle close to the skin (*fig 9*).

Then, closure of the deltotrapezius muscle fascia and wound closure are performed as described for acute cases.

■ *Postoperative care*

The arm is kept in a sling for 6 weeks, with physiotherapy starting after removal of the drain. Abduction and anteversion are limited to 90° for 6 weeks. To prevent heterotopic ossification, indomethacin (2 x 50 mg) is given for 2 weeks, and no heavy lifting, pulling or pushing is allowed for 3 months.

■ *Special circumstances or variations of the technical procedure*

If the transferred acromioclavicular ligament is too short, a release of the anterior fasciculus of the coracoacromial ligament provides more length. In elderly patients with only mild instability and an arthritic joint, a resection of the distal clavicle is performed as described by Mumford [10].

■ *Complications and results*

Apart from general complications such as wound infection, osteomyelitis or nerve injury, the following procedure-associated complications are reported: soft-tissue ossification, AC arthritis, loss of purchase of the fixation. Weaver and Dunn [15] reported 73% good results in their initial series in 1972, but they did not perform an additional CC augmentation. Rockwood [13] added a CC screw fixation, and Weinstein [16] performed a CC fixation with a heavy No. 5 suture to the Weaver-Dunn operation. These modifications are in principle similar to our procedure and achieved good and excellent results in 87% [4] and 77% [16].

■ *Conclusions, indications and limitations*

Reconstruction of acute AC joint dislocations gives overall good results [1, 6, 13, 17], regardless of whether or not CC or AC fixation is performed. A combination of both, together with a repair and imbrication of the deltotrapezius muscle fascia and a repair of the CC and AC ligaments, as described above, gives a solid reconstruction. The single unthreaded acromioclavicular K-wire secures the anatomical reposition of the AC joint and horizontal stability, and allows rotation. The CC fixation with a PDS cord through a drill hole in the clavicle and around the base of the coracoid provides stability without anterior displacement of the clavicle. Reconstruction of the CC and AC ligaments and the repair with imbrication of the deltotrapezius muscle fascia gives additional stability.

In chronic AC joint dislocations, when the symptoms are related to the persistent instability, a simple resection of the distal clavicle is not appropriate [4, 13]. A replacement of the CC ligaments, in addition to the transfer of the acromial attachment of the coracoacromial ligament into the distal clavicle, gives a stable AC reduction with 87% good results [4].

References

[1] Bannister GC, Wallace WA, Stableforth PG, Hutson MA. The management of acute acromioclavicular dislocation. *J Bone Joint Surg Br* 1975 ; 36 : 848-850

[2] Bateman JE. Athletic injuries about the shoulder in throwing and body-contact sports. *Clin Orthop* 1962 ; 23 : 75-83

[3] Bosworth BM. Acromioclavicular separation: new method of repair. *Surg Gynecol Obstet* 1941 ; 73 : 866-871

[4] Guy DK, Wirth MA, Griffin JL, Rockwood CA. Reconstruction of chronic and complete dislocations of the acromioclavicular joint. *Clin Orthop* 1998 ; 347 : 138-149

[5] Hessmann M, Gotzen L, Gehling H. Acromioclavicular reconstruction augmented with polydioxanonsulphate bands: surgical technique and results. *Am J Sports Med* 1995 ; 23 : 552-556

[6] Lancaster S, Horowitz M, Alonso J. Complete acromioclavicular separations. *Clin Orthop* 1987 ; 216 : 80-88

[7] Larsen E, Bjerg-Nielsen A, Christensen P. Conservative or surgical treatment of acromioclavicular dislocation. *J Bone Joint Surg Am* 1986 ; 68 : 552-555

[8] Lemos MJ. The evaluation and treatment of the injured acromioclavicular joint in athletes. *Am J Sports Med* 1998 ; 26 : 137-144

[9] Morrison DS, Lemos MJ. Acromioclavicular separation. Reconstrustion using synthetic loop augmentation. *Am J Sports Med* 1995 ; 23 : 105-110

[10] Mumford EB. Acromioclavicular dislocation. *J Bone Joint Surg* 1941 ; 23 : 799-802

[11] Nachtkamp J, Magin M, Paar O. Die operative Behandlung der ACG-Sprengung. *Aktual Traumatol* 1996 ; 26 : 42-47

[12] Phemister DB. The treatment of dislocation of the acromioclavicular joint by open reduction and threaded wire fixation. *J Bone Joint Surg* 1942 ; 24 : 166-168

[13] Rockwood CA Jr, Williams GR, Young DC. Injuries to the acromioclavicular joint. In : Rockwood CA Jr, Green DP, Buchholz RW, Heckman JD eds. Fractures in adults. Philadelphia : Lippincott Raven, 1996 : 1341-1413

[14] Shoji H, Roth C, Chuinard R. Bone block transfer of coracoacromial ligament in acromioclavicular injury. *Clin Orthop* 1986 ; 208 : 272-277

[15] Weaver JK, Dunn HK. Treatment of acromioclavicular injuries, especially complete separation. *J Bone Joint Surg Am* 1972 ; 54 : 1187-1194

[16] Weinstein DM, McCann PD, McIlveen SJ, Flatow EL, Bigliani LU. Surgical treatment of complete acromioclavicular dislocations. *Am J Sports Med* 1995 ; 23 : 324-331

[17] Zeiler G. Die operative Behandlung der akromioklavikulären Luxation. *Oper Orthop Traumatol* 1994 ; 6 : 38-45

Sternoclavicular dislocations

M Vastamäki

Abstract. – Operative treatment is seldom used in acute anterior sternoclavicular dislocations due to the risk of severe complications, but unreduced acute or chronic posterior sternoclavicular dislocations should be treated operatively. Old recurrent anterior dislocations are usually fairly asymptomatic, but occasionally may require operative treatment. There are two choices: stabilisation procedures and resection arthroplasty. It is important to improve the stability of the medial end of the clavicle. Operative treatment for spontaneous anterior sternoclavicular instability in young individuals is never indicated.

Keywords: shoulder, sternoclavicular dislocation, Speed's technique, resection arthroplasty, intra-articular disc ligament.

Introduction

The sternoclavicular joint is important for shoulder function. A joint which is too stiff may cause difficulties in the normal rotation of the clavicle and problems in the acromioclavicular joint. A joint which is too loose may be painful.

Sternoclavicular dislocations are classified on the basis of anatomy and aetiology into: traumatic (anterior and posterior or retrosternal) dislocations and atraumatic dislocations.

Anatomy

The sternoclavicular joint is a diarthrodial joint and the only true articulation between the upper extremity and the axial skeleton. The osseous stability of the sternoclavicular joint is only fair, because less than half of the medial clavicle articulates with the upper angle of the sternum. The stability of the joint is secured by various ligaments. The costoclavicular ligament, also called the rhomboid ligament, is short and strong and consists of an anterior and a posterior fasciculus (fig 1). The configuration of the two-part costoclavicular ligament is similar to that of the two-part coracoclavicular ligament. The interclavicular ligament connects the superomedial aspects of the clavicles. The capsular ligament representing thickening of the joint capsule covers the

Martti Vastamäki, M.D., Ph. D., ORTON Hospital, Helsinki, Finland.

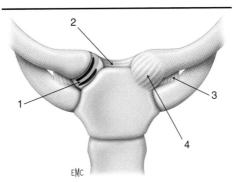

1 Ligaments of the sternoclavicular joint. 1. intra-articular disc ligament; 2. interclavicular ligament; 3. costoclavicular ligament; 4. capsular ligament.

anterosuperior and posterior aspects of the joint. The intra-articular disc or disc ligament is a very dense, fibrous structure that arises from the junction of the first rib to the sternum and passes through the sternoclavicular joint, acting as a checkrein against medial displacement of the inner clavicle [12].

Mechanism of injury

The mechanism producing sternoclavicular dislocation may be either a direct blow on the clavicle or a transmitted force. Posterior dislocation is uncommon and is almost always caused by a direct force pushing the clavicle posteriorly behind the sternum and into the mediastinum. Anterior dislocation is caused by a force applied to the anterolateral or posterolateral aspect of the shoulder. The most common causes of injury are vehicle and sports accidents [7].

Clinical and radiological assessment

The patient with an acute dislocation of the sternoclavicular joint has marked pain around the sternoclavicular joint, especially when the shoulders are pressed together by a lateral force. With an anterior dislocation, the medial head of the clavicle is visibly prominent – in contrast, with a posterior dislocation, the usually palpable medial end of the clavicle is displaced posteriorly. The corner of the sternum is more easily palpated. However, these patients may also have prominent anterior swelling [12]. Posterior dislocation of the sternoclavicular joint may be a serious injury, due to the vital structures behind the joint, such as the trachea and large vessels of the mediastinum, making the situation a true emergency (fig 2).

Routine chest radiographs may occasionally suggest sternoclavicular joint dislocation, but they are often hard to interpret. Therefore, special views have been developed, such as Rockwood's serendipity view of a 40 degree cephalic tilt [12]. However, to evaluate acute and chronic traumatic injuries of the sternoclavicular joint, the best imaging method is computed tomography.

It should not be forgotten that a prominence about the sternoclavicular joint may also be caused by a fracture of the medial end of

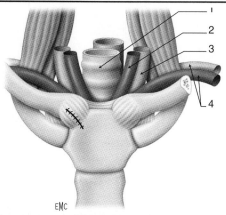

2 *Vital structures behind the sternoclavicular joint. Capsular incision used to check the intra-articular disc and joint surfaces. 1. Trachea; 2. common carotid artery; 3. internal jugular vein; 4. subclavian vein and artery.*

the clavicle or by a fracture-dislocation. In younger patients, physeal injuries are possible. The medial clavicular epiphysis does not ossify until age 18 to 20, and it fuses with the shaft of the clavicle some 5 years later [7].

Treatment

CONSERVATIVE TREATMENT

In acute anterior sternoclavicular dislocation, closed reduction is usually easily obtained by placing traction on the arm and direct pressure on the medial clavicle. If the sternoclavicular joint remains reduced, the shoulders can be stabilised with a soft figure-of-eight dressing for 6 weeks.

In posterior sternoclavicular dislocation, general anaesthesia is usually required for closed reduction. Before reduction, it is important to assess the neurovascular status of the upper extremity. With the patient supine, lateral traction is applied with the arm abducted in slight extension. If this fails, a sterile towel clip placed on the clavicle provides more leverage. After reduction, the shoulders should be held back for 4 to 6 weeks with a figure-of-eight dressing [12].

Spontaneous atraumatic anterior sternoclavicular instability is seen in hypermobile teenagers and young adults with generalised joint laxity. This condition is mostly painless and no treatment is indicated. It is important to reassure the patient and his parents that no harm is being done and that the prognosis for recovery is excellent. Operative treatment for spontaneous anterior sternoclavicular subluxation is rarely, if ever, indicated [11].

INDICATIONS FOR OPERATIVE TREATMENT

There is still controversy regarding the treatment of acute or chronic anterior dislocation of the sternoclavicular joint. Most acute anterior dislocations are unstable after reduction, and various procedures have been

recommended for repair or reconstruction of the joint. On the other hand, the operative complications may be severe and the end result unsatisfactory.

As stated above, operative treatment is seldom performed in acute anterior sternoclavicular dislocations due to the possibility of severe per- and post-operative complications. If operation is undertaken, the surgeon must be totally familiar with the anatomy immediately cephalic and posterior to the sternoclavicular joint. The subclavian vein is directly behind the clavicle and is easily torn, especially in posterior dislocations. The pleura is also easily entered. A thoracic surgeon should be available.

In selected acute anterior sternoclavicular dislocations, it may be beneficial to perform ligament repair and temporary fixation, as for almost all ligamentous injuries of other joints. In acute posterior sternoclavicular dislocations where closed reduction has failed, open reduction is always necessary.

Old recurrent anterior sternoclavicular dislocations are usually fairly asymptomatic and require no treatment, but they may occasionally become painful [2, 12]. When pain and disability persist, surgery might be indicated. Old posterior sternoclavicular dislocations should be treated surgically.

OPERATIVE TECHNIQUES

Basically, there are two choices of surgical procedures for sternoclavicular instability: reduction and stabilisation of the joint, or resection arthroplasty. The author prefers reduction and stabilisation if the joint surfaces are preserved, and particularly if the intra-articular disc ligament can be repaired. However, if the joint is destroyed, resection arthroplasty is advisable.

■ *Stabilisation procedure (modified Speed)* [8]

Make an incision along the medial 5 cm of the clavicle and over the sternoclavicular joint to the midline of the sternum. Elevate the soft tissue carefully, staying very close to the clavicle.

Expose the capsule of the sternoclavicular joint and open it along the line of its fibres to check the intra-articular disc ligament *(fig 2)*. If the disc is torn from its insertion on the medial head of the clavicle, reinsert it using no. 00 non-absorbable sutures. If the disc is too damaged and impossible to refix, it must be resected to avoid painful impingement. If the joint surfaces are severely damaged, consider resection of the medial end of the clavicle.

Expose the medial end of the first rib and its cartilage by detaching and retracting laterally and distally a part of the pectoralis major muscle. By subperiostal dissection performed very close to the bone, free about 3 to 4 cm of the first rib of soft tissue but keep its cartilage intact.

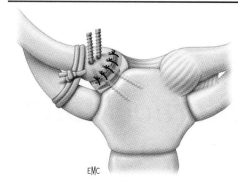

3 *Modified Speed technique to stabilise the sternoclavicular joint. Temporary K-wire fixation may be risky.*

Use an aneurysm needle having a curved blunt-pointed end with the eye at the point and pass it deep to the first rib. Thread through the eye of the needle a non-absorbable suture to which is attached a palmaris longus or, if that is lacking, a plantaris longus tendon. Draw the tendon deep to the rib [8]. Then expose the medial end of the clavicle by subperiostal dissection performed very close to the bone and pass the tendon deep to the clavicle in a similar manner. If the tendon is long enough (more than 15 cm long, i.e. when using the plantaris longus tendon), draw with the tendon an additional accessory suture and use it to form a double loop when repeating the procedure with the tendon. Then tighten the loop and tie the tendon to itself and secure the knots by no. 0000 non-absorbable sutures *(fig 3)*. At this stage, the joint should be fairly stable. Then, try to repair the elongated joint capsule by reefing.

Immobilisation of the sternoclavicular joint is problematic. Kirschner wires may cause severe complications due to migration [6, 12]. The pins, either intact or broken, may migrate to the heart, pulmonary artery, aorta or spinal cord. Because of the heavy leverage force applied to the pins that cross the sternoclavicular joint, fatigue breakage of these pins is common. Threaded pins can also migrate, causing serious complications including death. Thus, fixation of the sternoclavicular joint should not be considered.

However, the author has used two threaded 2.0 mm K-wires with bent ends from the clavicle to the sternum and immobilised the arm in a Velpeau® dressing for 5 to 6 weeks to avoid pin migration *(fig 3)*. After that, the pins are removed under local anaesthesia and mobilisation is started. The pins are easier to remove if they are not bent more than 50 degrees. The position of the pins may be checked postoperatively by computed tomography. Of course, it is important that a pin not perforate the posterior cortex of the manubrium. If pins are not used, the arm is immobilised in a Velpeau® dressing for 4 weeks, after which pendular excercises are started.

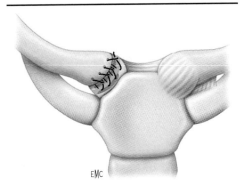

4   *Repair of intra-articular disc ligament.*

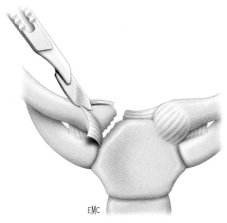

5   *Periosteal incision for sternoclavicular joint arthroplasty.*

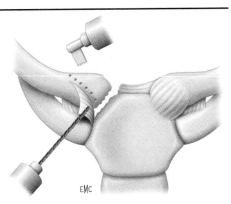

6   *Technique resecting medial end of clavicle.*

■ Intra-articular disc ligament

Patients occasionally present with a stable sternoclavicular joint associated with a reproducible and painful clicking or popping sensation after an injury such as falling on the shoulder or on the outstretched hand. These symptoms may be caused by injury to the intra-articular disc ligament [3, 12]. This injury should be considered in the differential diagnosis of any acute or chronic post-traumatic injury of the sternoclavicular joint, because it is relatively easy to treat surgically.

The biggest problem in sternoclavicular disc lesions is proving the diagnosis. History and clinical signs may give an idea, CT-arthrography may be helpful, but there also exist many "normal" disc abnormalities.

The procedure consists of exposing the sternoclavicular joint as presented earlier and repairing the disc (*fig 4*), or if this is impossible, resecting the disc. Close the capsule and the wound. Apply a sling for 3 weeks. Start pendular exercises on the first postoperative day.

■ Resection arthroplasty

Surgical resection of the medial clavicle is recommended by some authors as the method of choice for all kinds of sternoclavicular instabilities that require surgery [10]. As stated, after some poor experiences in the past, the author prefers stabilisation and ligament reconstruction in appropriate cases [4]. Also, in resection arthroplasty, it is important to create some

kind of stability of the medial end of the clavicle, because normally the costoclavicular ligament is not intact in these cases. If the ligament is intact, the resection line should be medial to it.

Expose the medial portion of the clavicle, as shown. Make an oblique incision through the periosteum of the medial portion of the clavicle from medial inferior to lateral superior, taking care to preserve the periosteum for later closure (*fig 5*). Excision of the medial portion of the clavicle is facilitated by placement of a series of holes through both cortices of the clavicle [5]. The osteotomy line is oblique in order to preserve the costoclavicular ligament and to excise the entire superior prominence (*fig 6*). Bevel the corners of the clavicle and repair the periosteal tube carefully around the residual portion of the clavicle. If the sternal attachment of the intra-articular disc ligament is intact, the clavicular end of the ligament may be fixed into the medullary canal of the medial end of the clavicle. Immobilise the arm in a sling for 6 weeks, allowing pendular exercises after 3 days and gentle active flexion and abduction after 3 weeks [10].

If the costoclavicular ligament is absent, some stabilising structure between the first rib and the clavicle is needed [1]. Neer [7] proposed a free tendon graft through drill holes in the first rib and clavicle. Rock-

wood [10] used 1 mm Dacron® tape, passing it around the remaining medial end of the clavicle and its periosteal tube, and then through the residual scar of the old costoclavicular ligament on the cranial surface of the first rib. On the other hand, Reilly [9] did not advocate the use of Dacron® tapes, due to the erosion and nonunion of the clavicle and the first rib caused by these tapes, but in his case the tape was passed around both bones.

Detachment of the clavicular head of the sternocleidomastoideus diminishes the cranial pull to the remaining medial end of the clavicle.

Results and complications

Results after stabilisation procedures have been acceptable, but there is a high risk of complications, including pleural perforation and damage of retrosternal vital structures (especially when using K-wires), and even death due to K-wire migration. However, by using meticulous technique and by proscribing early mobilisation, these complications should be avoided.

Results after resection arthroplasty have been poor in some cases [4], but satisfactory in many others, especially if stability of the medial end of the clavicle is secured [10]. The complication risks of this method are not as high as those of the stabilisation procedure.

References

[1] Abbott LC, Lucas DB. The function of the clavicle. Its surgical significance. *Ann Surg* 1954 ; 140 : 583-599

[2] De Jong KP, Sukul DM. Anterior sternoclavicular dislocation: A long term follow-up study. *J Orthop Trauma* 1990 ; 4 : 420-423

[3] Duggan N. Recurrent dislocation of the sternoclavicular cartilage. *J Bone Joint Surg* 1931 ; 13 : 365

[4] Eskola A, Vainionpää S, Vastamäki M, Slätis P, Rokkanen P. Operation for old sternoclavicular dislocation. Results in 12 cases. *J Bone Joint Surg Br* 1989 ; 71 : 63-65

[5] Freeman BL 3rd. Old unreduced dislocations. In : Canale ST ed. Campbell's operative orthopaedics. St Louis : CV Mosby, 1998 : 2662-2663

[6] Lyons FA, Rockwood CA Jr. Migration of pins used in operations of the shoulder. *J Bone Joint Surg Am* 1990 ; 72 : 1262-1267

[7] Neer CS 2nd. Shoulder reconstruction. Philadelphia : WB Saunders, 1990 : 355-362

[8] Phillips BB. Recurrent dislocations. In : Canale ST ed. Campbell's operative orthopaedics. St Louis : CV Mosby, 1998 : 1352-1354

[9] Reilly P, Bruguera JA, , Copeland SA. Erosion and nonunion of the first rib after sternoclavicular reconstruction with Dacron. *J Shoulder Elbow Surg* 1999 ; 8 : 76-78

[10] Rockwood CA Jr, Groh GI, Wirth MA, Grassi FA. Resection arthroplasty of the sternoclavicular joint. *J Bone Joint Surg Am* 1997 ; 79 : 387-393

[11] Rockwood CA Jr, Odor JM. Spontaneous anterior subluxation of the sternoclavicular joint. *J Bone Joint Surg Am* 1989 ; 71 : 1280-1288

[12] Wirth MA, Rockwood CA Jr. Acute and chronic traumatic injuries of the sternoclavicular joint. *J Am Acad Orthop Surg* 1996 ; 4 : 268-278

Osteosynthesis of intra-articular fractures of the proximal humerus

H Resch
P Povacz
R Schwaiger

Abstract. – In the case of displaced intra-articular fractures of the head of the humerus, vascularisation is always at risk when the whole of the anatomical neck is involved. In addition, reconstructing multiple segment fractures at this site is a challenging procedure. The technical difficulties involved can be exacerbated in elderly patients as a result of osteoporosis. Among other things, this can create problems of seating the implants with a consequent risk of loosening. For this reason, prosthetic management may be the procedure of choice in older patients. In younger patients, however, such procedures will only be indicated in exceptional cases, in view of the limited life of the prostheses. Reconstruction can be performed by open or percutaneous reduction. As long as the surgeon avoids damage to the soft tissues and makes sparing use of implants, necrosis rates are no higher for open reduction. However, the need for immediate postoperative exercise therapy to counteract scarring tendencies does require a high degree of stability of the repair. Percutaneous procedures demand powers of spatial imagination and experience on the part of the surgeon for both the fracture lines and the residual soft tissue linking the various fragments. In the latter case, the surgeon's knowledge is essential for exploiting the effects of ligamentotaxis. One advantage of percutaneous reduction is that postoperative management is similar to that for conservative methods, in that there is little risk of iatrogenic scarring. The types of fracture that have proved particularly amenable to closed procedures include two and three-part fractures and valgus impacted four-part fractures. Severely displaced four-part fractures, four-part fracture dislocations and head-splitting fractures are less suited to percutaneous reduction, because soft tissue connections between the various fragments are largely absent.

Keywords: arm, proximal humerus fractures, intra-articular fractures, avascular necrosis, classification, open reduction, minimal osteosynthesis.

Introduction

The aim of a fracture classification system is to describe fractures for comparative, therapeutic and prognostic purposes. In Neer's classification, all displaced fractures, i.e. fractures with more than 1 cm displacement or 45° angulation, have a poor functional prognosis and therefore require surgical repair [11, 12]. In the case of four-part fractures, there is an additional risk of compromised vascularisation in the humeral head. The risk is particularly high in the case of four-part fracture dislocations. For four-part fractures and four-part fracture dislocations, Neer accordingly recommends endoprosthetic replacement at primary surgery. Neer's definition of the relevant degree of displacement is an arbitrary value based on his own personal experience [11].

Herbert Resch, M.D.
P Povacz, M.D.
R Schwaiger, M.D.
General Hospital Salzburg, Unfallchirurgie, Müllner-Hauptstrasse 48, A-5020 Salzburg, Austria.

One common fracture, namely the valgus impacted humeral head fracture, is not included as a distinct type in his system of classification even though it can be distinguished from the four-part fractures on the basis of the necrosis rate alone [7, 13]. In the French system of classification by Duparc, which relates primarily to the risk of compromised vascularisation, a distinction is made between extra and intra-articular fractures [3]. In spite of the considerable risk of necrosis, he advises treating displaced intra-articular fractures with the fracture line passing along the anatomical neck ("col anatomique et cephalo-tubérositaire") using reduction techniques and osteosynthesis in younger patients, and prosthetic management in older patients [4]. In the AO/ASIF classification, a distinction is also made between extra and intra-articular fractures [9]. Both the Duparc and AO classifications treat the valgus impacted humeral head fracture as a distinct type.

There is a general consensus that displaced fractures left untreated have a poor functional outcome [8, 12, 16, 18]. Although there is a danger that reduction by open surgery may increase the risk of necrosis in four-part fractures and four-part fracture dislocations, it is essential to reduce the fragments. The risk of necrosis is increased still further by exposure of the fracture as required for plating osteosynthesis in comparison to that required for minimal osteosynthesis [5, 6, 10]. The use of a prosthetic implant in four-part fractures does not solve the problem, at least in young patients, because of the limited survival time of the implants [5, 6]. Open minimal osteosynthesis is therefore seen as the treatment of choice, at least in younger people with severe humeral head fractures. To avoid the additional risk of necrosis involved in open surgery, percutaneous reduction and fixation would therefore seem to be even more desirable.

Pre-operative radiographic assessment

Siebenrock and Gerber described low inter- and intra-observer reliability for the Neer and AO classification systems [15]. The same results were reported by Sidor et al for Neer's classification [17]. As a possible cause of the poor reproducibility of the results, the authors mention the absence of standardised radiographs in at least two planes. A CT scan in combination with 3D reconstruction would also be desirable but not always feasible. Visualisation in at least three planes as already recommended by Neer, i.e. AP, axial and transscapular radiographs (trauma series after Neer [12]), would seem to be a sine qua non for correct fracture assessment.

Indications for surgery to preserve the humeral head

– Intra-articular two, three and four-part fractures with more than 3-5 mm displacement (age dependent).
– Fracture-dislocations.

INDICATIONS FOR OPEN/PERCUTANEOUS REDUCTION

Basically, it is always possible to attempt reduction using closed procedures. However, in most cases, the following classification has proved meaningful.

■ *Open reduction*

– Severely displaced four-part fractures and four-part fracture-dislocations in which it must be assumed that no periosteal connections between the shaft and head segments are intact.
– Head splitting fractures.

■ *Percutaneous reduction*

– Two and three-part fractures.
– Valgus impacted four-part fractures.
– Moderately displaced four-part fractures.

Indications for primary prosthetic management

Two-part (anatomical neck) and four-part fractures and four-part fracture dislocations in elderly patients with porous bony substance.

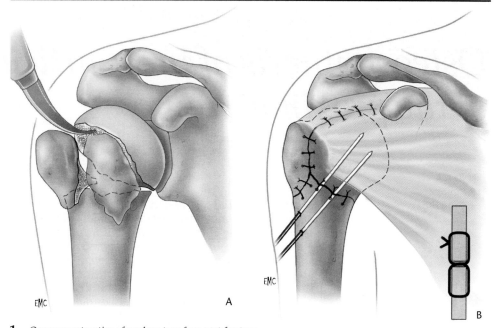

1 *Open reconstruction of a valgus type four-part fracture.*
A. Schematic drawing of reduction; the impacted humeral head is raised by means of an elevator.
B. Fixation of the fracture by minimal osteosynthesis; the tuberosities are fixed to each other and to the shaft fragment with numerous sutures in a figure eight.

Techniques for open surgical repair

INTRA-ARTICULAR TWO-PART FRACTURE

Using an anterior approach, access to the fracture is via the deltopectoral groove. A blunt elevator is introduced and advanced beneath the articular segment, which will normally be displaced medially and distally, in the region of the axillary recess. In order not to jeopardise the axillary nerve, the instrument must be advanced under the head fragment laterally and ventrally following the bone as closely as possible. The articular segment is then raised while traction is applied to the arm. Finally, fixation of the head fragment is performed with two small fragment cancellous bone screws or with K-wires only.

THREE-PART FRACTURE

An anterior incision is made to gain access to the fracture via the deltopectoral groove. The subcapital fracture is always reduced first. In the case of severely displaced subcapital fractures involving avulsion of the greater tuberosity, rotation of the head of the humerus, caused by the pull of the subscapularis muscle, must first be neutralised and the subcapital fracture fixed with K-wires. The greater tuberosity is then secured with one or two screws. In the case of porous bone, the tuberosity is also secured to the shaft using thread or wire cerclage.

FOUR-PART FRACTURES [13] *(fig 1, 2)*

The humeral head is exposed with an anterior approach via the deltopectoral groove. In the continuation of the intertubercular line of fracture, a 1 cm incision is made cranially in the rotator cuff

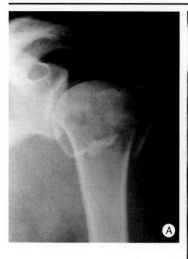
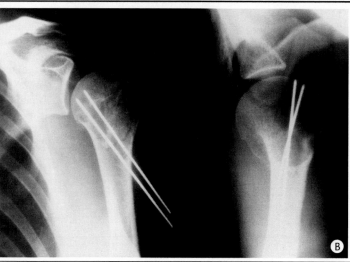

2 *A. Valgus impacted humeral head fracture.*
B. Minimal osteosynthesis with 2 K-wires and transosseous sutures of which the drill holes are visible.

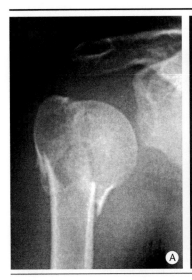
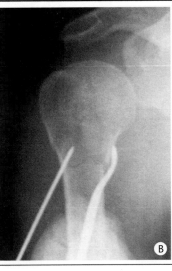

3 *Percutaneous treatment of a two-part fracture.*
A. Two-part fracture with medially displaced head.
B. The head is reduced by means of an elevator; fixation is performed with K-wires. Basically, the same technique is used as with open techniques.

in the direction of the fibres to expose the fragment with its cartilaginous covering. With an elevator, the articular segment is raised far enough to permit lateral approximation of the tuberosities. To secure the head segment to the shaft, two or three 2 mm K-wires are passed percutaneously through the shaft and into the head segment. The tuberosities are then relocated in their correct anatomical position, secured to each other, and anchored to the main distal fragment with numerous osteosutures. The holes for the sutures are drilled as close to the fracture margins as possible. Each pair of holes is sutured together with the sutures crossing the fracture line in a figure of eight to prevent subsequent inward or outward displacement of the fragments. The void created by raising the impacted head is filled with chips of autologous cancellous bone placed in the cranial area of the intertubercular line of fracture. The incision in the rotator cuff is sutured.

Techniques for percutaneous surgical repair [14]

Instruments: Reduction is performed with the help of a pointed hook retractor, an elevator and, if necessary, a 4 mm Steinmann pin. Screw fixation is performed with a cannulated screw fixation system (Oswald Leibinger). A cannula set with a blunt trocar helps minimise damage to the soft tissue.

Positioning of the patient: The operation is performed under regional anaesthesia. The patient is placed in a supine position with the upper body inclined at an angle of about 30°. The arm is draped to permit mobility. The C-arm is set to create a right angle between the central beam and the head of the humerus.

INTRA-ARTICULAR TWO-PART FRACTURE *(fig 3)*

The technique is basically the same as described for the open technique, without skin incision. The elevator is inserted

percutaneously via a stab incision. Anterior to the humeral head and in steady contact with the bone of the humeral head, it is guided to the anatomical neck which is pushed in a superior direction. The reduced head tensions the rotator cuff which causes the greater tuberosity to approximate to the normal anatomical site.

THREE-PART FRACTURES *(fig 4)*

This fracture often involves internal rotational displacement of the humeral head plus angulation to anterior and sometimes also to medial. First the subcapital fracture is reduced with the arm in adduction and internal rotation. Simultaneous traction is applied to the arm, with the surgeon using his thumb to apply counter-pressure posterolaterally in the area of the fracture. The fracture is then secured by means of three 2 mm K-wires drilled inferiorly to superiorly through the fragment of the humeral shaft. The arm is then carefully returned to the neutral position and the greater tuberosity reduced by means of the pointed hook retractor which is inserted into the subacromial space. The greater tuberosity is engaged at the insertion of the supraspinatus tendon and moved antero-inferiorly until the correct position appears to have been reached. After temporary fixation with a K-wire, the correct position of the tuberosity is checked by maximum external and internal rotation of the arm. Finally, the tuberosity is fixed by means of two cannulated titanium screws. In cases of pronounced rotational displacement, a hook is inserted, and the lesser tuberosity grasped at the insertion area of the subscapularis tendon to achieve derotation of the head. Where the humeral head is displaced medially and inferiorly, a blunt elevator is advanced towards the humeral head from anteriorly, following the bone as far as the anatomical neck, and the head segment raised. The sliding action along the bone without losing bone contact presents no threat to the neurovascular structures.

FOUR-PART FRACTURES AND VALGUS IMPACTED FRACTURE *(fig 5, 6)*

The principles of reduction are the same as with the open technique. Reconstruction involves raising the head segment, as that is the only way to restore the anatomy of the tuberosities. The patient's arm is held adducted in the neutral position by the surgeon's assistant. An incision is made on the border between the anterior and middle thirds of the head and, working under image intensifier control, an elevator is advanced towards the impacted articular segment. The segment is then raised to its anatomical position as indicated by the greater tuberosity. The reduced head segment is secured with two or three 2 mm K-wires drilled from inferiorly through the fragment of the shaft into the articular segment. The greater tuberosity, whose impaction usually causes a lateral tilt while its longitudinal position remains largely unchanged, normally automatically regains its correct anatomy when the articular segment is raised. It is held inferiorly by the residual periosteum and superiorly by the rotator cuff. The cannula of the screw fixation system with the blunt trocar is advanced towards the upper part of the greater tuberosity and a screw is inserted through the tuberosity into the upper part of the articular segment. Another screw is passed through the inferior part of the greater tuberosity into the fragment of the shaft so that the greater tuberosity has a bearing function between the shaft and the articular segment. Finally, the lesser tuberosity, which is mainly displaced medially, has to be reduced. For this purpose the patient's arm is held in 70° of abduction, and the image intensifier is set for an axial view. A small incision is made and the hook retractor advanced towards the lesser tuberosity, which is engaged at the insertion area of the subscapularis tendon and pulled laterally, until the articular incongruity seen medially disappears. Temporary fixation is provided with a K-wire, and a 40 mm screw is placed anteroposteriorly. Finally the K-wires initially drilled into the head segment are cut off and left just beneath the skin. Four weeks later they are removed under local anaesthesia. Where there is no contact between the articular segment and the glenoid, either because impaction is so severe that it is facing laterally or because it is not only impacted but also displaced laterally (true four-part fracture), reduction is more difficult. Again, the decisive factor is manipulating the articular segment, which has to be raised and reduced with the help of the elevator. The first step is to reverse the impaction of the head segment as described above and then to use the elevator to correct lateral displacement. The procedure is then as described above. In none of the four-part fractures was cancelleous bone grafting performed after raising the head segment.

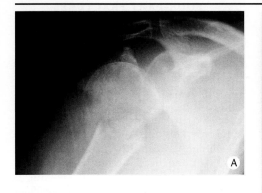

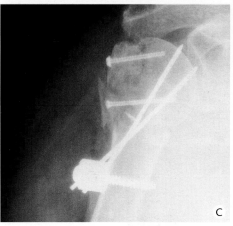

4 *Percutaneous treatment of a three-part fracture with very porotic bone quality.*
A. Three-part fracture in a 78 year old woman. Because of the fracture of the greater tuberosity the humeral head is rotated internally. The greater tuberosity is displaced into the subacromial space.
B. The internally rotated head has to be derotated by means of a hook grasping the head at the insertion of the subscapularis tendon and then fixed to the shaft with K-wires.
C. After derotation the head is fixed to the shaft by means of 2 K-wires which are fixed in a locking screw to avoid migration (prototype not yet available). The greater tuberosity is reduced by means of a hook and fixed with 2 screws (the K-wires intentionally penetrate the articular surface for a better grip in the porotic bone).

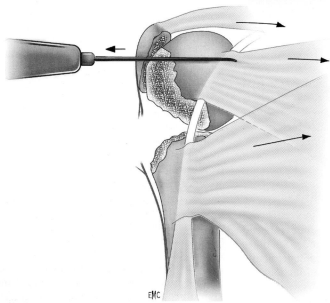

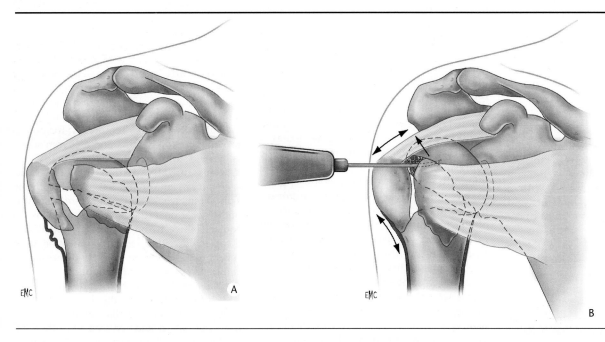

5 *Percutaneous treatment of valgus impacted fracture.*
A. Schematic drawing of a valgus impacted fracture.
B. Schematic drawing of reduction technique. Raising the head causes tensioning of the rotator cuff and of the periosteum between greater tuberosity and shaft.

POSTOPERATIVE TREATMENT

■ *Open technique*

The arm is immobilised against the body with light bandaging for 3 to 4 weeks (depending on the fracture type and bone quality). Passive exercising in the plane of the scapula without rotation is begun on the first postoperative day. After this time period, active motion including rotation is started.

■ *Percutaneous technique*

The arm is immobilised against the body with light bandaging for three weeks. Depending on the degree of stability achieved, passive exercising in the plane of the scapula without rotation is begun on the first day postoperatively. In the fourth week, therapy is extended to include rotation and active movement exercises.

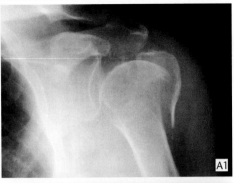
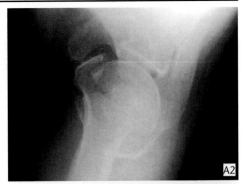
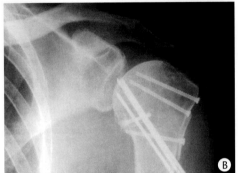
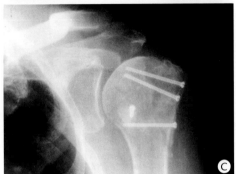

6   A. *Valgus impacted fracture of a 76 year old woman, AP (left) and axillary view (right).*
B. *After percutaneous reduction, fixation with K-wires and cannulated screws.*
C. *Six weeks after surgery the K-wires are removed.*

Results

OPEN TECHNIQUES [13]

The open technique, as described above, was applied between 1985 and 1991 before the percutaneous technique was used. Most of the cases were valgus impacted humeral head fractures. Over this time period, a total of 28 patients presenting pronounced valgus impaction (average impaction 38°) were operated on. The average age of the patients was 52 years (range 26 to 65 years).

On follow-up evaluation (minimum 18 months, average 36 months), one patient had sequestration of the head segment, and another had clinically asymptomatic partial necrosis (necrosis rate 9%). Slight arthrosis was present in two patients, and moderate arthrosis was present in one. Where anatomical reconstruction had been successful, the long-term functional outcome was almost identical to the non-traumatised side.

Constant score [2]: The Constant score was fully evaluated in 20 patients. The average score was 81; the range was 66 to 100 points. The average functional score in comparison with the non-traumatised side was 84% (72% to 108%). In the case of patients with perfectly restored anatomy, the average was 88% (77% to 108%).

PERCUTANEOUS TECHNIQUES [14]

Between 1990 and 1994, 27 patients with three and four-part fractures (9 three-part and 18 four-part fractures) were operated on using a percutaneous technique for reduction and screw fixation. Of the 18 patients with four-part fractures, 13 were of the valgus type without any significant lateral displacement of the articular segment, whereas 5 showed significant displacement. Good approximation to the anatomy of the humeral head was achieved with almost all fractures. The average follow-up period was 24 months (18 - 47 months). All the three-part fractures showed good to very good functional results (average Constant score 91%; range 84% - 100%) without signs of necrosis. As for the four-part fractures, good radiological results were achieved in the case of valgus impacted fractures with the exception of one patient who showed signs of partial necrosis of the humeral head. With regard to the four-part fractures with lateral displacement of the articular segment, revision surgery with a prosthetic implant was required in one patient because of head necrosis, and in another patient because of secondary redisplacement of the fracture. The overall head necrosis rate of all patients with four-part fractures was 11%. The average Constant score of all patients with four-part fractures and preserved head (without the 2 failures) was 87% (range 79% - 100%).

Until the end of 1997, a total of 67 cases with three and four-part fractures (most of them valgus impacted fractures) were treated according to this technique, confirming the results mentioned above.

Conclusion

In the case of a four-part fracture, a disruption of the greater and lesser tuberosities creates a situation in which the blood supply to the articular segment is maintained only via the periosteum extending to the medial part of the anatomical humeral neck [1]. This periosteum has to be preserved at the time of surgery. The low rate of necrosis in the openly reconstructed fractures proves that surgical intervention does not further compromise the circulation when careful surgical techniques are used and the use of implants is kept to a minimum. The necrosis rate in valgus impacted humeral head fractures is about the same as with percutaneously treated cases. The comparison between the open and closed group of valgus impacted four-part fractures shows that the functional results are slightly better with the percutaneous approach. Patients who were operated using the percutaneous technique were able to return to work significantly earlier than those who underwent open surgery (on average 11 weeks as compared to 14 weeks).

Important features of the percutaneous technique are:

– A crucial factor for the success of percutaneous reconstruction is the presence of soft tissue bridging the various fragments and thus offering support in the form of ligamentotaxis.

– In the case of three-part fractures and valgus impacted four-part fractures, the percutaneous reduction technique almost always produces good to very good functional results.

– Because of the reduced availability of soft tissue bridges between the fragments, four-part fractures with pronounced lateral displacement of the articular segment are clearly less suitable for the percutaneous technique than those without significant lateral displacement.

– The necrosis rate is, at least, not increased by this technique.

– In the absence of fracture exposure, adhesion within the surrounding gliding surfaces is reduced, and the rehabilitation period is shorter than in the case of open surgery.

– Due to the reduced development of adhesions in the surrounding gliding surfaces, no aggressive rehabilitation within the initial three weeks is necessary. In cases with porotic bone quality, the arm can be immobilised for at least 3 weeks without motion. This is in contrast to open surgical treatment where early movement of the shoulder is mandatory.

References ➤

References

[1] Brooks CH, Revell WJ, Heatley FW. Vascularity of the humeral head after proximal humeral fractures: an anatomical study. *J Bone Joint Surg Br* 1993 ; 75 : 132-136

[2] Constant CR, Murley AH. A clinical method of functional assessment of the shoulder. *Clin Orthop* 1987 ; 214 : 160-164

[3] Duparc J. Classification des fractures articulaires de l'extrémité supérieure de l'humérus. *Acta Orthop Belg* 1995 ; 61 (suppl 1) : 65-70

[4] Huten D, Duparc J. Classification et traitement des fractures de l'extrémité supérieure de l'humérus. In : Bonnel F, Blotman F, Mansat M ed. L'épaule. Paris : Springer Verlag, 1993 : 489-502

[5] Jaberg H, Jakob RP. Trümmerfrakturen des proximalen Humerus. *Orthopädie* 1987 ; 16 : 320-335

[6] Jakob RP, Ganz R. Proximale Humerusfrakturen. *Helv Chir Acta* 1981 ; 48 : 595-610

[7] Jakob RP, Miniaci A, Anson PS, Jaberg H, Osterwalder A, Ganz R. Four-part valgus impactes fractures of the proximal humerus. *J Bone Joint Surg Br* 610

[8] Mills EJ, Horne G. Fracture of the proximal humerus in adults. *J Trauma* 1985 ; 25 : 801-805

[9] Müller ME, Allgöwer M, Schneider R, Willenegger H. Manual der Osteosynthese. Berlin : Springer-Verlag, 1992

[10] Münst P, Kuner EH. Osteosynthesen bei dislozierten Humeruskopffrakturen. *Orthopäde* 1992 ; 21 : 121-130

[11] Neer CS. Displaced proximal humerus fractures, Part I. Classification and evaluation. *J Bone Joint Surg Am* 1970 ; 52 : 1077-1089

[12] Neer CS. Displaced proximal humerus fractures, Part II. Treatment of three-part and four-part displacement. *J Bone Joint Surg Am* 1970 ; 52 : 1090-1103

[13] Resch H, Beck E, Bayley J. Reconstruction of valgus impacted humeral head fractures: Indication, technique and long-term results. *J Shoulder Elbow Surg* 1995 ; 4 : 73-80

[14] Resch H, Povacz P, Fröhlich H, Wambacher M. Percutaneous fixation of three- and four-fractures of the proximal humerus. *J Bone Joint Surg Br* 1997 ; 79 : 295-300

[15] Sidor ML, Zuckerman JD, Lyon T, Koval K, Cuomo F, Schoenberg N. The Neer classification system for proximal humeral fractures. *J Bone Joint Surg Am* 1993 ; 75 : 1745-1750

[16] Siebenrock KA, Gerber C. The reproductibility of classification of fractures of the proximal end of the humerus. *J Bone Joint Surg Am* 1993 ; 75 : 1751-1755

[17] Stableforth PG. Four-part fractures of the neck of the humerus. *J Bone Joint Surg Br* 1984 ; 66 : 104-108

[18] Svend-Hansen H. Displaced proximal humeral fractures. *Acta Orthop Scand* 1974 ; 45 : 359-364

Shoulder prostheses: generalities and main designs

F Duparc
J Duparc

Abstract. – Shoulder arthroplasty has become more frequent, and real improvements have been made due to continuous development of the ideas set forth by CS Neer. The biomechanics of the shoulder joint have been studied, as well as the anatomy and kinematics which a prosthesis should aim to reproduce. These parameters are reviewed, the relationships between the humeral and glenoid components are discussed, and the main concepts in the design of shoulder prostheses are presented. These designs are often based on the concepts developed by Neer, but recent prostheses, such as the so-called anatomical, reversed or bipolar prostheses, are also presented.

© 2000, Editions Scientifiques et Médicales Elsevier SAS. All rights reserved.

Keywords: shoulder, prosthesis, designs, humeral implant, glenoid implant.

Introduction

During recent decades, the design of shoulder prostheses has undergone considerable changes. Before 1950, numerous constrained designs were described, but these showed a high rate of failure. In 1951, Charles Neer opened the modern era with his humeral prosthesis (fig 1), first used for humeral fractures. In a second period of development, Neer's prosthesis was completed by a glenoid implant, so as to be used for a non-constrained total shoulder arthroplasty (TSA) (fig 2). Neer's model has been widely used and reproduced, and remains the most significant reference and the gold standard for shoulder prostheses. Other derived implants and technical systems for implantation have been proposed to provide solutions for treatment of specific anatomical conditions (i.e., the reversed prosthesis, implants with acromial fixation).

The third and most recent period of research on shoulder prostheses has been guided by two main concepts: modularity and adaptability. To improve modularity, a greater range of implant sizes has been introduced, offering more numerous possibilities. Later, research on the adaptability of the implant to the bone gave rise to the so-called "anatomical prosthesis",

Fabrice Duparc, M.D., , C.H.U. de Rouen, Hôpital Charles Nicolle, Pavillon Felix Deve, 76031 Rouen, France.
Jacques Duparc, M.D., Honorary Chairman.
Chirurgie et Traumatologie, Hôpital Bichat Paris, France.

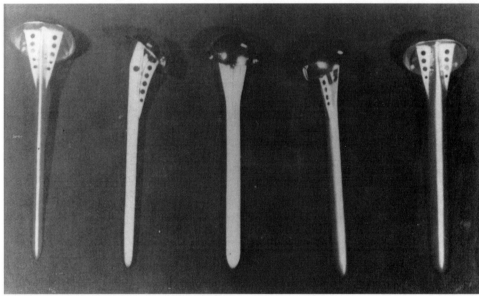

1 *The original Neer prosthesis made in 1951 had only one stem, but within four years it was made with five stem diameters and small holes in the flanges for ingrowth of bone.*

which takes into account the variable inclination and retroversion of the humeral head. The necessity for prostheses in cases of joint destruction associated with cuff ruptures has led to new designs and the development of bipolar prostheses or reversed prostheses.

Despite these recent improvements, the increasing number of implanted shoulder prostheses will necessarily lead to the development of revision shoulder implants.

This article reviews the requirements for a shoulder prosthesis, the anatomical and biomechanical conditions that influence the designs of implants, and the concepts of shoulder replacement; it also provides some examples of the prostheses now available to surgeons.

Requirements for a shoulder prosthesis

FUNCTIONAL AIM

The functional aim of a shoulder prosthesis is to restore or to reproduce the compromise between mobility and stability provided by

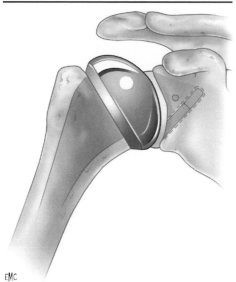

2   *The Neer total shoulder arthroplasty: a glenoid component was added.*

the normal kinematics of the glenohumeral joint. An optimal prosthetic reconstruction depends on the design of the prosthesis, but also on the implantation, the quality of the surgical reconstruction of soft tissues, the postoperative healing, the rehabilitation process, and the long-term biological response to the implant. Matching anatomy is difficult, and altering the anatomy by prosthetic reconstruction has biomechanical consequences [26].

PROSTHESIS DESIGN

The design will be influenced by anatomical and biomechanical factors. The main requirements for a prosthesis are:

– to reproduce the normal anatomy;

– to restore shoulder kinematics;

– to preserve the bone stock;

– to avoid mechanical debris between the implants;

– to obtain satisfactory mobility of the components without impingement;

– to allow early rehabilitation of the peri-articular soft tissues.

ANATOMY AND BIOMECHANICS OF THE ARTICULAR SURFACES

■ *Proximal humerus*

Most often, the head of the humerus is considered as the third of a sphere. The

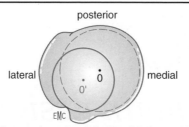

3   *The posterior and medial offset of the humeral head: the centre of the humeral head (0) is posteriorly and medially displaced in relation to the axis of the humeral shaft (0') (according to Walch and Boileau [32]).*

mean diameter is about 46 mm (36 to 56.9) [7, 19]. The radius of the sphere increases from the central part to the oval-shaped periphery. Its mean surface is 43.3 mm² (36.5 to 51.5) [5, 7].

The thickness and the radius are correlated values that allow the use of 8 to 12 sizes for the replacement [19].

The axis of the head is inclined 45° upwards in relation to the vertical axis of the humeral shaft. The inclined head is placed in retroversion. The angle of retroversion depends on the distal landmarks that are used for measurement. Mean values are about 17° to 30°, but the extreme values show significant variations (from 5° forwards to 60° backwards) [6, 7, 17, 27, 28].

The centre of the head is not placed on the axis of the humeral shaft, but presents a combined posterior offset of 3 to 5 mm and a medial offset of 6 mm [6, 28, 31] *(fig 3)*.

■ *Glenoid* *(fig 4)*

The glenoid is a pear-shaped surface, which is slightly curved: 50° in the transversal plane, and 70° to 75° in the frontal plane. It is oriented 3° to 5° upwards, and presents a variable retroversion: 7° (2°-12°) *(fig 4)*. The mean surface is 6.3 cm² (± 1.74) [18].

The superoinferior mean diameter is 39 mm ± 5, and the anteroposterior mean is 29 mm ± 3.2 [19, 21]. The curving radius is about 24 to 26 mm in the frontal plane.

The subchondral bone is quite flat; the cartilage, which is much thicker in the periphery, gives the curved aspect, which is increased by the labrum [12]. The depth of the anteroposterior dimension is 5 mm ± 1 and the superoinferior dimension is 2.9 mm (± 1) [24].

The distance between the base of the coracoid process and the glenoid surface is about 0 to 5 mm.

■ *Glenohumeral relationships: the essential role of soft tissues*

The congruence (equality of the radius of curvature of both the surfaces) is not complete, but rather acquired by the effect of concavity, which is not provided by the glenoid surface, but by the cartilage and the labrum. The conformity depends on the depth of the glenoid, the thickness of the cartilage and the size of the labrum; this limits the anteroposterior and superoinferior displacements of the humeral head in relation to the glenoid [30]. In cases of joint destruction, the surfaces will be destroyed, and the replacement by implant will have to provide stability as well as resistance to shearing and compression forces.

However, the design of most prostheses will not allow replacing the poor local condition of the surrounding soft tissues, except in the case of a reversed prosthesis. In deciding which type of prosthesis to implant, the surgeon must take into account the status of the cuff tendons as well as the bone stock of the glenoid.

Concepts of joint restoration

GLENOHUMERAL JOINT

The replacement of the glenohumeral joint with articular components aims to reproduce the global anatomy and mechanics of the joint. Selection of the shoulder prosthesis should take into account the lateral glenohumeral distance between the base of the coracoid process and the lateral edge of the greater tubercle: 43 to 68 mm [19] *(fig 5)*. The dimensions of the glenoid and the humeral head are correlated [19], and correspond to the optimal tension of the soft tissues: capsule, ligaments, tendons of the cuff. If the local conditions of the bone and soft tissues are good or may be corrected, a good functional result may be expected.

When the local anatomical conditions are disturbed (destroyed glenoid, retracted capsule, cuff tear without possibility of good

4   *Retroversion of the glenoid: the plane of the scapula is oriented 5° to 20° backwards in relation to the perpendicular plane of the axis of the scapula.*

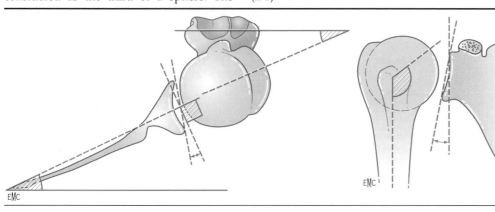

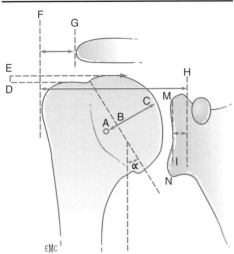

5 *The lateral offset of the glenohumeral joint. DH: the distance between the base of the coracoid process and the lateral edge of the greater tubercle measures the lateral offset of the glenohumeral joint; AC: shows the radius of the head; FG: the extra-acromial offset; ED: the height between the top of the head and the top of the greater tubercle; MN: the height of the glenoid; αα: angle of inclination of the head.*
All these parameters will have to be taken into account in deciding the type and size of the implants, as well as their position.

repair), the design of the prosthesis should facilitate the surgical correction of abnormalities. A non-anatomical reconstruction will not provide the optimal tension of soft tissues, because the lateral glenohumeral offset is not restored, and the shortening will create instability and weakness during movement. If the humeral implant is not centred in relation to the glenoid implant, the kinematics will be modified; the main risk will be elevation of the head, which will cause loosening of the glenoid. In such cases where anatomic reconstruction is impossible, special prosthesis designs are required.

HUMERAL IMPLANT

■ *The head*

The size of the head must be perfectly adapted: if it is too large, it will damage the cuff; if it is too small, the lateral glenohumeral offset will be decreased, as well as the lever arm of the tendons and muscles. The pressure on the glenoid will be increased. If the diameter is irregular (i.e. decreased in the upper part to respect the cuff above an oval-shaped head), the lever arm will also be shortened during elevation [16]. In some newer implants, the so-called anatomical implants, the section of the head closely follows the limit of the articular surface, and the cephalic component copies the diameter and thickness of the cephalic fragment. This modularity allows adaptation to the resection plane of the humerus, so as to optimise coverage of the bone section.

The humeral head must cover (but not "over-cover") the surface of the humeral

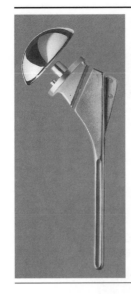

6 *The Aequalis® prosthesis (Tornier). Four diameters of humeral stem, four possibilities of inclination of the neck (125° to 140°), ten sizes of cephalic component, eight positions available allowing the head to cover the osteotomy.*

osteotomy. Good coverage will be obtained by using the correct diameter size for the prosthetic head, well-positioned with the correct inclination. The correct version and angle of inclination will be determined by the anatomical section or by the correctly-placed section guide system. Adaptation of the inclination using a system of variable necks may improve the positioning (fig 6, 7).

In order to reproduce the posterior offset, right and left implants may be available, or an eccentric fixation system such as the Aequalis® prosthesis (fig 8).

■ *The stem*

The stem must fill the humerus without excessive reaming parallel to the axis of the humeral shaft. The retroversion will be determined according to the insertion of the cuff tendons and in relation to the intertubercularis sulcus. The interest of an anatomical prosthesis (of which the dimensions are correlated to the bone section of the humeral head) is that it is independent of the prosthetic keel and therefore of the clinical measurement of retroversion. The length, as recommended by Neer [24], must be 6 times the diameter of the humeral shaft. Filling the diaphysis must be carried out without aggressive reaming; the diameter of the stem is often about 9 or 10 mm. Good contact between the stem and the cortical bone must be sought, to obtain a

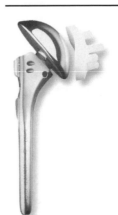

7 *The Anatomica® prosthesis (SulzerMedica): the trial components are assembled according to the anatomy of the sectioned upper extremity of the humerus; a special frame is guided by this trial implant so as to reproduce the definitive implant.*

press-fit effect in good alignment with the axis of the humeral shaft. Poor positioning of the stem (not strictly parallel to the shaft axis) will cause poor positioning of the head of the prosthetic component; a varus position, in particular, would incline the head inferiorly.

■ *Fractures*

In cases presenting fractures, two points should be especially studied:

– The height of the implant, which should be determined by measuring the length of the contralateral humerus. A low position in relation to the upper pole of the greater tuberosity would create an abnormal subacromial contact during elevation. A high position would damage the cuff.

– The retroversion of the implant, which will influence the stability of the glenohumeral joint in rotation and elevation, as well as the reattachment of the tuberosities.

The lateral keel provides stability in torsion, and holes allow fixation of the tuberosities when they are separated (fig 9).

Cement is recommended by most authors, particularly if the bone is brittle (rheumatoid arthritis, osteoporosis) [25]. This point will be further discussed.

THE GLENOID COMPONENT

The dimensions and the shape of the implant will influence the contact between the non-articular structures of the proximal

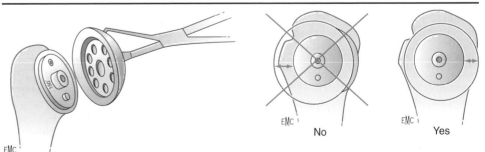

8 *The eccentric system for fixation allows good coverage of the humeral osteotomy. In this Aequalis system®, the prosthetic head is placed on the trial prosthesis in the position that provides the best coverage of the section of the bone, so as to reproduce the anatomy.*

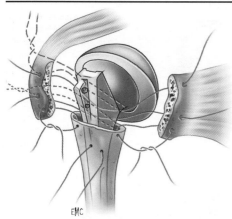

9 *Fixation of the tuberosities on the humeral implant: the prosthesis must not be too large; two holes are necessary.*

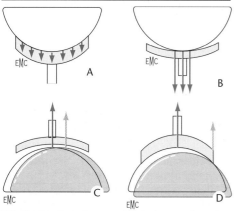

10 *Conformity and non-conformity between the articular surfaces:*
A. Conformity spreads the loading forces over the entire surfaces.
B. Non-conformity will increase the pressure forces applied on the glenoid, because the area of contact is reduced.
C. Non-conformity of the surfaces allows eccentric loading which remains applied on the articular surfaces of the smaller component.
D. In conformity, the eccentric loading will carry the applied forces to the edge of the smaller surfaces, causing the risk of loosening.

humerus and the cuff with the edge of the glenoid, in the extreme positions. The pear-shaped glenoid implant will improve the range of mobility before abnormal contacts occur between the humerus or the cuff and the glenoid.

The surface: the choice between conformity and non-conformity of the cephalic and glenoid components remains controversial. Conformity requires symmetry with the humeral head and provides a uniform distribution of the stresses and good stability. However, the stability stresses applied around the edge of the surface are transmitted to the fixation and to the interface with bone, which can cause loosening effects [3, 13, 29]. Most authors now advocate a non-conforming system.

In non-conforming systems, the curve of the glenoid is greater than that of the cephalic implant *(fig 10)*. The contact area becomes smaller and the pressure is increased. The translation of the prosthetic head

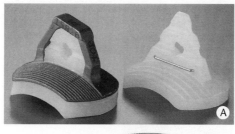

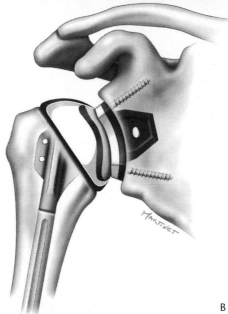

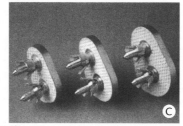

11 *Different types of glenoid components.*
A. Cemented polyethylene glenoid components with and without metal-backing.
B. Screw fixation of the glenoid component.
C. Expansion screw fixation system of hydroxyapatite-coated metal implant.

corresponds to decreased stability and increased eccentric stress applied on the edge in the extreme range of motion.

Fixation remains the main problem in shoulder total arthroplasty. The shear and compression forces are considerable on the surface and at the site of fixation. Different designs present plugs or a keel, metal-backed or not; the fixation may use cement or screws *(fig 11)*. The resistance to tear off is better with plugs than with a keel. The early radiolucent line often seen on radiographs is not always correlated with loosening of the implant, but has justified research on non-cemented fixation systems.

The use of a metal-backed keel may increase the lateral glenohumeral offset and create difficulties for cuff closure. In addition, the resulting decreased thickness of the polyethylene is not a good solution; the increased rigidity of the implant presents a greater risk of loosening under eccentric

loading. Also, the screw fixation may increase the number of polyethylene particles.

Most authors currently favour the use of uncemented non-conforming implants, but the quality of the glenoid fixation and the optimal degree of non-conformity are still under discussion [4, 8]. The cemented glenoid implants show frequent radiolucent lines around the keel that do not correspond to a real loosening. In uncemented systems with screw fixation, these radiolucent lines are not as frequent, but they do quite consistently reveal a loosening of the glenoid.

The ideal glenoid design (keel or plugs, mono-block polyethylene or modular metal-backed with inserts) remains to be determined, as well as the type of fixation.

CEMENTED OR UNCEMENTED PROSTHESIS

The same implants cannot be used for both cemented and uncemented implantation. The questions about the use of cement are different for humeral and glenoid implants.

■ *Cemented prosthesis*

Humeral side: The extremity of the bone is covered by the prosthesis. Inflammatory cells, particles of polyethylene or cement will not migrate.

Glenoid side: Radiolucent lines and real loosening are frequent.

■ *Uncemented prosthesis*

Complications are more frequent with uncemented prostheses.

Humeral side: Diaphyseal fractures, poor positioning of the articular surface, osteolysis around press-fitted implants without a porous-coated surface, migration, or bone damage during the removal of implants with a porous-coated surface have been reported in the literature. Nevertheless, good results have been reported with ingrowth total shoulder arthroplasty [9, 10].

Glenoid side: Complications include secondary cuff tears with superior or anterior instability because of the increased thickness of the implants, dissociation between the polyethylene and the metal tray, potential increased wear of the polyethylene against a metal-backed component because of the small amount of plastic. Nevertheless, the rate of radiolucent lines appears to be smaller [10]. No radiolucencies were observed in the hydroxyapatite coated implants around humeral or glenoid components.

According to Walch and Boileau [32], cemented shoulder prostheses remain the gold standard to which any new implant must be compared. Recent advances have been made in using metal-backed implants with hydroxyapatite and expansion screw fixation, but these must be evaluated.

The uncemented surface replacement shoulder arthroplasty proposed by S.A.

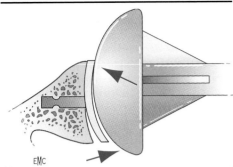

12 *The "rocking horse effect": when the cuff is ruptured or not efficient, the contraction of the deltoid will make the humeral prosthesis move upward and cause loading on the superior part of the glenoid component. These asymmetric constraints will induce the loosening of the glenoid implant.*

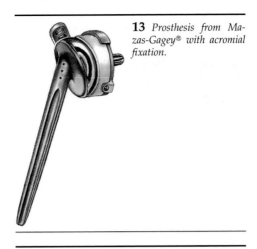

13 *Prosthesis from Mazas-Gagey® with acromial fixation.*

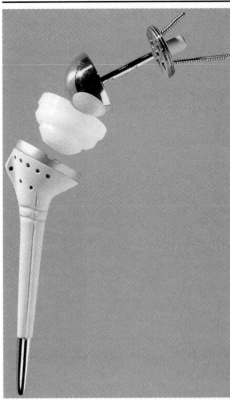

15 *The reversed prosthesis (P Grammont) (DePuy). The glenosphere articulates with the humeral component, the inversed retentive device allows the function of abduction, in maintaining the head centered and medialised, without upward migration.*

Copeland is an original concept to replace the damaged humeral surface by a cup coated with hydroxypatite, fixed by a screw or a plug, and the glenoid surface by a polyethylene implant fixed on a metal-coated base.

LOCAL CONDITIONS

The requirements for shoulder components in joint restoration may be influenced by local conditions. Good conditions are: a respected bone stock, an efficient rotator cuff, and no retracted or easily released capsule and ligaments. Destruction of the glenoid, large cuff ruptures and shoulder stiffness are unfavourable conditions.

The stability of a prosthetic joint is related to the design of the components and the constraints applied between the implants. The choice of the size and the placement of the implant must be optimal to avoid any impingement. Abnormal contact may cause premature wear of the component or loosening[29].

The prosthesis must also be designed so that it can be adapted to local conditions. In cases of rotator cuff ruptures, the constraints exerted on the glenoid implant are related to the superior translation of the humeral component, and will cause progressive loosening according to the "rocking-horse effect" described by Matsen[22] *(fig 12)*. For this reason, some authors have proposed other implants such as the semi-constrained prosthesis, bipolar prosthesis and reversed total shoulder arthroplasty. In cases of shoulder stiffness, an impaired capsular release will provoke asymmetrical wear of the glenoid, due to glenohumeral translation.

Semi-constrained total shoulder prostheses

Transacromial fixation has been thought useful to reinforce and preserve the stability of the glenoid implant. Apoil et al[2]

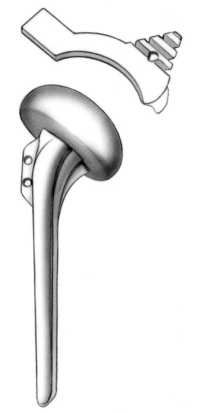

14 *A hooded glenoid component of the mid-1970s. The overhanging superior rim was intended to replace the action of the rotator cuff, but failed to do so. It interfered with closing the cuff and the greater constraint invited mechanical failure. This concept in design has been abandoned.*

proposed a fixation with cement on the glenoid and on the inferior side of the acromion, completed by screw fixation in the coracoid process.

Mazas and De La Caffinière[23] proposed a prosthesis with acromial contact and fixation that would limit the upper migration of the head and increase the fixation of the glenoid implant; this concept has been further developed in the Mazas and Gagey prosthesis *(fig 13)*.

The hooded glenoid, as described by Amstutz et al[1], was designed to control the high displacement of the humeral prosthesis *(fig 14)*.

Anatomical constrained total shoulder prostheses

The concept of a direct retentive articulation between the implants, in order to increase the stability of the prosthesis, has been proposed. Medialisation of the rotation centre has been advocated by a few authors, and Lettin and Copeland[20] have shown that the problem of these prostheses is the glenoid fixation, instead of the increased lever arm applied on the glenoid.

Reversed constrained total shoulder prostheses

Such prostheses have been described, but a great number of failures occurred because of the lateralisation of the centre of rotation. Grammont[14, 15] has used the concept of the medialisation and lowering of the fixed prosthetic centre of rotation, combined with improved fixation to limit the effects of loosening forces, to allow recovery of function with the deltoid alone.

The design of the implant creates the reverse of a glenohumeral joint *(fig 15)* and associates a "metaglene" which is fixed by screws on the glenoid, a spherical weight-bearing element ("glenosphere") which is fixed on the "metaglene", a humeral keel (cemented or not), a humeral concave cup that will be fixed on the humeral keel and articulated with the "glenosphere". The two sizes of the humeral cup may be used to increase the tension of the deltoid with a lateralisation effect.

Bipolar shoulder arthroplasty (BSA)

First described as a salvage procedure, the BSA has been proposed to increase the stability, range of motion and strength of the deltoid in patients who represent good classical indications for hemi-replacement, known to provide good relief of pain and satisfactory function [11]. Restitution of the lateral offset in cases where the cuff is ruptured will allow a stronger arm lever of the deltoid. The problems encountered with the glenoid implant are avoided (fig 16).

The shoulder revision prosthesis

In cases where the bone defect is important, and especially when the humeral bone stock

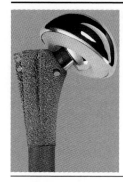

16 *The bipolar shoulder arthroplasty (Biomet).*

has been damaged, after the loosening of an implant or difficult conditions of removal, or after oncological resection, longer stems may be used. The intramedullary fixation will be stronger in the remaining humeral shaft, and reconstruction of the bone and soft tissues around the upper part of the implant can be performed.

Future developments and conclusions

This short review of the concepts and the main designs of shoulder prostheses cannot be exhaustive in presenting all the currently available implants. The main problem under study remains the fixation of the glenoid implant. The development of new implants, such as porous-coated components with expansion screws, creates hopes of finding a solution to the high rates of radiolucent lines and glenoid loosening, but these implants are still under evaluation. In addition, it must be noted that the designs of prostheses are not responsible for all failures, and the increased knowledge of the shoulder prosthesis will allow to better define the indications (total or hemi-arthroplasty), in order to limit the risk of loosening if it is foreseeable.

The problem of associated cuff ruptures is becoming more frequent. The semiconstrained implants are not yet widely used, and their reliability must be evaluated in coming years. The reversed prosthesis has not become widespread.

The bipolar shoulder prosthesis appeared as a new solution, but the results concerning shoulder function are now being debated and these prosthesis too will have to be evaluated.

References

[1] Amstutz HC, Thomas BJ, Kabo JM, Jinnah RH, Dorey FJ. The DANA total shoulder arthroplasty. *J Bone Joint Surg Am* 1988 ; 70 : 1174-1182

[2] Apoil A, Koechlin P, Augereau B, Honiger J. Prothèse totale d'épaule à appui acromio-coracoidien. Prothèse de résection humérale. Étude préliminaire. *Acta Orthop Belg* 1983 ; 49 : 571-575

[3] Ballmer FT, Sidles JA, Lippitt SB, Matsen FA 3rd. Humeral head prosthetic arthroplasty: surgically relevant geometric considerations. *J Shoulder Elbow Surg* 1993 ; 2 : 296-304

[4] Ballmer FT, Sidles JA, Lippitt SB, Matsen FA 3rd. Total shoulder arthroplasty: some considerations related to glenoid surface contact. *J Shoulder Elbow Surg* 1994 ; 3 : 299-306

[5] Boileau P, Walch G. Adaptabilité et modularité au cours des prothèses d'épaule. *Acta Orthop Belg* 1995 ; 61 (suppl 1) : 49-61

[6] Boileau P, Walch G. The three dimensional geometry of the proximal humerus: implications for the surgical technique and prosthetic design. *J Bone Joint Surg Br* 1997 ; 79 : 857-865

[7] Boileau P, Walch G. The combined offset (medial and posterior) of the humeral sphere. *J Shoulder Elbow Surg* 1994 ; 3, (suppl) : S65

[8] Brems J. The glenoid component in total shoulder arthroplasty. *J Shoulder Elbow Surg* 1993 ; 2 : 47-54

[9] Cofield RH. Uncemented total shoulder arthroplasty: a review. *Clin Orthop* 1994 ; 307 : 86-93

[10] Cofield RH, Daly PJ. Total shoulder arthroplasty with a tissue-ingrowth glenoid component. *J Shoulder Elbow Surg* 1992 ; 1 : 77-85

[11] Fenlin J, Romsey M, Allardyce T, Frieman B. Modular total shoulder replacement. *Clin Orthop* 1994 ; 307 : 37-46

[12] Frich L, Jensen N, Odgoard A, Pedersen C, Sejberg J, Dalstra M. Bone strength and material properties of the glenoid. *J Shoulder Elbow Surg* 1997 ; 6 : 97-104

[13] Fukuda K, Chen CM, Cofield RH, Chao EY. Biomechanical analysis of stability and fixation strength of total shoulder prostheses. *Orthopaedics* 1988 ; 11 : 141-149

[14] Grammont PM, Baulot E. Delta shoulder prosthesis for rotator cuff rupture. *Orthopaedics* 1993 ; 16 : 65-68

[15] Grammont PM, Baulot E, Chabernaud D. Résultats des 16 premiers cas d'arthroplastie totale d'épaule inversée sans ciment pour des omarthroses avec grande rupture de coiffe. *Rev Chir Orthop* 1996 ; 82 (suppl I) : 169

[16] Harryman DT, Sidles JA, Harris SL, Lippitt SB, Matsen FA 3rd. The effect of articular conformity and the size of the humeral component on laxity and motion after glenohumeral arthroplasty. A study in cadavera. *J Bone Joint Surg Am* 1995 ; 77 : 555-563

[17] Hernigou P, Duparc F, Filali C. Rétroversion humérale et prothèse d'épaule. *Rev Chir Orthop* 1995 ; 81 : 419-427

[18] Huber CE. Zur Form and Grösse der cavitas glenoidalis. *Anat Anz* 1991 ; 172 : 137-148

[19] Iannotti JP, Gabriel JP, Schneck SL, Evans BG, Misra S. The normal glenohumeral relationships: an anatomical study of one hundred and forty shoulders. *J Bone Joint Surg Am* 1992 ; 74 : 491-500

[20] Lettin AW, Copeland SA, Scales JT. The Stanmore total shoulder replacement. *J Bone Joint Surg Br* 1982 ; 64 : 47-51

[21] Mallon WJ, Brown HR, Vogler JB, Martinez S. Radiographic and geometric anatomy of the scapula. *Clin Orthop* 1992 ; 277 : 142-158

[22] Matsen FA 3rd, Lippitt SB, Sidles JA, Harryman DT. Practical evaluation and management of the shoulder. Philadelphia : WB Saunders, 1994 : 151-219

[23] Mazas F, De La Caffinière J. Une prothèse d'épaule non-rétentive. À propos de 38 cas. *Rev Chir Orthop* 1982 ; 68 : 161-170

[24] McPherson EJ, Friedman RJ, An YH, Chokesi R, Dooley RL. Anthropometric study of normal glenohumeral relationships. *J Shoulder Elbow Surg* 1997 ; 6 : 105-112

[25] Neer CS. Shoulder reconstruction. Philadelphia : WB Saunders, 1990 : 1-271

[26] Pearl ML, Kurutz SA. Geometric analysis of commonly used prosthetic systems for proximal humeral replacement. *J Bone Joint Surg Am* 1999 ; 81 : 660-671

[27] Randelli M, Gambrioli PL. Glenohumeral osteometry by computed tomography in normal and unstable shoulders. *Clin Orthop* 1986 ; 208 : 151-156

[28] Roberts SN, Folley APJ, Swallow HM, Wallace WA, Coughlan DP. The geometry of the humeral head and the design of prostheses. *J Bone Joint Surg Br* 1991 ; 73 : 647-650

[29] Severt R, Thomas BJ, Tsenter MJ, Amstutz HC, Kabo JM. The influence of conformity and constraint on translational forces and frictional torque in total shoulder arthroplasty. *Clin Orthop* 1993 ; 292 : 151-158

[30] Soslovsky LJ, Flatow EL, Bigliani LU, Mow JC. Articular geometry of the gleno-humeral joint. *Clin Orthop* 1992 ; 285 : 181-190

[31] Tillet E, Smith M, Fulcer M, Shanklin J. Anatomic determination of humeral head retroversion: the relationship of the central axis of the humeral head to the bicipital groove. *J Shoulder Elbow Surg* 1993 ; 2 : 255-256

[32] Walch G, Boileau P. Results of a new uncemented glenoid prosthesis. In : Walch G Boileau P eds. Shoulder arthroplasty. Berlin : Springer-Verlag, 1999

Hemi-arthroplasty

PM Rozing

Abstract. – Replacement of the humeral head is indicated when only the bone of the humeral head is destroyed, for example by a fracture, an osteonecrosis or a chronic dislocation, and when the glenoid bone and cartilage are still intact. If the cartilage is affected, such as in osteoarthritis or rheumatoid arthritis, the placement of a glenoid component may be considered. A contraindication for insertion of a glenoid component exists in those cases where there is a high risk of the implant loosening.
Most available shoulder systems have a range of stems for cemented and uncemented use and modular heads to reconstruct the normal anatomy of the proximal humerus.
The frequency of complications is comparable with that for hip and knee prostheses.

Keywords: shoulder, hemi-arthroplasty, osteoarthritis, rheumatoid arthritis, shoulder prosthesis.

Introduction

The main indication for shoulder arthroplasty is severe pain, limitation of motion and destruction of the glenohumeral joint. At surgery, in addition to replacing the glenohumeral joint, further procedures may have to be performed to deal with the specific pathology present. There is still some controversy as to whether glenoid resurfacing and/or repair of a ruptured rotator cuff at the time of shoulder arthroplasty will improve the end result [5]. In hemi-arthroplasty, only the humeral head is replaced and this procedure is recommended in those cases in which the bone and cartilage of the glenoid are intact, e.g. in avascular necrosis of the humeral head and proximal humeral fractures. In osteoarthritis, the cartilage of the glenoid is often thin or absent but the glenoid bone is undisturbed and strong. In those cases, a hemi-arthroplasty may be performed with good clinical results. In patients with rheumatoid arthritis, it is still controversial as to whether clinical results with regard to pain relief, range of motion and patient satisfaction are better with total arthroplasty than with hemi-arthroplasty. Only one randomised study has been published [2]. The disadvantage of total shoulder arthroplasty may be loosening of the glenoid component. The disadvantage of a hemi-arthroplasty is erosion of the bone of the glenoid by direct contact between the metal humeral head

Piet M Rozing, Prof. dr., Professor in Orthopaedics, Department of Orthopaedics, Leiden University Medical Center, Rjnsburgerweg 10, 2333 AA Leiden, Netherlands.

and the glenoid bone. This erosion may become painful [8].

A ruptured rotator cuff will eventually affect the postoperative range of motion and the clinical score. There is debate as to whether or not a repair of a thin or ruptured cuff should be considered at the same time as shoulder arthroplasty or a tendon transfer performed [6]. Technically, a cuff repair is not always possible; this provides a strong argument for resorting to shoulder arthroplasty at an earlier stage, before the cuff is ruptured, for example in the rheumatoid patient. A well functioning rotator cuff is a prime factor in the prevention of postoperative proximal migration of the humeral head.

Preoperative assessment

The patient usually presents with complaints of pain and loss of function and has high expectations of a shoulder prosthesis, especially when he has already been operated for a hip or a knee prosthesis. To prevent disappointment after surgery, it is important to inform the patient before the operation of the limitations of shoulder arthroplasty with regard to gain in range of motion and function.

PHYSICAL EXAMINATION

The physical examination reveals muscle wasting, decreased shoulder motion and diminished strength. The limitation of glenohumeral motion is best evaluated by putting one hand on top of the shoulder to stabilise the scapula, while the other hand grasps the elbow to move the humerus and to feel the glenohumeral contraction.

RADIOGRAPHIC EVALUATION

For good preoperative planning, good quality AP and axial radiographs are essential. A true anteroposterior view is obtained by directing the roentgen beam perpendicular to the plane of the scapula. On the AP view, the radiographic destruction of the humeral head and the glenoid can be judged and the status of the glenoid, in particular, will determine the need for a glenoid replacement. The AP view is used for radiographic templating to define the appropriate stem diameter and head size to be used (fig 1). If the humeral head is not well centred and there is an upward subluxation, a rotator cuff tear may be present. On the axillary view, anterior or posterior erosions of the glenoid may be seen to result in a anterior or posterior version of the glenoid (fig 2). In rheumatoid arthritis a subluxation of the humeral head is often combined with a superior-anterior erosion of the glenoid resulting in a superior tilt of the glenoid (fig 3). In severe cases, the inferior corner of the glenoid may be impinging against the humerus. If the glenoid is eroded beyond the base of the coracoid, glenoid replacement is not recommended (fig 4).

If severe bone deficiencies are present on the plain radiographs, computerised tomography is advisable to assess bone-stock and the need for a bone graft if the insertion of a glenoid component is considered. Arthrography or preferably an arthro-MRI can be carried out if knowledge of the status of the rotator cuff is required for surgical planning. If there is an irreparable rotator cuff tear, it is now recommended that only a hemi-arthroplasty be performed.

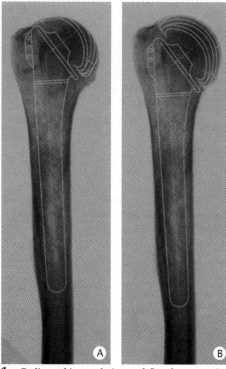

1 *Radiographic templating to define the appropriate stem size and head diameter.*
A. The stem placement is too proximal and the diameter and height of the modular head too small.
B. Correct positioning of the humeral head and the stem.

PREOPERATIVE PLANNING

Based on the functional demands of the patient and the data from the history, the physical examination and the radiographic examination, the surgeon will decide to perform a hemi-arthroplasty or a total shoulder replacement. Indications in favour of a hemi-arthroplasty are: young active persons and a minimal deformity or incongruity (fig 5) of the glenoid. A glenoid component cannot be used in cases with a high risk of loosening such as: severely eroded glenoid with loss of bone stock, fixed proximal migration of the humeral head, and an irreparable cuff tear.

Surgical approach

The most frequently used surgical approach for insertion of a shoulder prosthesis is a long deltopectoral incision. This approach gives good exposure to the humerus and is the preferred approach for hemi-arthroplasty. It is sometimes not sufficient for preparation and bone grafting of the glenoid surface and a complete capsulotomy must be performed to improve exposure. An alternative approach is the posterolateral approach which gives a better access to the glenoid.

Prosthesis

Most available shoulder systems have a range of stems for cemented and uncemented use with different sizes. The correct diameter can

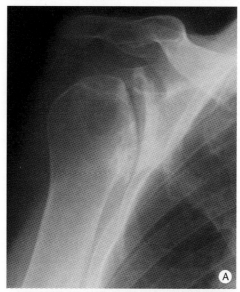

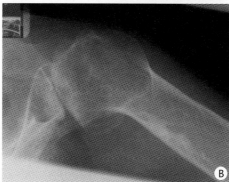

2 *Radiographs of an osteoarthritic shoulder.*
A. Erosion and flattening of the glenoid surface which make it incongruent with a humeral head prosthesis.
B. On the axillary view, a posterior erosion of the glenoid resulting in a posterior version.

be chosen by templating the preoperative radiographs. Non-cemented press-fit humeral components are preferred in younger patients but they function well in all patients. Cemented fixation is indicated when press-fit fixation is not achieved and in fractures of the proximal humerus in which the tuberosities provide no rotational stability. Cemented fixation may be indicated in poor bone stock of the proximal humerus caused by degenerative cysts or secondary to an underlying disease such as rheumatoid arthritis.

The modular system provides the surgeon with an opportunity to reconstruct the normal anatomy of the proximal humerus. This modularity helps balance the soft-tissue and facilitates revision procedures. In most shoulder systems, standard and offset humeral heads are available. In hemi-arthroplasty, the size and radius must duplicate that of the original humeral head because the replaced head will articulate with the non-replaced glenoid. To assess the proper head size, radiographs of the opposite shoulder may sometimes be needed. The preferred radius of the humeral head is chosen by templating the preoperative radiograph (see fig. 1). At surgery, the resected head can also be used as a reference

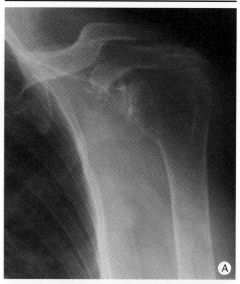

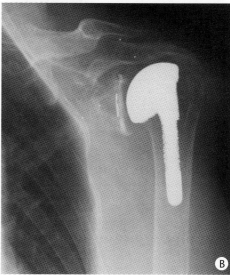

3 *Radiographs of a rheumatoid shoulder.*
A. Superior tilt of the glenoid by superior-anterior erosion of the glenoid resulting in proximal migration of the humeral head with intact rotator cuff.
B. Radiograph after replacement with a short stemmed prosthesis.

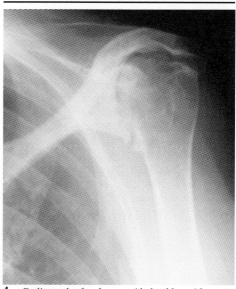

4 *Radiograph of a rheumatoid shoulder with severe erosion of the glenoid and impingement of the inferior corner of the glenoid.*

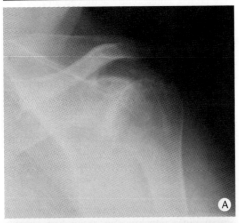

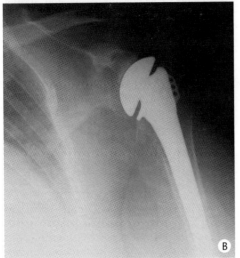

5 *Radiographs of the shoulder of a patient with osteoarthritis.*
A. Minimal and concentric erosion of the glenoid.
B. Good congruency of the shoulder after humeral head replacement.

for choosing the proper radius and thickness of the humeral head prosthesis. The head will cover the resection area of the proximal humerus and balance the cuff. If the chosen head is too thick, it will tension the cuff and limit motion postoperatively.

Patient positioning and preparation

The standard surgical approach for hemiarthroplasty is the deltopectoral incision. Preoperative prophylactic antibiotics are given intravenously at the time of anaesthetic induction. The surgery is performed under general anaesthesia and may be combined with regional anaesthesia, notably an interscalene block according to Winnie. If the procedure is expected to last longer than three hours, an urinary catheter may be considered; in hemi-arthroplasty this is seldom necessary. After completion of the anaesthetic, the patient is placed so that the arm to be operated rests on a short arm-board but can be hyperextended during surgery for accessibility to the humeral shaft. (Patient positioning is very important in total shoulder surgery.) The patient is placed in a semi-sitting or beach-chair position of about 30°

with the torso close to the edge of the table to permit hyperextension of the arm when the humeral component is inserted. The short arm-board is attached to the table to support the arm during surgery. A towel is placed under the medial border of the scapula to stabilise it and ease exposure of the glenoid. It is advisable to fasten the head securely with tape to a neurosurgical headrest or the table itself, so that movement of the extremity during surgery will not cause extreme movements of the neck or dislodge the endotracheal tube. The torso is also secured to the table. An adhesive plastic sterile drape is then applied to the neck to outline the area to be prepared and to keep the patient's hair outside the operating field. With a pencil the important landmarks of the shoulder are drawn, such as the coracoid, the acromioclavicular joint and the anterior tip of the acromion. Then the line of the incision is marked, beginning at the clavicle just lateral to the coracoid process and carrying down in a straight line lateral to the axilla, to the insertion of the deltoid. In this type of surgery, a skin incision of sufficient length has to be used and keyhole surgery is not appropriate.

By marking the anatomical structures and the incision, the area to be prepared is outlined. Skin preparation includes the lower part of the neck superiorly, the middle of the chest anteriorly, the breast inferiorly and as far as the towel posteriorly. The upper extremity should be prepared to the wrist, while an assistant holds the arm by the wrist and moves it in different directions to ease the skin preparation. The wrist, forearm and lower part of the arm are draped or covered with a stockinette and the torso is covered with a U-drape. An adhesive plastic drape is than applied to cover the shoulder, anteriorly and posteriorly, and the axilla; this drape will also secure the towels.

SOFT TISSUE APPROACH

The deltopectoral approach is used and a straight skin incision is made from the clavicle down across the tip of the coracoid (or just lateral to the coracoid) to the insertion of the deltoid muscle. The skin flaps are undermined to identify the deltopectoral groove. The cephalic vein is mobilised and retracted medially (some surgeons prefer to retract the vein laterally). The clavipectoral fascia is incised lateral to the coracoid muscles. A retractor is placed beneath the acromion and deltoid muscle and beneath the conjoined tendon of the coracoid muscles. The shoulder is externally rotated and the subscapular muscle can be seen. The insertion of the subscapular muscle lies medial to the bicipital groove; the inferior border is defined by the anterior circumflex humeral vessels and the superior border is below the tip of the coracoid process at the rotator cuff interval. The anterior circumflex humeral vessels are cauterised and the subscapular tendon with the capsule are released as one unit from the humerus. The inferior capsule may have to be released to dislocate the head anteriorly and to bring it out of the glenoid

fossa. The humeral head is dislocated by external rotation and extension of the humerus.

RESECTION OF THE HUMERAL HEAD

Before osteotomy, the area (particularly inferiorly) must be assessed for osteophytes which are common in osteoarthritis. These are removed with an osteotome or rongeur so that the normal anatomy of the humeral head is defined. Appropriate retractors are placed to expose the proximal humerus. The humeral head resection guide can then be fixed to the humeral shaft with two pins or held in place (some systems use a intramedullary guide). The humeral head is resected at 10°-30° retroversion which is determined by using the forearm as a goniometer with the elbow flexed at 90°. The osteotomy is performed using a oscillating saw, taking care not to remove excessive bone and risk jeopardising the insertion of the rotator cuff both superiorly and posteriorly.

HUMERAL CANAL PREPARATION

The humerus is extended and a starting hole is made laterally on the cut surface of the humerus in line with the humeral shaft. After reaming to the appropriate size and depth, the humeral canal is shaped using humeral rasps taking care to maintain the proper retroversion and aiming for the preoperatively chosen size of the prosthesis. If it does not fit, the alignment of the instruments must be checked to see if it is correct. Once the rasping has been completed the trial humeral prosthesis can be inserted.

The modular trial head with the preoperatively determined radius is put in place. The height of the head with regard to the greater tuberosity is checked and the superior surface of the head should be in line with the greater tuberosity. The shoulder is reduced, and the retroversion of the prosthesis is correct when the head faces towards the glenoid in neutral rotation. The tension of the cuff can be checked by translating the head posteriorly. If it is too tight, a thinner head with the same radius should be tried.

PROSTHESIS INSERTION

After the trial stem is removed, the selected humeral component is inserted. The appropriate head component is impacted in place by a series of small blows.

CLOSURE

The subscapular tendon is sutured to the bone or, if the tendon was previously divided or lengthened with a Z-plasty, closure using absorbable or non-absorbable number two suture material is carried out. A suction drain is inserted between the deltoid muscle and the rotator cuff and the deltopectoral interval is reapproximated using a few interrupted absorbable sutures. Subcutaneous fat and skin are closed in routine fashion. A sterile dressing is applied and the arm is protected in a sling.

Postsurgical care

The rehabilitation programme after surgery depends on the status of the soft tissues (security of the repair of the subscapular tendon and/or rotator cuff), and the stability of the implant. The underlying illness may restrict the exercise programme, such as in severe rheumatoid arthritis with involvement of the neighbouring joints of the shoulder. Sometimes, the goals of the rehabilitation programme must be limited in this type of patient. The success of shoulder replacement is closely related to adequacy of postoperative rehabilitation and patient expectation. The surgeon, therapist and patient must work together closely. For the first 24 hours after surgery the arm is routinely protected in a sling. Active motion of the elbow, wrist and fingers is encouraged early on and, in bed, the patient can take his arm out of the sling if it feels more comfortable alongside his body. Gentle passive range of motion is begun on the second day postoperatively. The patient is encouraged to use hand and arm for gentle everyday activities like eating, drinking, etc. The sling can be discontinued while the patient is lying in bed or sitting in a chair but used when ambulating. On the third or fourth postoperative day, passive and active assisted external rotation and forward flexion exercises are started. In the first weeks, it is necessary to achieve range of motion by passive and active assisted exercises. After three weeks, active and gradual strengthening exercises are started.

Complications

The function of the shoulder, more than that of the hip, knee or elbow, is highly dependent on the integrity and proper functioning of the shoulder muscles. A complication and/or revision operation will severely jeopardise the functional outcome.

Instability or subluxation of the prosthesis may be caused by a bone deficiency of the glenoid, a destroyed rotator cuff or a wrong version of the prosthesis [4]. Subluxation is mostly anterior and occurs in the rheumatoid shoulder because of anterosuperior bone loss of the glenoid in combination with a resection of the acromioclavicular ligament. A posterior subluxation may be seen in a osteoarthritic shoulder with bony erosion of the posterior rim of the glenoid. A superior subluxation will occur if a ruptured rotator cuff is present at the time of surgery or develops in the years after implantation [7]. Another cause of anterior subluxation is the postoperative disruption of the sutured subscapular tendon due to too much tension on the suture line during postoperative rehabilitation.

The frequency of infection after shoulder arthroplasty is about 1%. Predisposing factors are diabetes mellitus, rheumatoid arthritis or infections elsewhere. Treatment is not different from infections of other joint prostheses.

Many prosthetic fractures occur intra-operatively or postoperatively [1]. During surgery, they can be caused by forced manipulation of the humeral shaft to obtain good exposure for reaming and prosthesis insertion. A spiral fracture of the humeral diaphysis may be treated with a cerclage or a long stemmed prosthesis. Late peri-prosthetic fractures are mostly post-traumatic and the first choice of treatment is conservative, consisting of a (orthoplast) fracture brace with isometric exercises and early motion when pain and swelling subside. If a diaphyseal fracture with a stable prosthesis does not heal, the fracture must be addressed surgically, using rigid internal fixation leaving the fixed humeral stem in place and adding autogenous bone grafts. Poor bone quality requires additional procedures.

The incidence of loosening of the humeral component after five to ten years is approximately 5%. Revision may be considered if loosening is symptomatic or bone loss is progressing.

Results

Patients are normally evaluated by different shoulder scoring methods such as the Constant Score, the HSS score or the score of The American Shoulder and Elbow Surgeons. Important components of the score are pain, range of motion and function. With these scoring methods, no statistically significant difference has been found between hemi-arthroplasty and total arthroplasty in different diagnostic categories, but the published studies are mostly non-randomised and retrospective. In hemi-arthroplasty, pain relief may be less consistently achieved and 80% of the patients may have no or slight pain after surgery, in contrast to 90% after a total shoulder arthroplasty [2]. The range of motion after surgery varies greatly according to diagnosis: patients with osteoarthritis have better active abduction and elevation (average 140°) than patients with rheumatoid arthritis (100° or less) [3, 7]. However, the difference in active range of motion is not statistically significant between hemi- or total arthroplasty, although in some reports, rheumatoid patients with a hemi-arthroplasty experienced greater improvement in postoperative range of motion.

Hemi-arthroplasty has the following advantages: a technically easier and shorter operative procedure, less bone removal, less blood loss. The disadvantage is the risk of progressive glenoid erosion with pain which may necessitate revision (3%).

Total shoulder arthroplasty has the advantage that its pain relief is uniformly high. The disadvantages are: a technically more difficult and longer surgical procedure, more blood loss, high rate of glenoid loosening (± 50%) although the revision rate is low (3.6%).

Conclusion

Hemi-arthroplasty and total shoulder arthroplasty have their specific indications but there is a large area where either procedure can be performed. The main indications for hemi-arthroplasty are:
− Osteonecrosis of the humeral head.
− Malunions and non-unions of old proximal humeral fractures.
− Four-part fractures of the proximal humerus.
− Three-part fractures of the proximal humerus in the elderly.
− Chronic dislocations.
− Some forms of primary osteoarthritis.
− Some forms of rheumatoid arthritis.
− Elderly patients with non-union of the surgical neck.
− Cuff tear arthropathy.
The revision rate of hemi-arthroplasty is low and is comparable with hip and knee prostheses. The pain relief after hemi-arthroplasty is good, but the functional improvement is often moderate and depends on the preoperative condition of the shoulder.

References

[1] Campbell JT, Moore RS, Lannotti JP, Norris TR, Williams GR. Periprosthetic humeral fractures: mechanisms of fracture and treatment options. *J Shoulder Elbow Surg* 1998 ; 7 : 406-413

[2] Gartsman GM, Roddey TS, Hammerman SM. Shoulder arthroplasty with or without resurfacing of the glenoid in patients who have osteoarthritis. *J Bone Joint Surg Am* 2000; 82 : 26-34

[3] Kelly IG. Unconstrained shoulder arthroplasty in rheumatoid arthritis. *Clin Orthop* 1994 ; 307 : 94-102

[4] Lohr JF, Floren M, Schweijzer HK, Simmen BR, Gschwend N. Shoulder joint instability after primary arthroplasty. *Orthopade* 1998 ; 27 : 571-575

[5] Rodosky MW, Bigliani LU. Indications for glenoid resurfacing in shoulder arthroplasty. *J Shoulder Elbow Surg* 1996 ; 5 : 231-248

[6] Rozing PM, Brand R. Rotator cuff repair during shoulder arthroplasty in rheumatoid arthritis. *J Arthroplasty* 1998 ; 13 : 311-319

[7] Sjobjerg JO, Frich LH, Johannsen HV, Sneppen O. Late results of total shoulder replacement in patients with rheumatoid arthritis. *Clin Orthop* 1999 ; 366 : 39-45

[8] Sperling JW, Cofield RH. Revision total shoulder arthroplasty for the treatment of glenoid arthrosis (see comments). Comment on J Bone Joint Surg Am 1998 ; 80 : 860-867 in: *J Bone Joint Surg Am* 1999 ; 81 : 592

[9] Stewart MP, Kelly IG. Total shoulder replacement in rheumatoid disease: 7 to 13 year follow-up of 37 joints. *J Bone Joint Surg Br* 1997 ; 79 : 68-72

Total shoulder arthroplasty

IG Kelly

Abstract. – Total shoulder arthroplasty is a well-established procedure in the management of arthritic conditions of the shoulder. Glenoid resurfacing is not appropriate when there is severe glenoid bone loss or a deficient rotator cuff. Its place with regard to humeral head replacement alone has yet to be established, but it is essential in some circumstances. Insertion of the glenoid component can present surgical difficulties, but these can be overcome by good surgical exposure achieved by attention to soft tissue contractures. The surgeon needs to know techniques of soft tissue release and lengthening, and methods of managing problems with bone deficiency.

Keywords: shoulder, total shoulder arthroplasty (TSA), glenoid resurfacing, soft tissue tension, osteoarthritis, rheumatoid arthritis.

Introduction

Total shoulder replacement became a well-established procedure during the last quarter of the twentieth century. However, the necessity of resurfacing the glenoid has been challenged in certain situations [2]. To date, the only randomised prospective trial to have been published is that of Gartsman [7] concerning patients with osteoarthritis. It suggested that there was little to choose between total replacement and humeral head replacement. Although radiolucent lines around the glenoid component have been reported commonly, glenoid loosening is an infrequent occurrence [3].

Reports have shown that humeral head replacement is usually sufficient in the management of avascular collapse of the humeral head if the glenoid bone is not involved [5]. Gartsman and colleagues [7] have reported good early results for humeral head replacement in glenohumeral osteoarthritis, but recorded some problems with glenoid erosion with increased follow-up. Levine has demonstrated that glenoid resurfacing is necessary in the osteoarthritic shoulder with a flat glenoid face [10]. Although it has been suggested that glenoid resurfacing is necessary in rheumatoid shoulders [2], we

Ian G Kelly, BSc MD FRCS (Edinburgh and Glasgow), Consultant Orthopaedic Surgeon and Honorary Clinical Senior Lecturer, University of Glasgow, Glasgow Royal Infirmary, Castle Street, Glasgow G4 0SF, Scotland.

have encountered few problems in a mid-term study, although radiographic erosion is very common [9].

Given the current situation, the surgeon may have to base the choice of procedure on the relative risks of glenoid component loosening and glenoid bone erosion. However, since glenoid resurfacing is mandatory in certain situations, the shoulder surgeon must be able to perform this procedure which can be technically difficult.

Pre-operative assessment and planning

Before undertaking glenohumeral joint replacement, it is necessary to establish that the glenohumeral joint is the source of the patient's pain. This might not be a problem in the patient with osteoarthritis, but can be difficult in the polyarthritic rheumatoid patient. The mere radiographic involvement of the joint does not provide sufficient basis but must be supported by restriction of external rotation and injection test localisation of pain [8].

Good quality radiographs are required, preferably a Grashey anteroposterior projection and an axillary projection. If the shoulder motion is severely restricted, an alternative "lateral" projection will have to be considered. The author's preference is for the apical oblique projection of Garth, Slappey and Ochs [6]. If there is doubt about

the state and/or version of the glenoid, a CT scan should be performed. This can also be useful in post-traumatic shoulders to assess the proximal humerus. The author has not found routine preoperative MRI or ultrasound assessment to be of particular value. Good imaging will provide a pre-operative guide to the feasibility of using a glenoid component.

Most prosthesis manufacturers provide radiographic templates and these can offer useful guidance regarding the probable stem diameter and head size to be used. Inability to ream to the size predicted may suggest an incorrect entry point and knowledge of the diameter of the intramedullary canal should prevent over-reaming and fracture.

Table and patient position

The preferred patient position is the beach chair posture (fig 1). The use of a neurosurgical head rest facilitates access to the shoulder and an adjustable arm board permits abduction of the arm, making the role of the assistant easier.

The patient must be positioned so that the arm can be extended at the shoulder over the edge of the table (fig 1). A small folded towel placed at the medial border of the scapula aids access and stabilises the scapula during insertion of the glenoid component (fig 2).

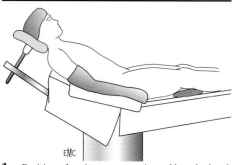

1   *Position of patient on operating table - the beach chair position. If a neurosurgical head rest is not available, a head ring can be used but a larger pad will be needed behind the shoulder. The patient must be positioned at the edge of the table to allow the arm to be extended at the side of the table.*

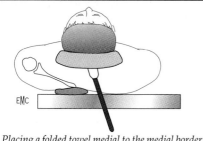

2   *Placing a folded towel medial to the medial border of the scapula facilitates access to the glenoid face and also stabilises the scapula.*

Incision and landmarks

A straight incision commencing anterior to the acromioclavicular joint and running distally, parallel to the axillary crease, for a distance of approximately 12 cm allows good access and heals well.

Soft tissue dissection and joint access

The deltopectoral groove is identified by virtue of the yellow band of fat which surrounds the cephalic vein. The vein may be left alone, excised or ligated proximally and distally before being reflected with the deltoid muscle. Proximal ligation should be where the vein perforates the clavipectoral fascia, to avoid bleeding if the thin vein is ruptured during the procedure and retracts beneath the fascia.

Elevation of the deltoid muscle off the underlying fascia using finger dissection, extending from the deltoid insertion superiorly into the subacromial space, allows for good and easy access to the proximal humerus at a later stage of procedure. Care must be taken to ensure that no fibres of the deltoid muscle are left attached to the fascia since this places the axillary nerve at risk.

A cobra retractor can be passed over the humeral head beneath the acromion, to retract the deltoid. The clavipectoral fascia is incised longitudinally and reflected using a blunt dissector. A further cobra retractor is passed beneath the coracoid muscles on the anterior surface of the subscapularis.

Additional exposure can be gained by incising the tendon of the pectoralis major insertion. It is usually only necessary to incise the proximal centimetre, but if the shoulder is particularly tight the entire tendon can be cut. In this situation it is useful to place stay sutures on each end of the cut tendon to facilitate later repair although this may be neither possible nor necessary, especially in rheumatoid patients.

Division of the pectoralis major tendon allows for easy access to the axillary region where the axillary nerve must be located. It often lies deep but is brought superficial with external rotation of the arm. There is often a plexus of fragile veins around the nerve and palpation must be performed with care. Once the nerve has been identified, it can be protected during the remainder of the procedure.

DIVISION OF THE SUBSCAPULARIS

The anterior circumflex artery with its two adjacent veins runs close to the distal border of the subscapularis tendon and should be coagulated prior to the opening of the joint.

The method of opening the joint is dependent on the degree of restriction of external rotation as well as on the diagnosis. With an external rotation of 10° or more, it is possible to place a dissector beneath the subscapularis tendon and divide it approximately 0.5 cm from its insertion to the lesser tuberosity, placing stay sutures in its medial portion. With external rotation of less than 10°, or an internal rotation contracture, it is preferable to open the joint by osteotomising the lesser tuberosity, reattaching this more medially on the neck of the humerus at the end of the operation *(fig 3A)*. An alternative is to elevate the insertion of the subscapularis to the lesser tuberosity by sharp dissection and to suture the tendon to the cut edge of the humeral neck at the close of the procedure *(fig 3B)*. Z-plasty opening of the subscapularis tendon *(fig 3C)* can also be considered but it does result in a weakened tendon.

In patients with rheumatoid arthritis the subscapularis tendon is frequently thin and somewhat elastic and extra length can be gained simply by releasing it from the neck of the scapula even when there is no external rotation.

If the subscapularis tendon is divided, the incision must be carried superiorly into the rotator interval dividing the coracohumeral ligament. The capsule is usually adherent to the deep surface of the subscapularis tendon and should be divided in the same line as the tendon. At this stage any intra-articular adhesions are divided.

To facilitate dislocation it is necessary to divide the inferior capsule. The axillary nerve is located and protected. Slight external rotation is applied to the humerus

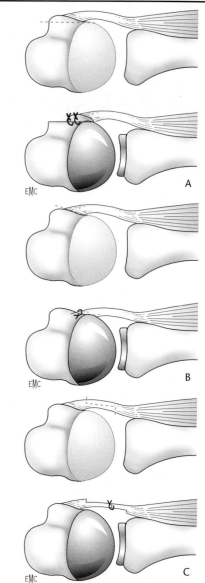

3   *A. When external rotation is very limited, access to the glenohumeral joint can be achieved by osteotomising the lesser tuberosity. This can be reattached to its bed, or more medially at the end of the procedure.*
B. The subscapularis tendon can be removed from the lesser tuberosity using sharp dissection and reattached more medially at the end of the procedure using suture anchors.
C. Z-plasty opening of the subscapularis and capsule will assist in the restoration of length of the subscapularis but also weakens the tendon.

and the inferior capsule is cut under direct vision. Further external rotation of the humerus allows for anterior dislocation of the humeral head. If any resistance is encountered, external rotation should be stopped and further capsular division undertaken.

At this stage the arm is extended at the side of the table and the head of the humerus is delivered into the wound using two retractors, one placed behind the humeral head beneath the acromion, and the other behind the humeral head within the glenohumeral joint. This is essential to permit adequate access to the humeral medullary cavity.

Humeral head resection

Various instrument systems are in existence for shoulder arthroplasty. Some require resection of the humeral head fragment using a guide, followed by reaming of the humeral canal whilst others use an intramedullary reamer as the basis for a head resection guide. Whichever system is used, attention must be paid to the height and version of the head resection. There may be considerable variation in the normal degree of retroversion of the humeral head and each shoulder must be evaluated individually. However, in most shoulders 30 to 35 degrees of retroversion in relation to the forearm will be appropriate. The resection line must not endanger the insertion of the rotator cuff - supraspinatus and infraspinatus - but should lie at the level of cuff insertion to avoid leaving the humeral head too prominent.

If reamers are to be introduced before resection of the humeral head, the point of entry lies midway between the anterior and posterior borders of the head at the margin of the articular surface. When there is marked deformity, entry approximately 5 mm posterior to the bicipital groove will usually prove to be correct. The reamers should be used until resistance is encountered. Particular care should be taken with osteoporotic bone.

Soft tissue release

At this stage of the procedure it is necessary to free the subscapularis from the anterior margin of the glenoid, the scapular neck and the undersurface of the coracoid process. This gains length. Any osteophytes on the anterior margin of the glenoid should be removed and osteophytes on the proximal humerus should also be resected. The posterior capsule should be freed from the posterior margin of the glenoid, especially where there has been some medialisation of the glenohumeral joint.

Insertion of trial stem

The diameter of the last reamer used dictates the diameter of the definitive stem. A trial stem is inserted with the appropriate amount of retroversion and the adequacy of the head resection is checked. In modular systems, a trial head is then positioned on the stem and the glenohumeral joint is reduced

The appropriateness of the retroversion of the humeral head can be checked in relation to the glenoid by holding the forearm in the position of neutral rotation. The humeral head should face the glenoid. If it does not, a decision will have to be made as to whether the adjustment should be made on the humeral side or in the orientation of the

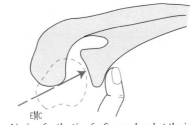

4 *Aiming for the tip of a finger placed at the junction of the glenoid and scapula blade allows correct alignment of instruments for the preparation of the glenoid face, especially when there is glenoid erosion.*

glenoid face. In the majority of cases, the adjustment will be made by altering the line of the humeral resection, although this may not apply when the glenoid is deformed.

Glenoid preparation

A humeral protector or trial prosthesis is inserted into the medullary canal to protect the cut surface and a cobra retractor is passed over the surface of the protector, posterior to the glenoid. A second cobra retractor is placed beneath the medially retracted subscapularis tendon on the neck of the scapula. The humerus is positioned in the appropriate degree of abduction and external rotation which gives the best access to the glenoid. If the soft tissue release described above has been performed, exposure is usually good. However, further capsular release (especially posteriorly) may be necessary. Remnants of the labrum and any fragments of synovium or capsule are removed. It is necessary to determine the extent of any remaining osteophytic ring, particularly inferiorly, to ensure that the implant is not offset in too low a position.

It can be very difficult to determine the degree of version of the glenoid at operation, but moderate deformity can be appreciated. Minor to moderate variations can be accommodated by reaming, but more severe deficiencies will require glenoid reconstruction (see below).

Whichever system is used and whichever type of glenoid prosthesis is chosen - cemented or uncemented - the glenoid face should be shaped to fit and support the back surface of the implant. In most cases, this involves creating a concave surface by using a reamer which is positioned by a pilot drill hole in the centre of the glenoid face. Palpation of the junction between the anterior surface of the scapular neck and the blade of the scapula provides the line to be followed (fig 4).

The further preparation of the glenoid depends upon the type of glenoid prosthesis. The cemented, keeled implant is probably the most widely used. With a slotted keel guide, three holes are drilled into the glenoid face, ensuring that the top of the slot is placed at the top of the glenoid. The holes are then linked using a drill or burr to outline the length and width of the

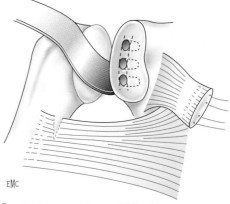

5 *Good exposure is essential for the correct preparation of the glenoid bone and insertion of the prosthesis. Division of the inferior capsule and the superior centimetre of the pectoralis major tendon greatly facilitates access. A retractor placed over the protected cut surface of the humerus and behind the glenoid is also required.*

keel of the glenoid prosthesis (fig 5). The cavity to accommodate the keel of the glenoid component is developed using angled curettes, attempting to excavate the cancellous bone at the base of the coracoid process and along the lateral border of the scapula. In many instances there is very little cancellous bone and this cavity must be developed cautiously using a burr. If the cortex is perforated it can be closed with cancellous bone taken from the resected humeral head.

GLENOID TRIAL

The fit of the glenoid component is tested using the trial component. The component must be absolutely stable and fully supported by bone. If there is insufficient glenoid bone to accommodate the keel of the glenoid component, a small portion of the polyethylene keel can be removed using heavy scissors.

CEMENT IMPLANT

The glenoid cavity is irrigated with saline. Haemostasis can be achieved by the use of hydrogen peroxide or chilled saline. Cementation can be difficult and several methods have been described. Low viscosity cement can be introduced using a syringe but can be difficult to retain in the small cavity. Neer has described a "double cementing" method in which a small amount of cement is introduced into the cavity and forced into the interstices of the cancellous bone with a sponge to control bleeding. This is followed by a plug of firmer cement from the same batch which is used to secure the implant. The glenoid component is held firmly in place with a glenoid pusher or the thumb. Excess cement is cleared at this stage, paying particular attention to the posterior portion of the joint. Once the cement has set, the fixation of the implant is tested and the joint is further irrigated with saline and any loose fragments of cement are removed. If the fixation is not firm the prosthesis must be removed and the cavity is prepared again.

Soft tissue tensioning and humeral implantation

The retractors are relocated and the arm is extended to deliver the proximal humerus into the wound. The humeral canal protector is then removed and the trial humeral component is inserted. When a modular device is being used, the appropriate trial humeral head is the one which:

– allows at least a one-third diameter humeral head translation against the glenoid;

– allows for 30° of external rotation after the reattachment of the subscapularis;

– allows 90° of internal rotation, with the arm at 90° of abduction.

Check that the head lies just superior to the tip of the greater tuberosity and that there is no contact between the glenoid and the calcar of the humerus, or the collar of the stem, especially during adduction and external rotation. If this is encountered, further resection of osteophytes on the humerus or inferior pole of the glenoid will be necessary.

The humeral component may be designed for cement, for press-fit use or for press-fit with bone ingrowth. If it is not to be cemented the appropriate definitive prosthesis is selected and introduced with the appropriate amount of retroversion. A secure press-fit must be obtained.

In some situations, it will not be possible to obtain a firm press-fit with some types of pathology, especially rheumatoid arthritis, where the quality of the cancellous bone may be poor, and a cemented insertion will be preferred. In this situation the humerus should be irrigated with saline and may be packed with a swab containing either hydrogen peroxide or chilled saline to achieve haemostasis. A cement restrictor should be used for low viscosity cement, but is not essential for standard cement. A suction tube is placed in the medullary canal and cement is inserted. If cement is to be injected, pressurisation should be avoided since it may result in cement extrusion, especially where the bone is thin and osteoporotic. The definitive prosthesis is then inserted using the introducer and, once it is in place, excess cement is removed.

In modular systems, a Morse taper will connect the head and the stem. It is essential that both parts of the Morse taper be absolutely clean and dry. Failure to ensure this will greatly weaken the bond and may result in dissociation of the components.

Closure

The shoulder is then reduced and the soft tissue tension is checked once more. The subscapularis is repaired according to its

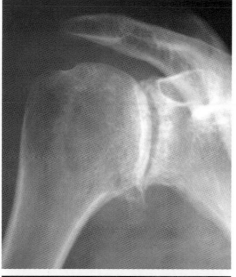
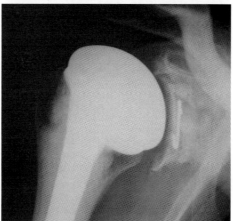
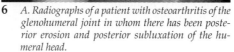
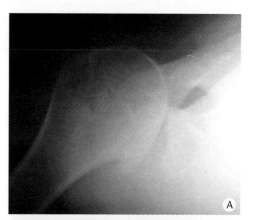
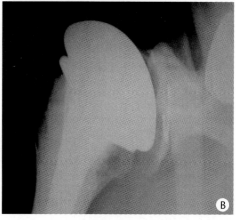

6 *A. Radiographs of a patient with osteoarthritis of the glenohumeral joint in whom there has been posterior erosion and posterior subluxation of the humeral head.*

B. Postoperative radiographs of the same patient showing the corrected position of the glenoid and the use of a glenoid component with a shortened stem. An apical oblique projection has been used [6].

mode of opening, with extra length being gained by displacement of the lesser tuberosity or suturing the stump of the tendon to the cut humeral neck. Suction drains are inserted deep to the deltoid and into the axillary recess. The deltopectoral interval can then be approximated using absorbable sutures. Skin is closed using an absorbable subcuticular suture or skin clips, if preferred. A shoulder immobiliser is then applied in most cases, although in special circumstances, some form of specialised brace may be required.

Special circumstances

CUFF RUPTURES

Small ruptures of the rotator cuff (supraspinatus) can usually be repaired easily. Large and massive tears require extensive mobilisation of the remaining cuff and reattachment to the greater tuberosity. The cuff is mobilised and bony sutures are placed before the humeral prosthesis is implanted.

DEFICIENT GLENOID BONE

Glenoid deficiency can have many causes. The most commonly encountered is probably the posterior glenoid loss seen in some forms of glenohumeral osteoarthritis (fig 6A). Anterior glenoid loss is seen with long-standing dislocations. Rheumatoid arthritis can result in extreme glenoid deficiency which is usually central but becomes more cephalic as it progresses. The inferior glenoid pole is frequently preserved in these patients and reaming away the preserved inferior glenoid pole is usually necessary to achieve an appropriately directed surface (fig 7).

Anterior and posterior glenoid loss can often be corrected by reaming the high side. However, only a small amount of bone can be removed or not enough will remain to support a glenoid prosthesis. With larger defects, other strategies have to be considered.

The glenoid component can be placed in an abnormal degree of version as determined by the glenoid bone and the humeral component version can be altered to allow a congruent joint. This method is limited by

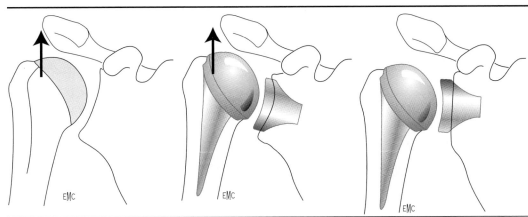

7 *In rheumatoid arthritis, the glenoid bone is frequently severely eroded in a cephalic direction as far as the base of the coracoid process whilst preserving the inferior pole. Glenoid implantation without correction will result in superior subluxation. Augmentation of the glenoid face is not usually satisfactory in the rheumatoid patient and resection of the inferior pole is recommended.*

the need to accommodate the keel of the component within the scapular neck (*fig 6B*). A bone graft taken from the resected humeral head or from the iliac crest can be used to augment the glenoid bone. It is fixed into place using two cancellous bone screws. Access for posterior augmentation can be difficult.

With superior wear such as that commonly encountered in rheumatoid arthritis, placing the glenoid component high on the glenoid with the keel engaging in coracoid bone can be useful. The extensive glenoid wear results in the base of the coracoid becoming continuous with the surface of the glenoid.

INSTABILITY

When arthroplasty is used for old posterior or anterior dislocations or posteriorly dislocated arthritic shoulders there will be excessive posterior or anterior capsular laxity. Reducing the retroversion of the humeral prosthesis has been described to cope with posterior laxity, but is unlikely to be effective without attention being paid to the soft tissues.

Any glenoid deficiency should be tackled as described above. This will determine the version of the humeral component. In the case of posterior instability (the most common situation) adequate lengthening of the subscapularis is essential (see above) and reefing of the posterior capsule may also be necessary. Postoperatively the arm should be held in either a hand-shake cast or a brace, immobilising the arm in neutral rotation. Mobilisation can commence early but must be passive and should avoid forward elevation for the first 3 weeks.

Postoperative management

At the end of the procedure, the arm is placed in a shoulder immobiliser, although

special braces or casts may be necessary in special circumstances.

If the humeral tuberosities have not been detached, rehabilitation of the shoulder can commence on the first postoperative day. A variety of regimes have been described, but nearly all of them are based on the regime described by Neer [11]. Passive elevation and external rotation are carried out with the patient being allowed to use his own muscles (active assisted) as he is able. Fully active motion then follows, with strengthening being introduced at about six weeks. Passive stretching continues throughout and is probably necessary during the first six months. Hydrotherapy can be very valuable, especially in patients with polyarthropathy.

Results

The results of total shoulder arthroplasty should be considered according to the diagnosis that was the indication for surgery. Pathology varies greatly, and the state of the soft tissues - especially the rotator cuff tendons - will influence the outcome of surgery. The published literature shows very little difference between the results for total replacement and humeral head replacement, although Gschwend has reported a significant difference in the number of patients receiving total replacements who felt much improved rather than only improved, compared to those receiving humeral head replacements [1].

On the basis of the few long-term studies available typical results are shown in Table I.

Several survivor analyses can be found in the literature for total shoulder replacement. Brenner [4] reported 73% survival rate for all diagnostic groups at 11 years, but 92% for arthroplasty in rheumatoid arthritis. More recently, Torchia [12] has reported a survival rate of 93% at 10 years and 87% after 15 years irrespective of diagnosis. However, Brenner used stricter criteria in defining the end point.

Conclusions

Total shoulder replacement is well documented as a successful procedure. Glenoid resurfacing is inappropriate in certain situations, such as when the rotator cuff is irreparable or when there is insufficient glenoid bone. However, proper preparation of the glenoid bone requires good exposure and this can be difficult. Medium term results of humeral head replacement indicating outcomes equivalent to those achieved with total replacement have resulted in many surgeons abandoning glenoid resurfacing. Currently, there is insufficient scientific evidence to guide our decision-making in routine cases. However, some situations demand glenoid resurfacing and all shoulder surgeons must be capable of performing this procedure.

Table I. – Rheumatoid arthritis and osteoarthritis results.

	N	FU	ABD	FLEX	ER	IR
Rheumatoid arthritis [12]	37	9.5y	-	90	38	B-T7
Osteoarthritis [13]	34	9.7y	-	143	55	B-T6

ABD = abduction; FLEX = flexion; ER = external rotation; IT = internal rotation.

References ➤

References

[1] Bell SN, Gschwend N. Clinical experience with total arthroplasty and hemiarthroplasty of the shoulder using the Neer prosthesis. *Int Orthop* 1986 ; 10 (4) : 217-222

[2] Boyd AD, Thomas WH, Scott RD, Sledge CB, Thornhill TS. Total shoulder arthroplasty versus hemiarthroplasty. Indications for glenoid resurfacing. *J Arthroplasty* 1990 ; 5 (4) : 329-336

[3] Brems J. The glenoid component in total shoulder arthroplasty. *J Shoulder Elbow Surg* 1993 ; 5 : 329-336

[4] Brenner BC, Ferlic DC, Clayton ML, Dennis DA. Survivorship of unconstrained total shoulder arthroplasty. *J Bone Joint Surg Am* 1989 ; 71 (9) : 1289-1296

[5] Dines DW, Warren RF, Altchek DW, Moeckel B. Posttraumatic changes in the proximal humerus: Malunion, non-union, and osteonecrosis. Treatment with modular hemiarthroplasty or total shoulder arthroplasty. *J Shoulder Elbow Surg* 1993 ; 2 : 11-21

[6] Garth WP, Slappey CE, Ochs CW. Roentgenographic demonstration of instability of the shoulder: the apical oblique projection - a technical note. *J Bone Joint Surg Am* 1984 ; 66 (A) : 1450-1453

[7] Gartsman GM, Roddey TS, Hammerman SM. Shoulder arthroplasty with and without resurfacing of the glenoid in patients who have osteoarthritis *J Bone Joint Surg Am* 2000 ; 82 (1) : 26-34

[8] Kelly IG. The source of shoulder pain in rheumatoid arthritis - the usefulness of local anaesthetic injections. *J Shoulder Elbow Surg Am* 1994 ; 3 : 62-65

[9] Kelly IG. The place of hemiarthroplasty in the rheumatoid shoulder. In : Vastamaki M, Jalovaara P eds. Surgery of the Shoulder. Amsterdam : Elselvier, 1995

[10] Levine WN, Djurasovic M, Glasson JM et al. Hemiarthroplasty for glenohumeral osteoarthritis: results correlated to degree of glenoid wear. *J Shoulder Elbow Surg Am* 1997 ; 6 (5) : 449-454

[11] Neer CsII. Shoulder Reconstruction. Philadelphia : Saunders, 1990

[12] Stewart MPM, Kelly IG. Total Shoulder Replacement in Rheumatoid Disease. 7 -to 13-year follow-up of 37 joints. *JBJS* 1997 ; (79B) : 68-72

[13] Torchia ME, Cofield RH, Settergren CR. Total shoulder arthroplasty with the Neer prosthesis: long term results. *J Shoulder Elbow Surg Am* 1997 ; 6 (6) : 495-505

Prosthetic treatment of fractures of the proximal humerus

M Randelli

Abstract. – The prosthetic treatment of fractures of the proximal humerus is indicated in complex cases: four-part fractures and fracture-dislocations, head-split and impression defects with more than 40% articular surface involvement, and some three-part fractures.
An accurate and meticulous technique is mandatory for obtaining successful results: proper humeral length and retroversion, secure reconstruction of the tuberosities and soft tissue tension restoration are the essential elements.
The importance of prolonged and well conducted functional rehabilitation is again emphasised.
The outcome is generally satisfactory regarding pain control, but more uncertain for the recovery of function, strength and movement.

Keywords: shoulder, joint prosthesis, hemi-arthroplasty, humeral prosthesis, arthroplasty, fractures of proximal humerus.

Introduction

Fractures of the proximal humerus are a relatively frequent occurrence, especially in elderly subjects having porous bones, although they are not rare in younger folk either.

Fortunately, in the large majority of cases (85%), such fractures do not pose any treatment problems. It has been schematically indicated that displacements of less than 1 cm or angulations of less than 45° do not require any reductive manoeuvre, being stable fractures that tend to heal spontaneously [13].

Classification criteria are essential in deciding the approach to treatment. "Each classification system should denote the morphology of the fracture, describe the biological and mechanical short term behaviour, provide therapeutic guidelines, and discuss expected long term clinical outcomes" [10]. In effect, "only a better anatomical approach allows for an improved final prognosis" [7]. Rather than considering the anatomical site (Kocher) or the trauma mechanism (Watson-Jones), it is useful to apply Codman's concept (1934), which

Mario Randelli, Direttore Dipartimento Patologia Apparato Locomotore, Istituto Clinico Humanitas, 20089 Rozzano, Italia.

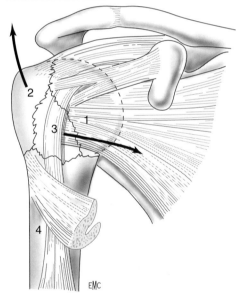

1 *The four segments of proximal humerus fractures. 1. Head; 2. greater tuberosity; 3. lesser tuberosity; 4. diaphysis.*

divides fractures of the proximal humerus into four main fragments following the former lines of epiphyseal union: the head, greater tuberosity, lesser tuberosity and diaphysis *(fig 1)*.

This classification principle was developed by Neer [13]. From a practical viewpoint, Neer's classification is still valid for leading to a correct indication and treatment.

Indications

FOUR-PART FRACTURES AND FRACTURE-DISLOCATIONS

These represent the prime indication.

The greater tuberosity, onto which the supraspinatus, infraspinatus and teres minor muscles are inserted, is shifted superiorly and posteriorly; the lesser tuberosity, because of subscapularis action, is shifted medially. The diaphysis, due to the combined action of the deltoid and pectoralis major, is pushed higher and medially; the humeral head, deprived of any vascular supply, may be variously dislocated *(fig 2)*.

In rare cases, the humeral head may be impacted into the metaphysis (valgus impacted fracture): such cases have a more benign prognosis and are amenable to reduction and osteosynthesis through minimum exposure *(fig 3)*.

Generally, in seriously displaced cases, the risk of vascular necrosis is very high. Then the treatment of choice, even in relatively young patients, is frequently primary replacement arthroplasty.

FRACTURES OF THE HUMERAL ARTICULAR SURFACE (HEAD-SPLIT AND IMPRESSION DEFECTS)

These lesions do not always show up clearly on standard X-rays, but are highlighted by CT scans *(fig 4)*. Should the fragments be

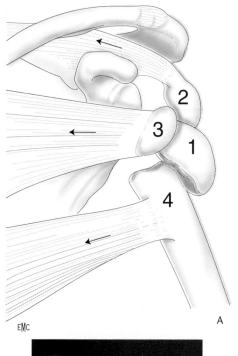

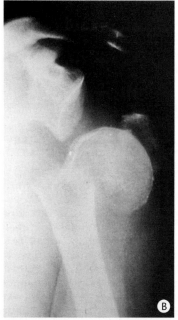

2 *A. Design. 1. Head; 2. greater tuberosity; 3. lesser tuberosity; 4. diaphysis.*
B. Radiograph of typical displacements in a four-part fracture.

sufficiently large, or the surface defect less than 40%, one can attempt reduction, synthesis and repair of the defect. If this is not the case, it is better to proceed directly to prosthetic replacement.

THREE-PART FRACTURES

This indication is limited to elderly patients or when the bone-stock is deficient (osteoporosis), as it is difficult in these cases to obtain a valid osteosynthesis. If possible, prosthetic treatment is avoided in younger subjects.

Surgical technique

ANAESTHESIA

General or regional (interscalene block) anaesthesia may be used. The latter is

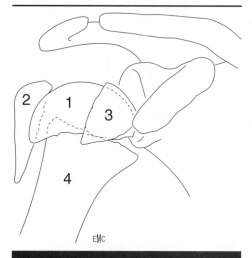

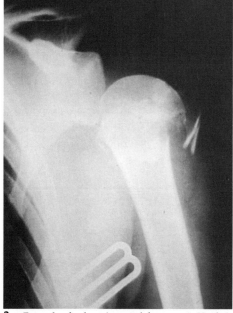

3 *Example of valgus impacted fracture. 1. Head; 2. greater tuberosity; 3. lesser tuberosity; 4. diaphysis.*

generally preferred because, apart from allowing excellent analgesic control during the operation, its effect extends into the post operative period.

POSITIONING

The patient is placed at the lateral edge of the table, in such a way as to allow complete mobility of the injured limb. Positioning is semi-reclined ("beach-chair"), with the trunk flexed at 30° and the knees at 45° *(fig 5)*. The head is in a neutral position, fixed to a headrest.

Preparation of the field should amply expose the shoulder, with the arm draped free.

In particular, there should be free extension of the arm to facilitate exposition and reaming of the medullary canal.

SURGICAL APPROACH

A long anterior deltopectoral incision that begins below the clavicle and extends towards the humeral insertion of the deltoid is used *(fig 6)*. The cephalic vein is identified

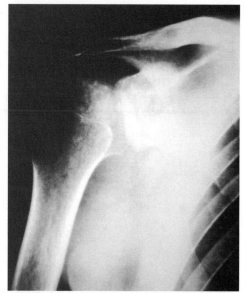

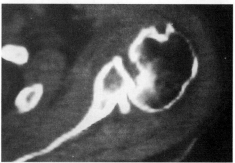

4 *Plain radiograph and CT scan of posterior dislocation of the shoulder. Observe, in the coronal view, the difficulty of showing up the head's dislocation.*

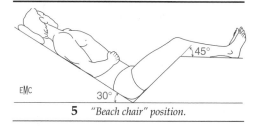

5 *"Beach chair" position.*

in the deltopectoral interval and retracted medially or laterally. In some cases it may be tied, without any particular consequences to the peripheral circulation. In order to improve access, it is sometimes necessary to partially release the humeral insertion of the deltoid, or to section about 2 cm of the pectoralis major tendon *(fig 7)*. The conjoined tendon (coracobrachialis and short head of the biceps) is retracted medially, it not being generally necessary to carry out an osteotomy of the coracoid process. The long head of the biceps tendon is then identified, usually undamaged, and followed proximally, it leads to the interval between the two tuberosities *(fig 8)*.

FRACTURE EXPOSURE AND PREPARATION

The two tuberosities are thus identified. Medially to the long head of the biceps, the lesser tuberosity onto which the subscapularis tendon is inserted is exposed.

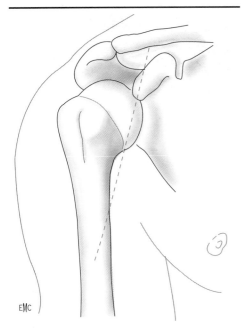

6   *Long anterior deltopectoral incision.*

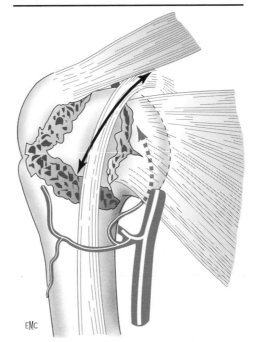

8   *The long head of the biceps is identified and followed proximally.*

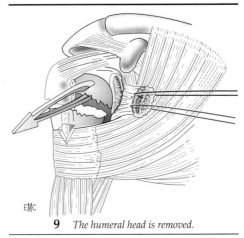

9   *The humeral head is removed.*

Laterally, is the greater tuberosity with the supraspinatus, infraspinatus and teres minor muscles. With the two tuberosities separated and mobilised, the humeral head is found and removed together with any small bone fragments *(fig 9)*. It can be difficult to remove the humeral head in anterior fracture-dislocations: it is therefore necessary to proceed with a cautious manoeuvre of retraction and rotation, being careful not to damage the neighbouring neurovascular bundle. It is appropriate then to inspect the rotator cuff, which in these cases is generally intact, to ensure it is regularly inserted into the tuberosities.

The proximal extreme of the humeral diaphysis is now exposed and regularised *(fig 10)*. Attention is paid to any fracture lines extending into the diaphyseal cortex and weakening it. In such an event, it is important to prevent possible secondary displacement by applying some cerclage wires.

PROSTHESIS PLACEMENT

(Reference is made to Neer's prosthesis). With manual instruments, the medullary canal is prepared using reamers of progressively larger diameters *(fig 11)*, evaluating the need for a press-fit or cemented implant. In the former case, the reaming has to allow for good fixation of the prosthesis against the cortex of the humerus: this carries a possible risk of splits. With the proper size of stem established, before the definitive implant, it is necessary to determine the proper retroversion angle and height for the prosthesis.

The advised retroversion angle is 35°- 45° [4], but more recent studies suggest an anatomical angle of 20° [2]. It is evaluated by making use of the forearm as one limb of a goniometer *(fig 12)*. In these fractures, in fact, it is rarely possible to refer to the bicipital groove. Where possible, the fin of the prosthesis is positioned 5-10 mm posterior to the groove.

A second essential element to be evaluated is the proper depth of the prosthesis into the medullary canal. A prosthesis seated too deeply would entail a weakness of the soft tissue with possible inferior subluxation. A too prominent prosthesis would give rise to an impingement against the acromion with joint stiffness and consequent damage to the cuff. It is difficult to establish the proper height of the prosthesis: as a general rule it is good to make the head of the prosthesis correspond with the glenoid surface, obtaining a proper tension of the soft tissues (in particular, the biceps tendon).

It is useful at this point to prepare some sutures on the humeral shaft which will subsequently be used to stabilise the tuberosities, and then proceed with the definitive implant *(fig 13)*. The stability of the press-fit stem is often insufficient and it is therefore necessary to resort to cementing, preserving the established height and retroversion. Excess cement is carefully removed. Neer's prosthesis has two head thicknesses available (15 mm and 22 mm) with just one radius of curve (44 mm). The more modern prostheses make use of several thicknesses and diameter options. In any case, the choice is governed by the bone parameters of the removed humeral head, and seeking the most suitable tension for the soft tissues.

SYNTHESIS OF THE TUBEROSITIES

This is an essential surgical phase, because its purpose is to fix the insertions of the cuff, the true "engine" of the prosthetic implant. Heavy, non-absorbable sutures are placed at the bone tendon junction of the two tuberosities, considering that sparse resistance is offered by the osteoporotic bone of the tuberosities. The tuberosities are then

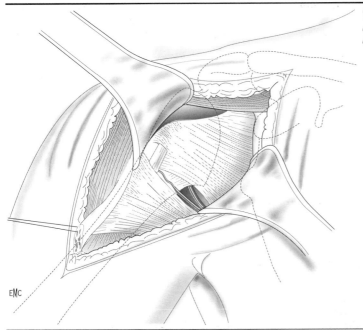

7   *To improve access, the deltoid tendon is partially cut and released.*

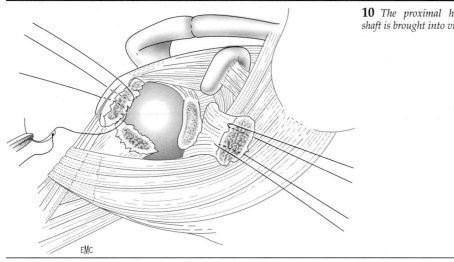

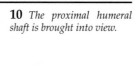

10 *The proximal humeral shaft is brought into view.*

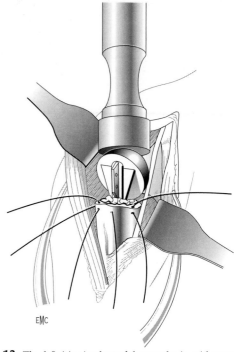

13 *The definitive implant of the prosthesis, with some sutures already prepared on the humeral shaft.*

Pendulum exercises may be started fairly early on (10-15 days). From the sixth week, self-assisted active elevation exercises (with pulleys) will begin and also isometric exercises and activities of daily living. From the tenth week, resistance exercises are commenced and continued for 4-6 months [3].

Complications

The onset of complications is rather frequent following prosthetic treatment of an acute fracture. In a review of the literature, Muldoon and Cofield [12] report 71 complications in 203 treated shoulders (35%). Septic complications (early and delayed) and intra-operative fractures of the humeral diaphysis are relatively rare. More frequent are complications linked to bad positioning of the prosthesis and greater

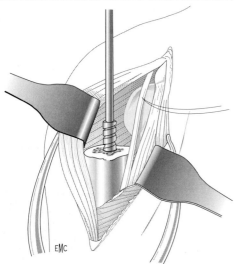

11 *The medullary canal is prepared using a reamer.*

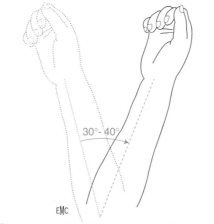

12 *To evaluate the angle of retroversion, the foream is used as one limb of a goniometer.*

repositioned around the prosthesis and fixed below the prosthetic head with two series of sutures: horizontal (between the two tuberosities and through the holes in the prosthetic fin) and vertical (to the humeral shaft, and between subscapularis and supraspinatus to close the rotator interval) *(fig 14)*. During the suturing, the limb is kept in slight abduction and external rotation (about 20°). It may sometimes be necessary to set some cancellous bone grafts from the humeral head to fill in the space between the tuberosities and the stem.

The long head of the biceps tendon may be variously treated: either preserved and incorporated between the two tuberosities, or sectioned and fixed in the bicipital groove.

At this point, drainage is applied, and then closure of the deltopectoral interval by layered suturing is performed.

Rehabilitation

This is critical for obtaining a good functional outcome. The arm is kept in a sling and swathe or a 45° abduction cushion for 4-6 weeks, until the healing process of

the tuberosities is at an advanced stage. Right from the early postoperative days, once the painful phase surpassed, passive physiotherapy should be initiated to maintain joint mobility. The limits on movement are established by the surgeon, based on the intraoperative evaluation of joint stability, the validity of the tuberosity synthesis and the status of the cuff. Passive elevation exercises are particularly useful, as is external rotation limited to 20-30°.

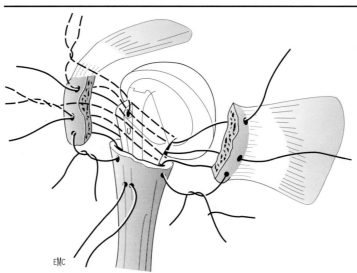

14 *The accurate suturing of the tuberosities is an essential step for obtaining good motor control of the prosthesis.*

tuberosity displacement, considering that such problems are connected and inter-dependent [2]. Other complications involve nerve injury (sometimes a consequence of the trauma), anterior and posterior instability of the prosthesis, the formation of ectopic bone (that rarely involves some functional limitations); and secondary rotator cuff tears.

Results

Evaluating the results from the literature is a somewhat contrasted affair. While there seems to be a general consensus on satisfactory pain control, there is much more uncertainty about the functional outcomes. Some series report excellent or satisfactory results in 90% of cases; others do not reach 50% [5, 8, 9, 11, 14, 16, 17]. The reason for such diversity, as well as taking the differing assessment criteria into account, is surely to be found in relation to the accuracy of the surgical technique and postoperative rehabilitation. Most of the causes of failure are technical in nature and preventable [1].

Conclusions

Prosthetic treatment appears to be perfectly indicated in complex fractures of the proximal humerus, especially in cases where grave comminution and bone stock deficit involve difficulties for osteosynthesis and a serious risk of osteonecrosis.

In order to optimise the outcome, some basic rules have to be observed:

– Operating quite early (within 2 weeks of the injury);

– An accurate and precise surgical technique, with special attention paid to the positioning of the prosthesis and to secure fixation of the tuberosities with rotator cuff repair;

– A long and well conducted period of rehabilitation and physical therapy.

References

[1] Bigliani LU, Flatow EL, McCluskey GM, Fischer RA. Failed prosthetic replacement for displaced proximal humerus fractures. *Orthop Trans* 1991 ; 15 : 747-748

[2] Boileau P, Tinsi L, Lehuec JC, Mole D, Sinnerton R, Walch G. Results of shoulder arthroplasty in acute fractures of the proximal humerus. In : Walch G, Boileau Peds. Shoulder arthroplasty. Berlin : Springer-Verlag, 1999 : 331-345

[3] Compito CA, Self EB, Bigliani LU. Arthroplasty and acute shoulder trauma. *Clin Orthop* 1994 ; 307 : 27-36

[4] Craig EV. Prosthetic replacement for four-part fractures of the proximal humerus. In : Paulos LE, Tibone JEeds. Operative techniques in shoulder surgery. Gaithersburg : Aspen, 1991 : 187-196

[5] Dines DM, Warren RF. Modular shoulder hemiarthroplasty for acute fractures. *Clin Orthop* 1994 ; 307 : 18-26

[6] Duparc J. Classification des fractures articulaires de l'extrémité supérieure de l'humérus. *Acta Orthop Belg* 1995 ; 61 (suppl 1) : 65-70

[7] Duparc J, Largier A. Les luxations-fractures de l'extrémité supérieure de l'humérus. *Rev Chir Orthop* 1976 ; 62 : 91-110

[8] Goldman RT, Koval KJ, Cuomo F, Gallagher MA, Zucker-man JD. Functional outcome after humeral head replacement for acute three- and four-part proximal humerus fractures. *J Shoulder Elbow Surg* 1995 ; 4 : 81-86

[9] Green A, Barnard WL, Imbird RS, Providence RI. Humeral head replacement for acute four-part proximal humerus fractures. *J Shoulder Elbow Surg* 1993 ; 2 : 249-254

[10] Jakob RP, Kristiansen T, Mayo K, Ganz R, Mueller ME. Classification and treatment of fractures of the proximal humerus. In : Bateman JE, Welsh RPeds. Surgery of the shoulder. Burlington : Decker, 1984 : 330-343

[11] Moeckel BH, Dines DM, Warren RF, Altchek DW. Modular hemiarthroplasty for fractures of the proximal part of the humerus. *J Bone Joint Surg Am* 1992 ; 74 : 884-889

[12] Muldoon MP, Cofield RA. Complications of humeral head replacement for proximal humeral fractures. *AAOS Instr Course Lect* 1997 ; 46 : 15-24

[13] Neer CS. Displaced proximal humeral fractures. Part I and II. *J Bone Joint Surg Am* 1970 ; 52 : 1077-1103

[14] Nicholson GP, Flatow EL, Bigliani LU. Shoulder arthroplasty for proximal humeral fractures. In : Friedman RJed. Arthro-plasty of the shoulder. Stuttgart : Thieme, 1994 : 183-193

[15] Patte D. Traitement chirurgical des fractures de l'éxtrémité supérieure de l'humérus de l'adulte. *Encycl Méd Chir* (Éditions Scientifiques et Médicales Elsevier SAS, Paris), Techniques Chirurgicales - Orthopédie-traumatologie, 44-290, 1987 : 1-15

[16] Tanner MW, Cofield RH. Prosthetic arthroplasty for fractures and fracture-dislocations of the proximal humerus. *Clin Orthop* 1983 ; 179 : 116-128

[17] Zyto K, Wallace WA, Frostick SP, Preston BJ. Outcome after hemiarthroplasty for three- and four-part fractures of the proximal humerus. *J Shoulder Elbow Surg* 1998 ; 7 : 85-89

Recurrent anterior shoulder instability: the Bankart procedure

SA Copeland
R Emery

Abstract. – The Bankart repair attaches the avulsed anterior capsule and/or glenoid labrum, together with the inferior glenohumeral ligament to the anterior rim of the glenoid fossa. Described originally in 1923, both the original technique of the surgical re-attachment, and the technique of capsular reconstruction have undergone many modifications. The standard technique is described, together with the author's preferred modifications. The role of suture anchors and shortening of the subscapularis in patients with large Hill-Sachs defect are discussed. The shoulder function following this procedure can be expected to be near normal, with a recurrence rate of less than 5%.

Keywords: shoulder, shoulder instability, recurrent anterior instability, Hill-Sachs deformity, Bankart procedure, suture anchor method, Copeland repair.

Introduction

Since the original description of the Bankart "lesion" [1], the classical Bankart repair has undergone many modifications over the years. However, the aim of the operation remains the same: to restore shoulder stability by securing an avulsed anterior capsule back to bone, into the anterior rim of the glenoid fossa [2]. The indications, operative procedure and results have been well described by Rowe [5, 6]. The Bankart procedure has the advantage of repairing the underlying pathological anatomy in an anatomical way without transferring tendons. However, in the classical description, as popularised by Rowe, the anterior capsule is overlapped and tightened and hence has the capacity to reduce external rotation. It is known that the long-term incidence of osteoarthritis is related to a marked loss of external rotation.

Indications

The Bankart procedure is indicated for traumatic anterior recurrent antero-inferior glenohumeral instability. The Bankart defect may be confirmed pre-operatively by an

S.A. Copeland *FRCS, Consultant Orthopaedic Surgeon, Royal Berkshire Hospital, London Road, Reading, Berkshire RG1 5AN, United Kingdom.*
Roger JH Emery, *FRCS, Consultant Orthopaedic Surgeon, St Mary's Hospital, Praed Street, Paddington London W2 1NY, United Kingdom.*

MRI scan, double contrast arthro CT or arthroscopy. It is the author's preference to arthroscope every unstable shoulder immediately, prior to stabilising surgery. The main elements of shoulder instability can then be assessed: i.e. size of the Hills-Sachs deformity, presence or absence and size of Bankart lesion, glenoid lip fractures, anterior capsular stretching, capsular volume and avulsion of the capsule from the humeral side (HAGL lesion) can also be excluded.

Operative technique

Under general anaesthesia, with a laryngeal mask or endotracheal intubation, the patient may be given additional interscalene brachial block for post-operative analgesia. The patient is placed in the semi-sitting beach-chair type position on the operating table, with an arm board positioned at the level of the elbow and the head on a neurosurgical headpiece. This allows the shoulder to be draped freely and posterior access gained. A preliminary arthroscopy can be made via a posterior viewing portal and the intra-articular damage verified. Without breaking to re-scrub, the surgeon can stand between the arm and the main trunk and the assistant to the lateral side of the shoulder. The coracoid is palpated and the arm passed across so that the hand touches the opposite axilla. The apex of the axillary skin crease is now marked with a skin marker. The skin incision is made from this mark vertically down into the anterior

axillary fold. *(fig 1)* The anterior skin and subcutaneous tissues are very mobile and hence the incision can be made very inferiorly, and then rotated superiorly using a retractor in the superior apex of the wound and subcutaneous tissues separated from the muscle layer. A line of fat within the deep fascial layer marks the deltoid pectoral interval, the upper extent of which is close to the coracoid process. The muscles are separated with scissors and finger to the medial side of the cephalic vein so that the vein is protracted laterally with the deltoid muscle. A self-retaining retractor is inserted and the coracoid now palpated. The conjoint tendon is identified at its origin on the coracoid process. Approximately one centimetre distal to the coracoid process, a one centimetre lateral incision to release the muscles is made. This small easing incision greatly facilitates access. A self-retaining retractor is then placed deep to the coracoid muscles to display the subscapularis *(fig 2)*.

The coracoid process can be predrilled and removed and then screwed at the end of the procedure. This is sometimes required if extra access is needed but often contributes to complications post-operatively with non-union and loosening of screw. It is only very rarely required. If the tip of the coracoid is removed, this must never be retracted distally as this can put traction on the musculocutaneous nerve. The subscapularis tendon is now identified and the musculocutaneous junction noted. The finger is placed at the superior border of the subscapularis to identify the rotator interval.

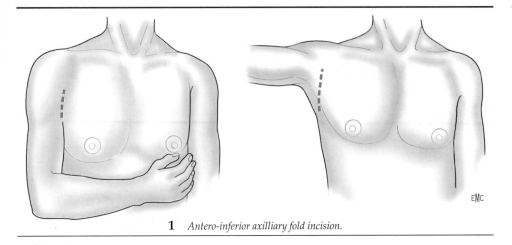

1   *Antero-inferior axilliary fold incision.*

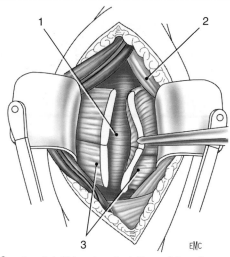

3   *Arm is held in external rotation and the subscapularis divided vertically down to capsule. 1. Anterior capsule; 2. conjoined tendon; 3. supscapularis.*

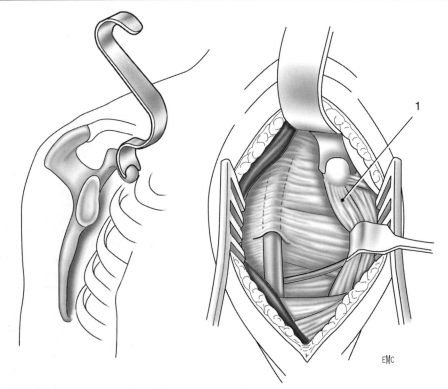

2   *Proximal margins of the wound retracted using a Copeland coracoid lever retractor (Ashbourne Surgical Limited). 1. Short head of biceps.*

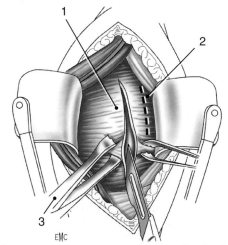

4   *Vertical incision 0.5 centimetres lateral to the glenoid rim. 1. Capsule; 2. glenoid rim, 3. Allis forceps.*

Sometimes this can be torn and may be widened in patients with excessive capsular laxity. The circumflex humeral vessels at the inferior margin of the subscapularis are identified and left intact. Visualisation is purely to identify the inferior margin of the subscapularis. Rowe advocated ligating these vessels and then sharply dividing the subscapularis approximately one centimetre lateral to the bicipital groove. However, Rockwood recommends cutting only the upper three-quarters of the subscapularis tendon so that the lower part of the subscapularis can remain to protect the axillary nerve, and also to identify the true length of the subscapularis at the time of closure [6]. The assistant now pushes the elbow into the side of the patient with the forearm straining the shoulder into external rotation. This puts the fibres of subscapularis under tension and they are divided down to the capsule *(fig 3)*. Stay sutures are placed in

the cut edge of the subscapularis to prevent retraction medially behind the brachial plexus. At this stage it is useful to put a periosteal elevator on a gauze swab and push the muscle medially to separate it from the capsule. This is more easily done at the inferior part than the superior part of the muscle, as it becomes more firmly embedded with the muscle itself at the superior margin where it runs into the rotator interval. The subscapularis is pushed medially so that the anterior glenoid rim can be easily palpated through the capsule. A vertical incision is made through the anterior shoulder capsule 0.5 cm lateral to the edge of the glenoid rim *(fig 4)*. A humeral head retractor is then inserted to push the humeral head posterolaterally.

Alternatively, the subscapularis may be split in the line of its fibres horizontally as described by Jobe [4], *(fig 5)*. He describes a

transverse capsular incision, with an extension superiorly and inferiorly, to create a T-shaped incision in the anterior capsule. This method allows the creation of superior and inferior flaps which overlap to achieve a capsular shift effect.

Re-attachment of the capsule to the glenoid rim

Classically, this has been described using holes through the bone of the anterior glenoid rim. A single spiked Hohmann retractor is placed on the anterior glenoid neck, approximately 1 centimetre medial to the rim retracting the medial capsule and the glenoid labrum. The retractor is reinserted from a superior to an inferior position as different holes are made in the glenoid rim. The anterior glenoid neck is decorticated using a gouge and small osteotomes with bone nibblers, to create a bleeding cancellous surface. The cortex of the scapular neck is perforated by a

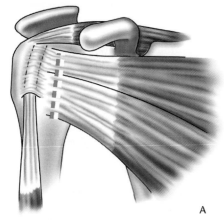

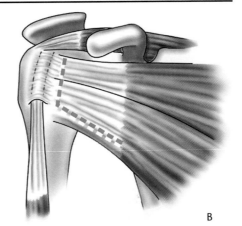

A

B

5 *Alternative methods of division of subscapularis.*
A. Classical lateral division.
B. Vertical division but leaving the inferior one quarter of subscapularis to protect the axillary nerve and preserve length of subscapularis.
C. Jobe type transverse separating fibres of subscapularis.

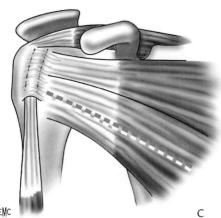

C

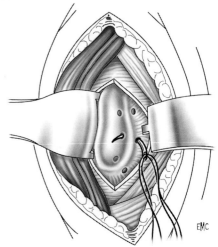

8 *A double suture is passed through the holes in the glenoid rim.*

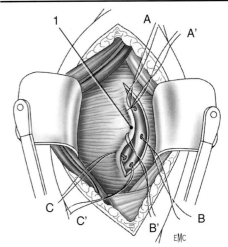

9 *Lateral capsular flap attached to anterior glenoid rim. 1. Edge of lateral capsule.*

Capsuloplasty

If a T-shaped incision has been made in the capsule, the inferior flap is pulled upwards and attached to the middle or upper holes in the glenoid rim, but this flap is overlapped by the superior flap which is pulled downwards and attached to the middle and/or lower holes (*fig 10*). The arm is positioned in internal rotation and the knots holding the capsule to the glenoid rim are then tied. Any remaining defects in the anterior capsule are sutured.

Closure of the subscapularis

The subscapularis tendon is returned and secured to its original insertion. If a horizontal split has been made in the subscapularis, then only its lateral tendinous portion should be sutured. If a coracoid osteotomy has been made then this is re-attached either with the pre-drilled screw attachment or with sutures through drill holes in the coracoid. Additional sutures can be passed through the coraco-acromial

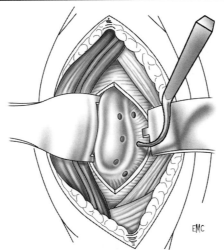

6 *"Classical" method of repairing Bankart defect by making holes in the anterior glenoid rim. 1. Humeral head retractor; 2. glenoid rim, 3. scaphoid gauge.*

7 *The hole is completed using a curved hand awl.*

scaphoid gouge or drill (*fig 6*). A curved spike is then used to complete the hole on the anterior aspect of the rim as well as the articular surface. The holes are placed 4-5 millimetres from the corner of the glenoid rim and are completed with a curved hand awl (*fig 7*). The holes are placed at approximately 2, 4 and 6 o'clock for the right shoulder and reverse for the left. A crochet hook is used to pass one of two strands of suture through each hole. The humeral head retractor is removed and a self-retainer re-inserted. The three pairs of double sutures are passed through the lateral flap of the capsule and tied (*fig 8*). There are now three

pairs of double sutures, one in the upper hole A and A1, one in the middle hole B and B1 and on in the lower hole C and C1. After sutures A1 and C1 are cut and discarded, a curved needle is used to pass the suture pair A through the medial flap of the capsule. Suture B is then passed through the corresponding medial flap of the capsule and then A and B sutures are tied. Sutures B1 and C are similarly passed through the medial flap of the capsule and then tied (*fig 9*) [6]. This procedure overlaps the medial lap of the capsule thus reinforcing the capsule repair. Shoulder motion is checked by externally rotating the arm in the neutral position. It should be possible to achieve 30° of external rotation.

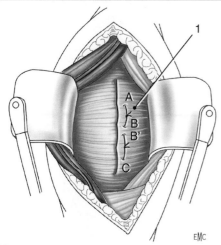

10 *Medial capsule double breasted over fixed lateral capsule, order of tying sutures shown. 1. Edge of medial capsule.*

ligament and insertion of the pectoralis minor muscle. The delta-pectoral interval is closed using interrupted fine absorbable sutures. Suction drain is usually not necessary if haemostasis has been carefully achieved. Subcutaneous and then subcuticular skin closure are carried out, sterile dressing is applied, and an immobilising sling used, with a body belt holding the arm down by the side.

Alternative methods of repair of Bankart defect

The authors prefer not to make holes in the articular surface of the glenoid as they feel this contributes to the possibility of late osteoarthritic change.

SUTURE ANCHOR METHOD *(fig 11)*

The capsule is exposed in exactly the same way by division of the subscapularis either vertically or horizontally. Once the Bankart defect is seen and identified, a Hohmann spike retractor is placed to keep the subscapularis pushed medially to demonstrate the defect. The defect is decorticated in the usual way and instead of drilling holes in the anterior lip, three anchor sutures can be used in the same positions. *(fig 12)* These anchors may be either absorbable or non-absorbable. These sutures with needles attached are then passed through the lateral flap and then the medial flap so that the anterior capsule is double breasted and the Bankart defect obliterated. The sutures are tied in the same order as in the description for the classical Rowe type repair.

COPELAND METHOD

This method also does not employ drill holes in the articular surface of the glenoid, nor suture anchors. The subscapularis is divided in the usual way but the capsule is

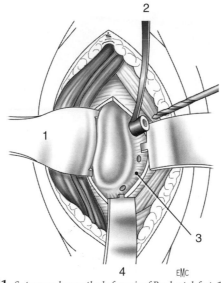

11 *Suture anchor method of repair of Bankart defect. 1. Point retractor; 2. drill guide; 3. scapular neck; 4. point retractor.*

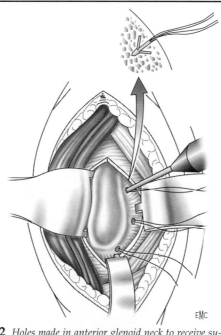

12 *Holes made in anterior glenoid neck to receive suture anchors.*

opened laterally. A vertical incision is made approximately half a centimetre from its insertion into the humeral neck. A horizontal capsular incision is now made so that there is a T-shaped opening in the capsule *(fig 13)*. The horizontal component of the capsulotomy goes down to the Bankart defect. The Bankart defect is decorticated in the usual way. The aim is to achieve healing of the anterior capsule against the glenoid neck. This can be achieved by closing the medial capsule around the glenoid neck using a vertical mattress suture. Usually one is adequate, but sometimes another may be necessary. The principle of this is demonstrated in *(fig 14)*. If the glenoid is considered a convex surface and the anterior structures are tightened, then, by definition, they must come to lie in apposition to the decorticated area. The suture is passed from

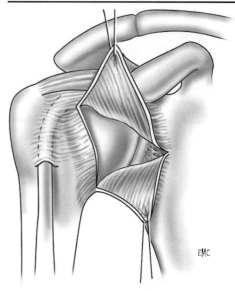

13 *Copeland method: horizontal capsular incision.*

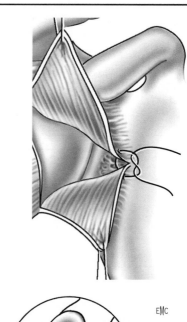

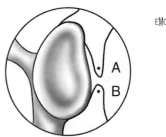

14 *Copeland method of repairing Bankart defect. Apex of the transverse capsulotomy enters the Bankart defect. The vertical suture shortens the distance AB.*

the outside of the superior flap to the inside. If any labrum is still present, the suture is passed through this and then out through the inferior flap. If there is no soft tissue structure on the anterior lip of the glenoid then the suture is just passed from outside in on the superior flap, and inside out on the inferior flap and the suture is tied. As the suture is tied the whole anterior capsule is seen to snug down firmly on to the decorticated anterior glenoid neck. If this is not adequately firm, a further suture may be used *(fig 15)*. If there is also an element of

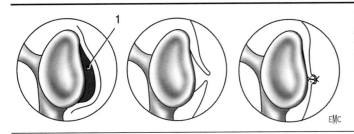

15 *Principle of the Copeland repair. Tightening the anterior capsule snugs the capsule against the decorticated anterior glenoid neck. 1. Bankart defect.*

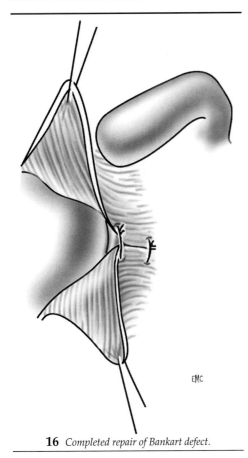

16 *Completed repair of Bankart defect.*

capsular stretching, then this can be corrected by a capsuloplasty. The inferior capsule is taken superiorly and the superior capsule taken inferiorly (*fig 16*).

Repair of the subscapularis

The decision whether to repair the subscapularis at anatomical length or to overlap it needs to be taken at this stage. If a large Hills-Sachs lesion (hatchet deformity) has been noted then it is wise to deliberately limit external rotation by shortening the subscapularis. If the bony hatchet deformity in the head is not a problem then the subscapularis does not need to be shortened and may be re-sutured anatomically. The advantage of this type of repair with the horizontal capsulotomy closure of the Bankart defect is that there is no overlapping of the anterior capsule, and hence no restriction of external rotation. It external rotation needs to be restricted this can be done by the method of subscapularis closure. Therefore, all aspects of the instability are controllable.

Postoperative management

In the classic Rowe repair, the sling is removed two days after surgery and pendulum exercises are begun. The patient is allowed to use the arm as tolerated and to use the sling for comfort as needed. He is instructed in the use of the extremity, graduated exercise and shoulder motion are gradually resumed. There is no formal physiotherapy. At three months, resisted exercises are started, rowing and swimming are begun. By six months after surgery, the patient can return to contact sports. The author's preferred method of post-operative management, following either suture anchor repair or glenoid neck capsular reefing, is to keep the patient in a sling and body belt for three weeks and then a free sling for a further three weeks. During the first three weeks the patient is encouraged to move the elbow, hand and wrist and the shoulder is mobilised by pendulum motion only. At three weeks, resisted external rotation and abduction exercises are started and resisted internal rotation is only started at six weeks.

Results

Rowe [5] has reported a recurrence rate of approximately 3.5% although others have failed to achieve such excellent results. Consequently, a recurrence rate of 5% is probably more general. His series reports on 161 patients (162 shoulders) with an average follow-up of six years although 97 (67%) were followed-up for only one to five years. It is also interesting to note that only 69% of those examined had complete elevation and external rotation. This outcome, together with the published description, suggests that he performed more plication, than practised by either Bankart or contemporary surgeons.

Discussion

As with all operations the success rate is dependent not only on the operative technique of the surgeon but the indication for which the operation was done. Rowe and Zarins [6] have reported carrying out a Bankart repair in patients who do not have a Bankart defect. This, in effect, is just an anterior capsular plication and perhaps can be achieved by other means. We prefer to talk in terms of doing a Bankart repair when there is a demonstrable anatomical Bankart defect. This usually implies that the patient has had a true anterior traumatic dislocation of the shoulder, which is not associated with hyperlaxity or transient subluxation, dead arm syndrome etc. However it must be realised that the Bankart defect is only one element of the damage sustained by the shoulder during traumatic dislocation. We believe that the Bankart defect must indeed be repaired but other elements of the instability must be addressed, i.e. capsular stretching, muscle avulsions, fractures, rotator interval disruption etc. It is only when all these elements of instability are addressed that the true recurrence rate can be minimised.

References

[1] Bankart AS. Recurrent or habitual dislocation of the shoulder joint. *Br Med J* 1923 ; 1 : 1123-1124

[2] Bankart AS. The pathology and treatment of the recurrent dislocation of the shoulder joint. *Br J Surg* 1939 ; 26 : 23-39

[3] Copeland SA. Operative shoulder surgery. New York : Churchill Livingstone, 1995 : 1-107

[4] Jobe FW. The unstable shoulder in athletes. *AAOS Instr Course Lect* 1985 ; 34 : 228-231

[5] Rowe CR, Patel D, Southmayd WW. The Bankart procedure: a long-term end-result study. *J Bone Joint Surg Am* 1978 ; 60 : 1-16

[6] Rowe CR, Zarins B. Recurrent transient subluxation of the shoulder. *J Bone Joint Surg Am* 1981 ; 63 : 863-872

[7] Wirth MA, Blatter G, Rockwood CA. The capsular imbrication procedure for recurrent anterior instability of the shoulder. *J Bone Joint Surg Am* 1996 ; 78 : 246-259

Treatment of recurrent anterior instability: Latarjet-Bristow procedure

G Walch
P Boileau

Abstract. – *The Latarjet-Bristow procedure was first described in the literature in 1954. The term "bone block" is not appropriate; the success of the intervention is explained by a triple effect.*
– Stable screw fixation of the horizontal limb of the coracoid process which is laid flat in a subequatorial position, flush to the anterior margin of the glenoid. This graft creates a reconstruction or an enlargement of the anteroposterior glenoid surface.
– Preservation of the musculotendinous fibres of the inferior third of the subscapularis which is maintained at the lower part of the joint by the conjoined tendon.
– Suturing of the lateral capsular flap to the medial 1 cm of the coracoacromial ligament which remains attached to the coracoid.
Precise surgical technique is crucial to avoid complications related to the use of metal within the joint.

© 2000, Editions Scientifiques et Médicales Elsevier SAS. All rights reserved.

Keywords: shoulder, anterior instability, coracoid transfer, Latarjet-Bristow procedure.

Introduction

In Europe in 1918, Eden [6] suggested the use of a preglenoid bone graft, which exhibits much better mechanical characteristics than capsular flaps, to prevent anterior migration of the humeral head. Then, Oudard and Noesske [10] began to use the coracoid process with two different techniques: Oudard split its horizontal portion into which he embedded a bone graft, whereas Noesske osteotomised the base of the coracoid to lower its tip, which was sutured to the anterior muscles. In 1954, Trillat [13] improved the stability of the osteotomised coracoid by securing the coracoid to the glenoid with a nail, and recommended routine exploration of the joint through an arthrotomy. Latarjet [7], in 1954, rationalised the coracoid bone block technique, suggesting that the horizontal limb of the coracoid process be fixed with a screw flush to the anteroinferior margin of the glenoid, making an horizontal incision through the fibres of the subscapularis.

Anglo-Saxon surgeons will more readily refer to the Bristow technique described by Helfet [3] in which the tip of the coracoid process is sutured to the capsuloperiosteal

Gilles Walch, M.D., Clinique Sainte Anne Lumière, 85 Cours Albert Thomas, 69003 Lyon, France.
Pascal Boileau, M.D., Professor of Orthopaedic Surgery, Hôpital Universitaire Larchet, 151 Route de Saint Antoine de Ginestière, BP 079, 06202 Nice Cedex 03, France.

elements through a short horizontal incision made in the subscapularis. In 1961, McMurray [9], like Latarjet, secured the coracoid to the anterior margin of the glenoid with a screw. May [8] explained that the efficiency of the coracoid bone block was attributable to the bracing role played by the coracobiceps tendon and the subscapularis tendon in abduction-external rotation, rather than the bone block itself.

Therefore, the terms "buttress" or "bone block" are not appropriate; the success of the intervention is explained by a triple effect. Patte proposed the term "triple blocking" to better describe the efficacy of the procedure [11, 12]:

– Stable screw fixation of a bone block laid flat in a subequatorial position, flush to the anterior margin of the glenoid. The bone block is the horizontal limb of the coracoid process.

– Preservation of the musculotendinous fibres of the inferior third of the subscapularis.

– Suturing of the lateral capsular flap to the medial 1 cm of the coracoacromial ligament which remains attached to the coracoid.

This technique is a combination of all the advantages of the Latarjet, May and Bankart procedures, plus some enhancements such as the preservation of the continuity of the subscapularis fibres. This has a double advantage: first, range of motion exercises in external rotation can be begun

immediately after the operation, and second, the integrity of the fibres of the subscapularis tendon is preserved. Damage to the tendon fibres is precisely what Rowe did not like about bone blocks, because it makes surgical revision (when necessary) more difficult. Furthermore, we have selected to use a fixation method which seems to provide good stability and solid fusion and to avoid secondary osteolysis of the bone graft.

Surgical procedure

PREOPERATIVE REQUIREMENTS AND IMAGING STUDIES

This procedure is proposed in cases of traumatic or atraumatic recurrent anterior instability (recurrent dislocation or subluxation) and painful shoulder with bony lesions proving the instability.

Preoperative imaging should include A.P. views in neutral, internal and external rotation and comparative Bernageau profile views of the glenoid [1] to detect bony lesions (Hill-Sachs, bony Bankart).

PROCEDURE

■ *Anaesthesia and patient postioning*

The procedure is performed under general endotrocheal anaesthesia. The patient is

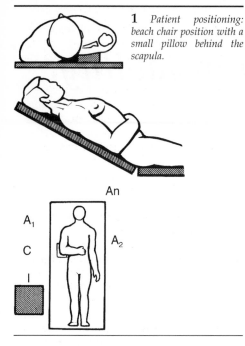

1 *Patient positioning: beach chair position with a small pillow behind the scapula.*

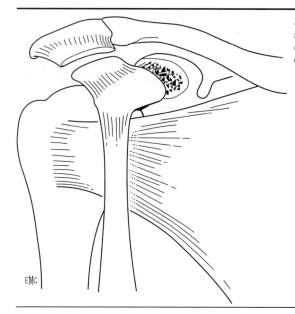

3 *Harvesting of the bone block that corresponds to the horizontal part of the coracoid process, retaining the conjoined coracobrachial tendon and coracoacromial ligament.*

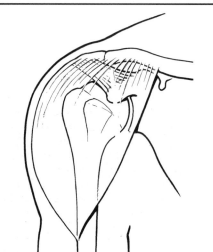

2 *Vertical incision under the tip of the coracoid process.*

secured in a beach chair position with a small pillow behind the scapula in order to have the glenoid surface perpendicular to the operating table (*fig 1*). The neck, chest, axilla and entire arm are sterilised and draped free.

■ *Incision, deltopectoral approach*

The skin is incised 4 to 7 cm under the tip of the coracoid process (*fig 2*). The deltopectoral interval is opened and the cephalic vein is taken laterally with the deltoid. A self-retaining retractor is placed in the deltopectoral interval and a Hohmann retractor is placed on the top of the coracoid process.

■ *Harvesting of the bone block*

With the arm abducted and externally rotated, the coracoacromial ligament is sectioned 1 cm from the coracoid. With the arm in adduction and internal rotation, the pectoralis minor is released from the

coracoid. The basis of the coracoid is exposed with a periosteum elevator in order to see the "knee" of the coracoid process. Then, either with an osteotome, or even better with a small angulated saw, an osteotomy of the coracoid process is performed from medial to lateral at the junction of the horizontal and vertical parts (*fig 3*). With the arm in abduction and external rotation, the coracohumeral ligament is released from the lateral part of the coracoid.

■ *Preparation of the bone block*

The bone graft is grasped with Museux forceps and carefully released from its deep attachments; dissection of the conjoined tendon should not exceed 30 mm to avoid damage to the musculocutaneous nerve. The bone graft is everted and its deep surface is decorticated using Liston forceps or a saw. Two holes are drilled parallel to each other in the deep surface of the bone graft, using a 3.2 mm drill. After measuring the thickness of the bone graft with a calliper, the graft is positioned under the pectoralis major pending subsequent use, and held there with the self-retaining retractor which maintains the deltopectoral interval open.

■ *Division of the subscapularis, capsulotomy and exposure*

With the upper limb in full external rotation, the inferior and superior margins of the subscapularis tendon are identified. The muscle is divided at the superior two-thirds/inferior one-third junction, in line with its fibres, using electrocautery and then Mayo scissors. Haemostasis is performed carefully, step by step. Division is slowly carried down to the white capsule, and then extended medially by inserting a compress with a marker wire into the cleavage plane, thus exposing the subscapular fossa. Laterally, it is extended as far as the lesser tuberosity. A Hohmann retractor is placed in the subscapularis fossa.

Placing the upper limb in neutral rotation provides full exposure of the capsule. The capsule is incised 1.5 cm vertically at the level of the anteroinferior margin of the glenoid which has been previously identified with an instrument. Placing the arm in full internal rotation allows insertion of a humeral head retractor which rests on the posterior margin of the glenoid. The superior two-thirds of the subscapularis are retracted superiorly with a Steinmann pin impacted at the superior part of the scapular neck. The inferior part of the subscapularis is retracted inferiorly with a Hohmann retractor pushed under the neck of the scapula between the capsule and the subscapularis. Exposure of the anteroinferior rim of the scapula is now completed. It is then possible to inspect the labrum, cartilage and insertion sites of the glenohumeral ligaments. The medial capsular flap is resected, as well as any damaged portion of the labrum or fracture fragments. The anteroinferior margin of the glenoid is exposed using a scalpel, and then decorticated with a curette or an osteotome (*fig 4*).

■ *Fixation of the bone block with screws*

The bone block is inserted through the soft tissue and positioned flush to the anteroinferior margin of the glenoid. It is easy to check its correct positioning with the limb in internal rotation. Whereas lateral overhang must be avoided, a slight medial positioning (no more than a few millimetres) is acceptable. The 3.2 mm drill is inserted into the glenoid neck through the inferior hole of the bone graft in an anterior-posterior and upward direction. It is important to check the orientation of the articular surface and to direct the drill parallel to this plane. The bone block is temporarily reflected to allow measurement of the drilling depth with a depth gauge. An AO malleolar screw driven into the posterior

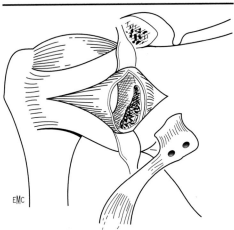

4   *The procedure is carried out by dissociation of the subscapularis (two-thirds superior, one-third inferior). The anteroinferior glenoid rim is exposed (capsulo-ligament or bone resection in cases of fracture) and decortication.*

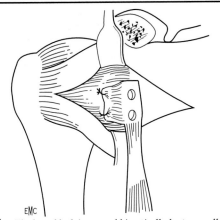

5   *The bone block is secured bicortically by two malleolar screws. Suture of the outer capsular flap to the remainder of the coraco-acromial ligament.*

cortex secures the bone block to the glenoid; this screw is loosely tightened to allow for easy rotation and proper positioning of the superior part of the bone block which is fixed with a second AO malleolar screw through the superior hole. Both screws are then firmly tightened (*fig 5*).

■ *Closure*

The remnant of the coracoacromial ligament is repaired to the lateral capsular flap using 2 interrupted absorbable sutures. Suturing is performed with the limb in external rotation. The compress previously placed in the subscapular fossa is removed. The arm is moved through all ranges of motion for assessment of mobility. The cut surface of the coracoid is coated with Orsley wax. A suction drain is placed and the superficial soft tissue layers are reapproximated and sutured.

■ *Surgical recommendations*

Osteosynthesis is crucial to avoid complications:

– put the coracoid process in the "lying position" rather than in the "standing" position to ensure better contact between the bone interface and to avoid pseudarthrosis;

– use a drill bit of 3.2 mm for both the coracoid and the scapula and malleolar screws to ensure good compression;

– the two screws must be bicortical;

– do not use a washer in order to avoid impingement with the humeral head;

– never accept a lateral overhanging of the coracoid in the joint, which is responsible for rapid degenerative joint disease. On the contrary, if the coracoid is 1 or 2 mm medial, there is no harmful effect.

POSTSURGICAL CARE

The patient wears a sling during the first 15 days for the activities of daily living, but immediately starts rehabilitation twice a day to recover full range of motion (elevation, external rotation) as soon as possible.

After 15 days, the patient may resume swimming and activities of daily living, with progressive strengthening exercices and complete recovery of motion, and resumption of working activities.

After 3 months, the patient may resume all types of sports activities including contact sports.

Results

Between 1985 and 1997, we carried out 1098 "triple blocking" procedures in cases of chronic anterior instability, which allowed us to acquire total confidence when applying the procedure.

The series reported here included 160 interventions with an average follow-up of 3 years. The patients had been diagnosed as having chronic anterior instability that did not include multidirectional hyperlaxity with a sulcus of over 2 cm and external rotation at the side superior to 90°.

The study included 79% male patients. Mean age at intervention was 28 years (18-40). The dominant side was involved in 66% of the cases; 88% played sports. Instabilities were classified as: recurrent dislocation (84%), recurrent subluxation (12%) and isolated painful shoulder (4%).

Radiographic lesions were demonstrated in 95% of the cases, either Malgaigne lesions (Hill-Sachs) (73%) or glenoid lesions (fracture or abrasion) (87%).

CLINICAL RESULTS

Stability was excellent in 72% of the cases, although 22% of the patients were apprehensive during sports activities and 5% in daily living; there was 1% recurrence.

Pain was present in 41% of the patients, generally during sports activities, seldom during activities of daily living. In one half of the cases, this pain was caused by an overhanging coracoid block. The patients often suffered from arm fatigue. Rotation was limited in 38% of the cases, more often in internal (25%) than in external (13%) rotation, but limitation was moderate. A total of 83% of these patients were able to resume their sports activities at the same level; 9% switched to another type of sport or practised at a lower level because of their operated shoulder. In total, 81% of the patients were very satisfied, 17% were satisfied and 2% were disappointed. The latter group included patients who had shoulder pain during sports or were apprehensive during activities of daily living. In total, 38% of results were excellent, 38% were good, 17% were fair and 7% were poor.

RADIOGRAPHIC RESULTS

Pseudarthrosis represented 2.4% of the cases; it was favoured by unicortical screws but had no influence on the outcome. Fractures represented 2.4% of the cases; they always occurred within months and were the result of preoperative overtight screws. In our series, they had no influence on the clinical result. Partial resorption of the coracoid occurred more frequently (9%), with varying extensions. Only those cases having more than two-thirds resorption of the coracoid led to persistence of apprehension and lowering of sports level; the position of the coracoid had no incidence on partial resorption. No narrowing of joint space was observed, although an inferior humeral osteophyte was present in 11.6% of the cases (< 7 mm). This correlated with an overhanging coracoid.

Conclusions

The above-cited retrospective study confirms that the Latarjet-Bristow procedure is a reliable operative technique, as has already been reported [2, 4, 5, 11, 14]. Nine out of ten patients were satisfied. Pain is reduced by a rigorous technique that imperatively rules out overhanging, which is also the prime condition to avoid arthritis.

References ➤

References

[1] Bernageau J, Patte D. Diagnostic radiologique des luxations récidivantes de l'épaule. *Rev Chir Orthop* 1979 ; 65 : 101-107

[2] Delaunay C, Lord G, Blanchard JP, Marotte JH, Guillamon JL. Place actuelle du traitement des luxations récidivantes et des instabilités antérieures de l'épaule par l'intervention de Latarjet. *Ann Chir* 1985 ; 39 : 293-304

[3] Helfet AJ. Coracoid transplantation for recurring dislocation of the shoulder. *J Bone Joint Surg Br* 1958 ; 40 : 198-202

[4] Hill JA, Lombardo SJ, Kerlan RK, et al. The modified Bristow-Helfet procedure for recurrent anterior shoulder subluxations and dislocations. *Am J Sports Med* 1981 ; 9 : 283-287

[5] Hovelius L, Korner L, Lundberg B, et al. The coracoid transfer for recurrent dislocation of the shoulder. Technical aspects of the Bristow-Latarjet procedure. *J Bone Joint Surg Am* 1983 ; 65 : 926-934

[6] Hybbinette S. De la transposition d'un fragment osseux pour remédier aux luxations récidivantes de l'épaule; constatations et résultats opératoires. *Acta Chir Scand* 1932 ; 71 : 411-445

[7] Latarjet M. À propos du traitement des luxations récidivantes de l'épaule. *Lyon Chir* 1954 ; 49 : 994-1003

[8] May VR. A modified Bristow operation for anterior recurrent dislocation of the shoulder. *J Bone Joint Surg Am* 1970 ; 52 : 1010-1016

[9] McMurray TB. Recurrent dislocation of the shoulder (proceedings). *J Bone Joint Surg Br* 1961 ; 43 : 402-405

[10] Noesske ?.. Zur habituellen schuulterluxation. *Zbl Chir* 1924 ; 51 : 2402-2404

[11] Patte D, Bancel P, Bernageau J. The vulnerable point of the glenoid rim. In : Surgery of the shoulder. New York : Marcel Dekker, 1985

[12] Patte D, Debeyre J. Luxations récidivantes de l'épaule. *Encycl Méd Chir* (Éditions Scientifiques et Médicales Elsevier SAS, Paris), Techniques chirurgicales - Orthopédie-traumatologie, 44-265, 1979

[13] Trillat A. Traitement de la luxation récidivante de l'épaule. Considérations techniques. *Lyon Chir* 1954 ; 49 : 986-993

[14] Walch G. La luxation récidivante antérieure de l'épaule. *Rev Chir Orthop* 1991 ; 77 (suppl 1) : 177-191

Recurrent anterior instability: the arthroscopic techniques

R Minola
G Zambonin

Abstract. – Our arthroscopic treatment of anterior shoulder instability is based on the use of three anchors: one knotless and two GII®. First, the anterior labrum is debrided and liberated from the anterior capsule to allow good capsular retensioning especially of the inferior glenohumeral ligament (IGHL). We think that a good capsular retensioning is the key to success of the procedure. We use the knotless anchor to retension the IGHL, positioned at five o'clock. The two GII® anchors are then inserted in the three o'clock and one o'clock positions respectively. We use these anchors with two Ethibond® sutures to provide an additional soft tissue repair. The first GII® anchor is used to repair the middle glenohumeral ligament and the anterior labrum; the second anchor is used to repair the superior part of the anterior capsule and labrum, including the superior glenohumeral ligament. If a superior labrum anterior to posterior (SLAP) lesion is present, it is treated with this last anchor.

Keywords: shoulder, recurrent anterior instability, arthroscopic repair, suture anchors, capsular shift, Bankart lesion.

Introduction

Although open procedures in the treatment of recurrent anterior instability are very reliable and predictable for the prevention of instability, arthroscopic techniques are gaining more and more consensus among orthopaedic surgeons. Compared to open procedures, arthroscopic treatment of anterior shoulder instability gives the surgeon the possibility to visualise the glenohumeral pathology directly and tailor an appropriate treatment. Other advantages include decreased postoperative pain, surgical morbidity and anatomical distortion, a negligible loss of external rotation and the possibility of performing the operation as an outpatient procedure. Despite these advantages, the rate of failure reported is not uniform and the results vary greatly from one study to another. This difference can be explained by the various techniques used to treat the pathology and the different criteria for selecting patients. Many arthroscopic techniques have been described to treat anterior shoulder instability including transglenoid suturing,

Riccardo Minola, M.D, Department of Orthopaedic Surgery, Humanitas Clinical Institute, Via Manzoni 56, 20089 Rozzano Milan, Italy.
Giovanni Zambonin, M.D.
Department of Orthopaedic Surgery, Ente Ecclesiastico Ospedale "F. Miulli", via Maselli Campagna 106, Acquaviva delle Fonti (Bari), Italy.

arthroscopic stapling and, more recently, techniques that use suture anchors. Over the years, we have used different techniques to treat shoulder instability including the Caspari and Morgan technique [7] or the use of Suretac® devices. We are currently using capsuloplasty with suture anchors in our institution. The advantage of this method compared to others is the possibility either of achieving a Bankart lesion repair or of shifting the anterior capsule superiorly to reduce the joint volume which is always increased in recurrent anterior instability, and, if left untreated, can be a cause of failure.

Surgical procedure

PATIENT SELECTION

At the beginning of our experience, we performed arthroscopic Bankart repairs in only a few selected cases. Currently, we perform closed capsuloplasty with anchors in almost all cases. In our opinion, the only contraindications are the presence of pathologies that alter the collagen quality or an extensive fracture of the anterior glenoid rim.

PREOPERATIVE REQUIREMENTS, IMAGING, PLANNING

Before starting the operation, the following examinations are required:

– X-ray evaluation: we usually recommend an AP view of the glenohumeral joint with the arm; 1) in neutral position; 2) internally rotated; 3) externally rotated; 4) an axillary view; 5) a West Point view.

– CT arthrogram: this exam is crucial because it can identify the alterations of the capsule and anterior labrum. In fact, when the radio-opaque agent distends the joint, it shows all the pathological alterations of anterior shoulder instability: increased capsular volume, detached anterior labrum or capsular damage.

EQUIPMENT

The technique we use to treat anterior shoulder instability is capsuloplasty with bone anchors. We employ two different suture anchors: 1) a knotless suture anchor and 2) a GII® easy anchor. The first does not require tying a knot since it has a no. 1 Ethibond® loop that is first passed in the tissue with the help of a no. 2/0 white Ethibond® suture and then is hooked onto the fork-like tip of the anchor. The GII® anchor is provided by the manufacturer with one no. 2 Ethibond® suture but we use it with an additional suture to obtain a second capsular bite and a stronger repair. We believe that non-absorbable sutures are better than absorbable ones because they allow a much more stable repair. Resorbable sutures can loosen before complete capsular healing on bone has taken place. The only problem we have with non-absorbable sutures is that they cannot be passed directly in the stitching instrument, usually a suture hook. There are many ways to solve this problem: an expensive one is to use the Shuttle Relay® which is a nylon-coated multistrand wire with a loop at its midpoint used to load the suture and pass it retrogradely or anterogradely. We prefer to use a less expensive doubled no. 2/0 PDS® wire. Once it is passed in the tissue, the no. 2 Ethibond® is loaded in its loop and passed anterogradely. To pass a suture retrogradely, it is necessary to use a second PDS® carrier.

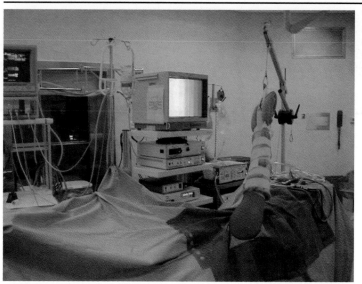

1 *Patient positioned and sterilely draped with the arm in traction ready for operation.*

PATIENT POSITION AND SURGICAL APPROACH

The operation is performed as an outpatient procedure. Before entering the operating room, the patient undergoes an interscalene block that has the advantage of being a good postoperative analgesia. The patient is positioned in a lateral decubitus position, posteriorly rolled 30 degrees so that the glenoid surface is horizontal. To hold the patient in position, we use a Vacupac® beanbag. A standard surgical preparation and draping are used. The operative arm is placed in sterile foam for shoulder traction and rotation and is subsequently held in the correct position by the shoulder traction apparatus. For this kind of operation, the right position is between 30 to 45 degrees of abduction and 15 degrees of forward flexion with 3 to 5 kilos of skin traction according to patient size *(fig 1)*. When the joint is opened by the traction, it is helpful to outline bony landmarks with a sterile marking pen. The distal clavicle, acromioclavicular joint, acromion, the coracoid process and the path of the coracoacromial ligament are outlined. It is very important to identify skin landmarks before starting the operation because once the periarticular tissues are impregnated with saline solution, it is very easy to lose orientation. Under these conditions, the possibility of committing errors dramatically increases. During the operation, we use an arthroscopic pump system to distend the joint, maintain constant intra-articular pressure and minimise bleeding. The standard pressure used is 40 mm Hg. To perform the operation, three standard arthroscopic portals, as described by Wolf [12], are used: posterior, anterosuperior and anteroinferior. The posterior portal is placed in the soft spot between the infraspinatus and teres minor which is approximately 1 to 2 cm distally and 1 to 2 cm medially from the posterolateral corner of the acromion, but it varies with patient size. The anterosuperior portal is created using an inside-out technique. Under visual control, the arthroscope is pushed anteriorly towards the triangle formed by the glenoid, the biceps tendon and the humeral head, until its tip is firmly in contact with the capsule of the superior portion of the rotator

interval. Then the arthroscope is removed and a switching stick is inserted in the scope sleeve and pushed through the capsule subcutaneously laterally and cephaladly to the coracoid process. An incision is made over the tip of the stick to establish the portal. Then, a small cannula is inserted over the stick and retrogradely pushed into the joint. The anteroinferior portal is created using an outside-in method. This is the operative portal and its position must be perfectly placed. We use a spinal needle to check the position that enables us to reach all the structures to be operated on at the correct angle. This point is roughly placed just superior to the intra-articular portion of the subscapularis tendon and 2 cm lateral to the glenoid. When the right point is found, a superficial skin incision is made and the 8 mm operative threaded cannula which is required to pass the suture hook is inserted in the joint. It is important that the distance between the two anterior portals be the maximum possible to avoid instrument impingement.

PROCEDURE

Before starting the repair, the joint is systematically evaluated through the posterior and anterosuperior approaches using the 15 point evaluation described by Snyder [11] to confirm the preoperative diagnosis and exclude other pathological conditions.

The most common pathological alteration found in recurrent anterior shoulder instability is the detached anterior labrum *(fig 2)* as described by Bankart [3] and the anterior labrum periostal sleeve avulsion (ALPSA) lesion *(fig 3)* as described by Neviaser [8]. Another pathological alteration associated with a Bankart or an ALPSA lesion is the humeral avulsion of the glenohumeral ligaments (HAGL) [1, 13] and intraligamentous lesions of the anterior capsule. The HAGL is a subtle lesion that must be excluded before starting any arthroscopic repair. We routinely search for

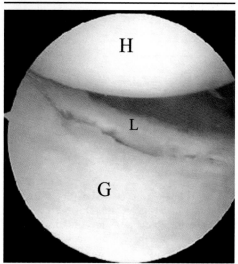

2 *A Bankart lesion. In this pathology, the anterior labrum is detached from the anterior glenoid rim. The entity of the detachment can be so wide as to completely involve the anterior labrum, from 6 o'clock to 12 o'clock. H. humeral head; L. anterior labrum; G. glenoid surface.*

it with the arthroscope inserted in the posterior portal and directed inferiorly between the humeral head and the posterior capsule, with the light directed upwards to visualise the humeral insertion of the posteroinferior portion of the inferior glenohumeral ligament (IGHL). The anteroinferior part of the IGHL can be visualised with the arthroscope inserted in the anterosuperior portal. If during the diagnostic phase, a major humeral avulsion of the ligaments or intraligamentous lesion of the anterior capsule are found, the procedure is suspended and the patient reprogrammed for an open procedure. On the contrary, minor lesions do not affect the outcome. Once the pathological basis of the instability is well understood, the procedure can be carried out.

For a classic Bankart lesion, the anterior detached capsulolabral complex is sharply separated from the adherences on the glenoid neck with the help of a sharp instrument inserted in the anteroinferior portal *(fig 4)*.

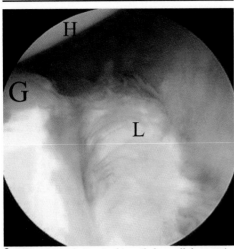

3 *An ALPSA lesion. In this pathology, all the anterior labrum has been detached by the traumatic event and has subsequently healed medially and inferiorly. In this new position, the anterior capsulolabral complex is not able to keep the humeral head in place, with a resulting anterior instability. H. Humeral head; G. glenoid surface; L. anterior labrum healed in pathological position.*

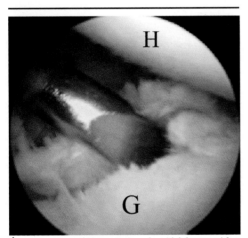

4 *Liberation of the anterior glenoid labrum with a sharp instrument. This phase is very important: it is only possible to perform an effective superior capsular shift if the capsulolabral complex is well liberated from the surrounding scar tissue adherences. G. Glenoid surface; H. humeral head.*

For the ALPSA lesion where there is medial retraction of the capsulolabral complex, we use a liberator elevator or VAPR® instrument with a 90 degrees hook electrode, because in this lesion there is a strong adhesion of the damaged labrum to the glenoid neck (fig 5). We routinely free the capsule until we see the underlying subscapularis muscle and until the anterior capsule automatically returns to the level of the anterior glenoid rim. When this occurs, a good capsule preparation has been performed. Once the capsulolabral complex is well divided from the surrounding scar tissue, we start to debride the anterior scapular neck and capsule: the arthroscope is inserted in the anterosuperior or posterior portal and the shaver inserted in the anteroinferior portal (fig 6). This step also creates slight bleeding from the bone and capsule that is useful for improving tissue healing. The shift of the inferior glenohumeral ligament is then checked from inferior to superior using a

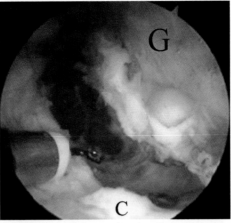

5 *Liberation of the anterior glenoid capsule and labrum from the anterior scapular neck using a VAPR® instrument. G. Glenoid surface; C. anterior capsule.*

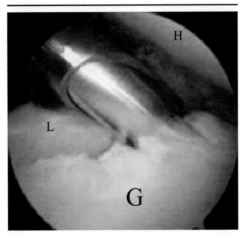

6 *Anterior glenoid debridement using a shaver. This step allows for slight bleeding which enhances tissue repair. G. Glenoid surface; L. anterior labrum; H. humeral head.*

soft tissue clamp. This step of the operation is crucial because it allows ligament retensioning and reduction of capsular volume. When the capsule can be easily shifted superiorly, and in the case of the ALPSA lesion also laterally, the first anchor is ready to be inserted (fig 7). It is important to place the anchor in a position that is superior to the point of the capsule to be grabbed with the first stitch, so that a good proximal shift of the capsule can be obtained. A good superior capsular shift is vital for the success of the operation. In fact, labral detachment is very often accompanied by capsular stretching [4] that if left untreated can lead to recurrence of instability. A correct operation should treat either the detached labrum or the increased capsular volume.

The first anchor is placed in the 5 o'clock position. We use a knotless anchor for this position which allows a very good capsular shift and capsular adhesion to the glenoid bone. To place the anchor correctly, it is necessary to drill the anchor hole at about 45 degrees to the glenoid surface and exactly on the edge of the glenoid. If the hole is placed too medially, a poor reconstruction of the labrum and a residual capsular laxity will result. Once the drill hole is correctly

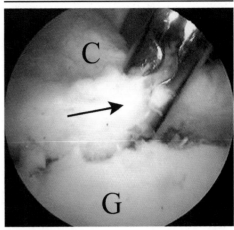

7 *Superior shift of the anteroinferior capsule using a soft tissue grasper. The arrow indicates the direction of the capsular shift. G. glenoid surface; C. anterior capsule.*

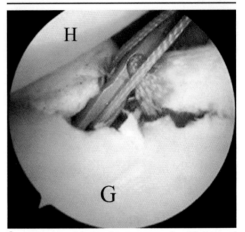

8 *Insertion of the knotless suture anchor. H. humeral head; G. glenoid surface.*

placed (from the anterior mid-glenoid cannula), a suture hook loaded with a doubled no. 2-0 PDS® (carrier wire) is inserted in the anterior mid-glenoid cannula while a soft tissue clamp is inserted in the superior cannula and the arthroscope in the posterior cannula. With the clamp, the anterior capsule is pulled superiorly (fig 7) while with the suture hook we take the amount of inferior glenohumeral ligament and labrum desired. During this step, the arm traction is reduced to obtain an easier and better superior capsular shift. The two free ends of the PDS® wire are passed through the suture hook into the joint and grasped with a clamp and pulled out through the superior cannula, leaving the closed loop of the PDS® wire exiting from the mid-glenoid cannula. The white carrier wire of the knotless anchor is passed through the closed loop of the PDS® wire that is subsequently pulled out from the anterosuperior cannula, allowing the no. 1 Ethibond® wire loop of the knotless anchor to pass anterogradely in the tissue previously hooked with the suture hook. The Ethibond® loop of the anchor is caught with the fork-like tip of the anchor, and the anchor-wire complex is inserted in the previously drilled hole (fig 8), obtaining the closure of the stitch without knots, the

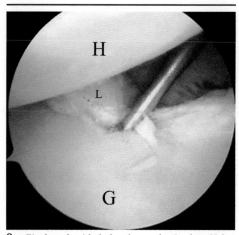

9 *Final result with the knotless anchor in place. H. humeral head; G. glenoid surface; L. anterior capsule and labrum superiorly shifted and repaired.*

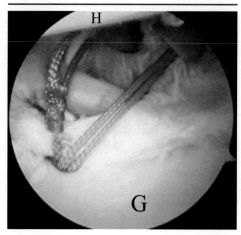

10 *The GII® anchor inserted. Note: the first dark Ethibond® has already been passed in the anterior capsule. The knot has already been tied.*

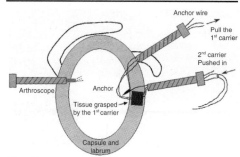

11 *The first carrier is passed in the tissue and exits with the closed end from the anteroinferior cannula and the open end from the anterosuperior cannula. The two limbs of the anchor wire exit one from the anterosuperior cannula and the other from the anteroinferior cannula. Since the Ethibond® limb that exits from the anterosuperior cannula must be passed retrogradely, a second PDS® carrier is passed in the loop of the first PDS® carrier limb pulled anterogradely in the anterosuperior cannula.*

anterior labrum repair and superior capsular shift *(fig 9)*. The more this anchor is hammered into the hole, the tighter the tissue adhesion to the bone, since the anchor can be pushed deep into the drilled hole. The second anchor is placed in a 3 o'clock position. We prefer to use a GII® anchor with two no. 2 Ethibond® wires preloaded on it. We use the first Ethibond® suture to reinforce the inferior glenohumeral ligament repair, while the second suture is used to plicate the capsule recreating the anterior glenoid labrum. To place the anchor, the hole is drilled from the anteroinferior cannula using the same precautions as described for the first anchor. Using a suture hook inserted in the anteroinferior cannula, we take a small amount of the capsule that will be used to recreate the anterior labrum, sometimes together with the middle glenohumeral ligament. Subsequently the two free limbs of the PDS® wire are passed through the suture hook into the joint. These two limbs are grasped with a clamp and pulled out through the superior cannula, leaving the closed loop of the PDS® wire exiting from the mid-glenoid cannula. A free Ethibond® wire is then inserted in the closed loop of the PDS® carrier which is pulled from the superior cannula, with one limb blocked outside the anteroinferior cannula with a clamp, so that the Ethibond® suture passes through the tissues.

The Ethibond® limb exiting from the anterosuperior cannula is pulled out of the anteroinferior cannula and inserted in the GII® anchor obtaining an anchor with 2 Ethibond® loaded sutures: one free and the second already inserted in the tissues *(fig 10)*. Then the GII® anchor is inserted in the 3 o'clock hole. The other two free limbs of the Ethibond® are pulled out of the anterosuperior cannula to allow a safe knot tying procedure from the mid-glenoid cannula. The second anchor wire is then passed in the capsule. To do this, one of the two free limbs of the Ethibond® is pulled out of the anterosuperior cannula and using a suture hook inserted in the anteroinferior cannula, a good bite of the inferior

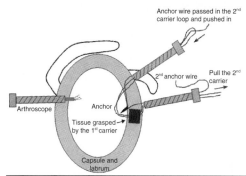

12 *The second carrier is pulled from the anteroinferior cannula, allowing the anchor wire to pass in the tissues retrogradely, from the anterosuperior to the anteroinferior cannula.*

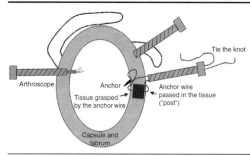

13 *Final result: both anchor limbs exit from the anteroinferior cannula. The limb that passes in the tissue is called the "post", and the knot must be tied.*

glenohumeral ligament is taken (always inferiorly with respect to the anchor) to obtain a further capsular shift. The no. 2 PDS® carrier is passed in the joint and pulled out of the anterosuperior cannula with a grasping clamp. Since the Ethibond® limb that exits from the anterosuperior cannula must be passed retrogradely, a second PDS® carrier is passed in the loop of the first PDS® carrier limb pulled anterogradely in the anterosuperior cannula *(fig 11)*. Finally, the Ethibond® is passed in the loop of the second PDS® carrier and pulled out the anteroinferior cannula through the capsule *(fig 12, 13)*. Before tying the knot, it is important to avoid twists in the sutures. An easy way to accomplish this is to place one limb of the suture in the knot pusher and push it down the cannula while visualising it with the arthroscope. If unwanted twists are found, they can be easily removed with a ring clamp. Normally, the wires do not slide in the tissues, so we

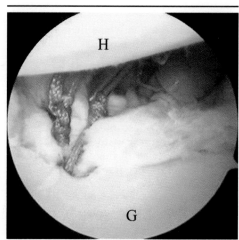

14 *Final result with both the knots tied. H: humeral head; G: glenoid surface.*

routinely use five half hitch knots: two over-under, one under-over, one over-under and again one under-over *(fig 14)*. We generally insert a third anchor (GII® with 2 Ethibond® wires) placed at 1 o'clock to repair the anterosuperior capsule and the superior glenohumeral ligament *(fig 9)*. If a superior labrum anterior to a posterior (SLAP) type 2 lesion is present, it is treated at this time with one of the two anchor wires. If the SLAP lesion also extends posteriorly, the detached posterior labrum is treated with another GII® anchor, this time with only one Ethibond® wire. Then the skin is closed with 2-0 resorbable stitches and a drain is inserted in the anterosuperior portal. The drain is removed a few hours after the operation and the patient is allowed to go home.

POSTSURGICAL CARE

As this is an outpatient procedure, the patient leaves the same day. The operated arm is kept in a shoulder immobilising device that must be worn day and night for four weeks. This device has a pillow spacer between the arm and the body that limits excessive internal and external rotation of the arm. The patient is allowed to perform exercises for the elbow, wrist and hand, and pendulum exercises as soon as pain diminishes, normally a few days after the operation. Starting from the third postoperative week, passive self-assisted mobilisation exercises are started: forward flexion with the arm internally rotated and external rotation exercises from the arm internally rotated to neutral or 10 degrees external rotation. The goal is to reach 80% of forward flexion of the shoulder within the first six postoperative weeks. At the third week, internal rotation strengthening exercises using a rubber band are started, while any active external rotation or passive external rotation beyond 10 degrees is still forbidden. Nine weeks after the operation, active forward elevation exercises can be started with the rubber band but not exceeding 90% of the full range of movement. Full range of motion and strengthening exercises are allowed, except for external rotation with the arm in 90 degrees abduction, which can be started 12 weeks after surgery, including a progressive return to throwing activities. We recommend returning to strenuous, full activity including throwing sports, six months after surgery.

VARIATIONS OF THE SURGICAL PROCEDURE

In a few patients with recurrent anterior instability, the only pathological alteration found is an increased capsular volume [10, 11]. The only arthroscopic findings in this pathology are an increased capsular volume and the pass-through sign where the arthroscope can easily be passed from the

posterior approach anteriorly through the joint, between the humeral head and the glenoid surface. Among this category of patients, we only treat arthroscopically those adults or young adults in whom the instability has occurred after a trauma. In these cases, we perform multiple arthroscopic plication at the level of the anterior and posterior bands of the inferior, middle and superior glenohumeral ligaments. If the patient is a teenager in whom the instability is due to anterior capsule overstress associated with generalised ligament laxity, we perform an open capsular retensioning.

Complications and results according to the international literature

COMPLICATIONS

Like other surgical procedures, the arthroscopic treatment of shoulder instability is also associated with a number of complications. Some of these are related to regional anaesthesia including phrenic or recurrent laryngeal nerve block or direct nerve damage during its administration. Other rare complications are related to the arm traction device, such as injury of the superficial radial nerve if a padded arm holder is not used. Risks of neurological or vascular damage are present when placing the portals. During the development of the posterior portal, there is a risk of damaging the descending branch of the suprascapular nerve if the trocar is directed too medially. When developing the anterior mid-glenoid portal, the cephalic vein or the musculocutaneous nerve can be damaged if the access is too medial, while the axillary nerve can be injured if the access is too inferior. Other complications are related to the use of bone anchors that can break during their bone insertion or, if improperly applied, can dislodge after the operation, resulting in an intra-articular loose body or in soft tissue swelling due to fluid extravasation which can injure several nerves [9].

RESULTS

Reported results of arthroscopic treatment of anterior shoulder instability with suture anchors, associated with arthroscopic knot tying, are mixed. They can vary from 7% failure or less at 1.5 to 3 years follow-up [2], which are similar to results obtained by

open procedures, to a failure rate as high as 30% after two to five years follow-up [6]. Interestingly, a higher success rate was seen in patients with a maximum of five dislocations before the operation. These differences could be related to the different surgical techniques, the different fixation devices used to repair the lesion or to the different criteria used to select patients, such as the number of dislocations before surgery or the kind and level of sporting activity. In our series, we have found a failure rate of 7% after two to five years follow-up. In our opinion, it is very important not only to perform the repair of the primitive lesion, but also to shift the capsule superiorly to reduce the global capsular volume because, in recurrent anterior instability, it is always stretched and increased.

Conclusions, indications and limitations

Arthroscopic treatment of anterior shoulder instability is an interesting alternative procedure. When compared to open procedures, closed treatment has several advantages but also some disadvantages. Advantages include less operative time, less postoperative pain, and negligible loss of external rotation which is a very important factor in patients who practice overhead sporting activities. Disadvantages include a higher failure rate and for this reason, the open Bankart repair for anterior instability is still the gold standard to which other new procedures must be compared [5].

Our current indications for arthroscopic treatment of instability are: five or fewer episodes of dislocation and the absolute certainty that the patient is able to comprehend the particularities of arthroscopic treatment and to follow our postoperative indications exactly, without damaging the repair. If the patient does not fully satisfy our requests or practices contact sports or has had more than five episodes of dislocation, he is selected for an open capsuloplasty and Bankart repair. In borderline cases, we perform a diagnostic arthroscopy first so that the best indication can be properly selected. No matter which treatment is chosen, the operative procedure is always carried out several weeks later, in order to give the patient the right amount of time to agree with our decision. The limitation of this procedure is the impossibility to treat all unstable shoulders, especially in patients in whom the anterior capsule is too damaged (usually if more than five dislocations have occurred), or if there is a severe glenoid rim fracture. In these instances, if an arthroscopic procedure is selected, results are often disappointing.

References ➤

References

[1] Bach BR, Warren RF, Fronek J. Disruption of the lateral capsule of the shoulder. *J Bone Joint Surg Br* 1988 ; 70 : 274-276

[2] Bacilla P, Field LD, Savoie FH. Arthroscopic Bankart repair in high demand patient population. *Arthroscopy* 1997 ; 13 : 51-60

[3] Bankart AS. Recurrent or habitual dislocation of the shoulder. *Br Med J* 1923 ; 26 : 23-29

[4] Bigliani LU, Pollock RG, Soslowsky LJ, Flatow EL, Pawluk RJ, Mow VC. Tensile properties of the inferior glenohumeral ligament. *J Orthop Res* 1992 ; 10 : 187-197

[5] Gill TJ, Micheli LJ, Gebhard F, Binder C. Bankart repair for anterior instability of the shoulder. Long term outcome. *J Bone Joint Surg Am* 1997 ; 79 : 850-857

[6] Koss S, Richmond JC, Woodward JS. Two to five years follow up of arthroscopic Bankart reconstruction using a suture anchor technique. *Am J Sports Med* 1997 ; 25 : 809-812

[7] McIntyre LF, Caspari RB. The rationale and technique for arthroscopic reconstruction of anterior shoulder instability using multiple sutures. *Orthop Clin North Am* 1993 ; 24 : 55-58

[8] Neviaser TJ. The anterior labroligamentous periostal sleeve lesion: a cause of anterior instability of the shoulder. *Arthroscopy* 1993 ; 9 : 17-21

[9] Pitman MI, Nainzadeh N, Ergas E, Springer S. The use of somatosensory evoked potentials for detection of neuropraxia during shoulder arthroscopy. *Arthroscopy* 1988 . 4 : 250-255

[10] Rowe CR, Patel D, Southmayd WW. The Bankart procedure: a long-term end result. *J Bone Joint Surg Am* 1978 ; 60 : 1-16

[11] Snyder SJ. Diagnostic arthroscopy of the shoulder: normal anatomy and variations. In : Shoulder arthroscopy. New York : McGraw-Hill, 1994 : 23-39

[12] Wolf EM. Anterior portals in shoulder arthroscopy. *Arthroscopy* 1989 ; 5 : 201-208

[13] Wolf EM, Cheng JC, Dickson K. Humeral avulsion of the glenohumeral ligaments as a cause of anterior shoulder instability. *Arthroscopy* 1995 ; 11 : 600-607

Recurrent anterior instability of the shoulder: the capsuloplasties

M Mansat

Abstract. – The selective capsular repair is a versatile procedure for treating recurrent antero-instability. It can be adapted according to the location and type of the capsulolabral pathology and allows the correction of excessive capsular laxity.
The repair addresses all the elements of the pathology encountered, without distorting the surrounding anatomy and gives a high percentage of successful results, achieving not only stability but also pain relief and near normal range of motion and function.

Keywords: shoulder, recurrent anterior instability, unstable shoulder, capsuloplasties.

Introduction

The challenge in instability surgery of the shoulder is to correct the specific pathology for each case, restoring normal anatomy and function. The principle is to reconstruct anatomically the disrupted anatomy of the avulsed or stretched antero-inferior capsulolabral structures. Neer et al described in 1985 [7] the reinforced capsular cruciate repair for recurrent anterior dislocations, a modification of the inferior capsular shift [8], and emphasised the importance of correcting excessive capsular laxity at the same time as repairing labral detachment. In our experience, selective capsular repair is the procedure of choice which addresses the whole spectrum of anterior instability, while restoring function.

Surgical technique

ANAESTHESIA AND PATIENT POSITION

Our anaesthesiologists prefer general endotracheal anaesthesia, but a regional inter-scalene block can also be used. The patient is secured in a modified beach chair position, the arm at 45° abduction on an adjustable, well padded arm board, the humerus in the plane of the scapula. Prior to the skin preparation, the shoulder is examined under anaesthesia to determine

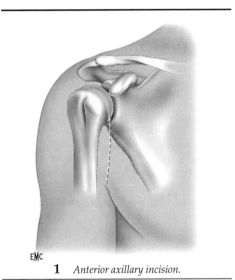

1 *Anterior axillary incision.*

the degree and all directions of instability, and to give information about laxity in different positions of abduction and rotation. Bony landmarks are marked: lateral clavicle and anterior acromion, coracoid process and axillary skin folds.

INCISION, SUPERFICIAL DISSECTION *(fig 1)*

The skin is prepared and different plastic drapes are applied. The skin incision, 6 cm long, starts at the anterior margin of the axilla and extends upward in the axillary crease towards the coracoid process (Leslie-Ryan approach) [5]. The area of the deltopectoral interval is exposed up to the inferior aspect of the clavicle. The deltopectoral interval is opened and the cephalic vein is moved laterally with the deltoid. A self-retraining retractor is placed in the deltopectoral interval to expose the underlying clavi-pectoral fascia. The fascia is incised along the lateral border of the muscle belly of the short head of the biceps. Sharp dissection continues superiorly to the coraco-acromial ligament. After the biceps tendon has been identified, the proximal 1 cm of the tendon of the pectoralis major insertion can be released and tagged for later repair. We do not recommend coracoid osteotomy or complete detachment of the conjoined tendon. A small wedge of the lateral aspect of the coraco-acromial ligament is usually resected to allow for better visualisation of the upper part of the capsule and subscapularis tendon.

THE SUBSCAPULARIS TENDON

A blunt retractor is placed gently under the conjoined tendon and retracted medially to expose the underlying subscapularis tendon and to avoid injury of the musculocutaneous nerve. The axillary nerve should be carefully palpated and protected during the procedure *(fig 2)*. The arm is then externally rotated for better visualisation of the subscapularis; the upper and lower borders are identified and the anterior circumflex vessels are ligated and divided. The tendon is incised at 1 cm medial to its insertion on the lesser tuberosity, and a careful blunt dissection is performed to elevate the subscapularis medially and to avoid entering the underlying capsule. Three or four non-absorbable N°1 sutures are placed

Michel Mansat, M.D., Department of Orthopaedic Surgery, C.H.U. Hôpital Purpan, 31059 Toulouse, France.

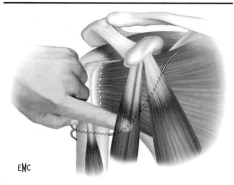

2 *Subscapularis incision. The location of the axillary nerve is noted by direct palpation.*

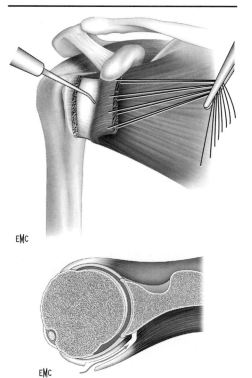

3 *Elevation of the subscapularis from the capsule. Sutures are placed at the edge of the tendon for traction.*

in the subscapularis tendon for retraction, and the retractor beneath the conjoint tendon is placed deep to the subscapularis *(fig 3)*.

THE CAPSULE

The capsule is now visible from its lateral insertion to the anterior glenoid rim. The "cleft" [6] between the middle and superior glenohumeral ligaments is identified, and sutures are placed in the superior edge for later repair. The capsule is incised laterally, near its insertion, 1 cm medial to the stump of the subscapularis and anterior to the intra-articular portion of the long head of the biceps under direct visualisation *(fig 4)*. The edge of the capsular flap is progressively tagged with sutures. As the humerus is externally rotated and flexed, the capsule is incised around the neck of the humerus while protecting the axillary nerve. The inferior extent of the capsular incision depends on the magnitude of the inferior capsular laxity. A finger may be placed in

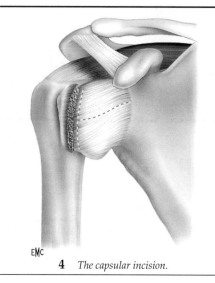

4 *The capsular incision.*

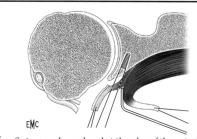

5 *Suture anchors placed at the edge of the anterior glenoid rim for fixation of the capsule.*

the inferior pouch [2] to assess how much redundant capsule needs to be released before shifting. When tension on the sutures in the capsular edge obliterates the pouch, capsulotomy is complete.

The degree of capsular takedown will vary in each case. In a unidirectional anterior case, only the anterior capsule is mobilised. The horizontal limb of the "T" is made between the inferior and middle glenohumeral ligaments and the corners of the capsular flaps are tagged with stay sutures.

A Fukuda ring retractor is inserted behind the posterior labrum to hold the humeral head back and to expose the glenoid surface and the antero-inferior labral attachment to the capsule.

If a "Bankart lesion" is encountered, with avulsion of the glenohumeral ligaments and labrum, they are re-attached to the freshened glenoid rim. The capsulolabral attachment is stripped medially and a 2 or 3 pronged retractor is placed into the bone to retract the capsule. The antero-inferior portion of the glenoid neck is decorticated with a small osteotome. Suture anchors are secured into the bone at 2, 3, and 5 o'clock, adjacent to the articular cartilage, to bring the labrum and capsule right to the rim as a buttress. Sutures are brought through the capsule from inside-out and tied down over the capsule. It is important to repair the lesion anatomically, without any capsular shortening in a medial direction *(fig 5)*.

In the rare instance where the glenoid margin is compromised by a glenoid rim fracture or wear, and if the defect is larger than 25%, and there is no avulsed bone to be repaired, a coracoid transfer is performed with attached muscles in the defect, outside the anterior capsule (extra-articular) and beneath the subscapularis tendon. A screw and washer are generally used, and complete closure of the capsule is delayed until the screw is in place. The aim is to act as a glenoidoplasty and deepen the socket, not as a bone block.

The shoulder is then placed in a position of at least 30° of external rotation, 60° of abduction and 10° of forward flexion during the capsular shift. The position of abduction and external rotation is determined individually, based on the patient's functional requirements [10].

The inferior flap is shifted superiorly and laterally as desired, and the capsule is repaired to its lateral stump *(fig 6A)*.

The arm is then repositioned in 0° abduction with the same flexion and external rotation, and the superior flap is brought inferiorly over the inferior flap *(fig 6B)*.

If there is a large "cleft", with a pre-operative sulcus sign and symptomatic inferior instability, it must be closed as part of the capsular shift. When there is a large defect, only a lateral incision is made in the

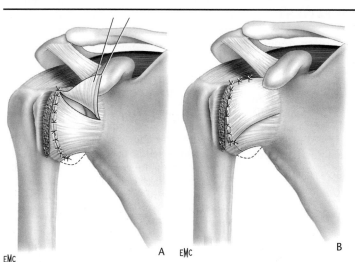

6 *Capsuloplasty.*
A. The inferior flap is shifted superiorly, reducing the inferior pouch.
B. After closing the superior cleft between the superior and middle glenohumeral ligament, the superior flap is shifted inferiorly.

capsule, and the entire flap is brought superiorly to close the capsule.

SUBSCAPULAR REPAIR AND CLOSURE

The subscapularis is then repaired anatomically to its stump on the lesser tuberosity with non-absorbable sutures. The tendinous portion of the pectoralis major may be repaired if necessary, one or two sutures are placed to approximate the deltoid and pectoralis major muscles, and the skin is closed in a subcuticular fashion. A shoulder immobiliser is applied with the elbow supported to prevent humeral extension.

Postoperative programme

The patient is discharged when she or he is comfortable, with the arm in a removable sling, generally 3 or 4 days after surgery. There are no general protocols, each one is modified on an individual basis, the aim being to protect capsular healing and to improve motion over several months, especially in patients with generalised joint laxity. Range of motion at the elbow, wrist and hand is encouraged immediately. Pendulum exercises are started after the second day with limitations based on the repair. From 10 days to 2 weeks, isometric exercises, with external rotation to 10° and elevation to 90°, are performed. From 2 to 4 weeks, external rotation is progressively increased to 30° and elevation to 140°. From 4 to 6 weeks, external rotation is increased to 40° and elevation to 160° and resistive exercises are begun. After 6 weeks, external rotation is increased to 50° and terminal elevation stretching allowed. After 6 months, terminal external rotation stretching is added. Careful and frequent follow-up is needed and the protocol is adapted. At 3 months the patient is permitted to swim, with ground strokes in tennis and a short game of golf at five months. Contact sports are not advised for about 6 to 9 months, after a specific reconditioning programme.

Results

The results of selective capsular repair for anterior glenohumeral instability have been gratifying. Pollock et al [9] reported 90% of successful results in 151 shoulders with a recurrence rate of 5%. In another series of 63 athletes with a similar procedure [1], 94% of patients had satisfactory results: 58 out of 63 (92%) returned to their major sports, 47 patients (75%) returned at the same competition level. In our series, out of 47 patients presented in 1993, the mean age was 26 years with an average follow-up of 27 months. 100% of our patients were stable with 7% of residual apprehension, 86% pain

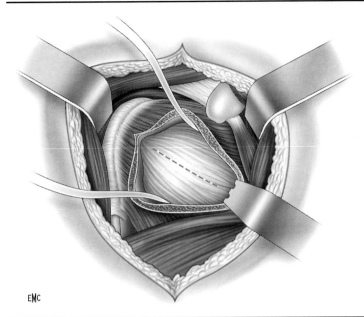

7 *Split of the subscapularis and location of the capsulotomy.*

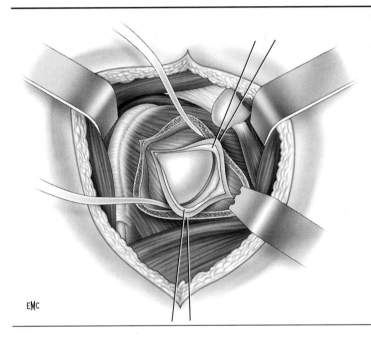

8 *Horizontal anterior capsulotomy with exposure of the scapular neck.*

free and 14% with mild pain. The mobility was identical to the opposite side in 86% of cases and in 10% the external rotation was less than 10°.

Other techniques of capsuloplasty

ANTERIOR CAPSULOLABRAL RECONSTRUCTION (F.W. JOBE) [3]

This technique is a modified, anterior capsular shift in which the subscapularis is split transversally in line with its fibres (fig 7) at the junction of the upper two thirds with the lower third. An horizontal anterior capsulotomy is then performed (fig 8). With manual distraction of the glenohumeral joint, a humeral head retractor is placed across the joint to retract the humeral head laterally. With sharp dissection the capsule

and periosteum are elevated from the anterior scapular neck. The inferior flap must be dissected inferiorly in the 6 o'clock position. This allows for sufficient superior advancement to eliminate the inferior capsular pouch.

Three holes are then created along the anterior rim 2 to 3 mm from the articular margin at 2, 4 and 5 o'clock and suture anchors are used (fig 9). The inferior capsular flap is advanced superiorly and secured into position using double stranded number 2 absorbable sutures. The superior capsular flap is then shifted inferiorly, overlying the inferior capsular flap and is secured into position using the same double-stranded sutures.

The arm is then positioned in 90° of abduction and 70° to 80° of external rotation and the remaining capsulotomy is closed in a vest over pants fashion with non-absorbable sutures (fig 10). The

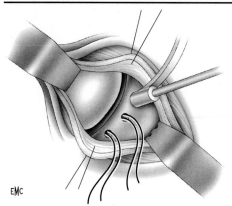

9 *Drill holes and suture anchors 2 mm medial to the glenoid rim.*

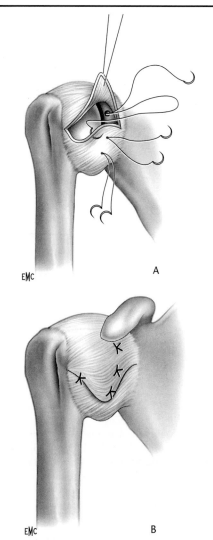

10 *A. Sutures passed through the inferior capsular shaft.*
B. Superior flap tied down with closing of the remainder of the capsulotomy.

subscapularis is then re-approximated and routine wound closure is carried out.

The patient is placed in a shoulder arm postoperative orthosis that maintains the arm at 90° of abduction, 45° of external rotation and 30° horizonal adduction (scapular plane).

Kvitne et al [4] obtained 97% good or excellent results in competitive athletes with

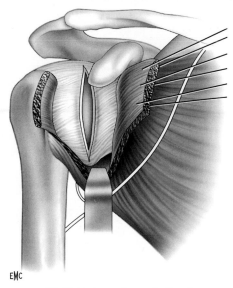

11 *Vertical capsulotomy (midway).*

81% of patients returning to the same level of competition. 100% of the patients were satisfied with the operation.

CAPSULAR IMBRICATION PROCEDURE (C.A. ROCKWOOD)

This technique not only addresses the repair of the capsule to the anterior labrum, but also the capsular laxity. The subscapularis is divided and reflected off the capsule that is entirely exposed. The capsule is then divided vertically, midway between its attachment on the glenoid rim and the humeral head *(fig 11)*. The joint is inspected for labral tear and stripping of the labrum capsule and periosteum off their normal attachments.

If stripping is noted, the capsule *(fig 12)* is reattached using sutures, followed by imbrication of the anterior capsule. The extent of antero-inferior capsular laxity determines the degree of imbrication necessary to reduce the glenohumeral joint

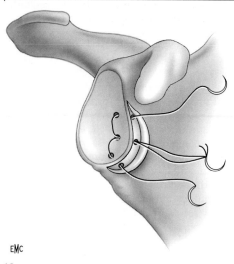

12 *Reattachment of the capsule using sutures after decortication.*

volume. The medial aspect of the capsule is overlapped laterally and superiorly under the lateral aspect, and secured with the arm held in 30° of external rotation *(fig 13)*. The lateral aspect of the capsule is advanced superiorly and medially over the medial aspect creating a double thickness of the weakened capsule. The subscapularis tendon is then anatomically repaired.

In a study of 132 patients [11], 93% had good or excellent results at a minimum follow-up of 2 years with a loss of external rotation of 7° compared with the contralateral side, and a 96% success rate on apprehension testing.

Conclusion

The selective capsular repair is a variation of the inferior capsular shift introduced by C.S. Neer [8] for multidirectional instability.
The procedure is logical, the aim being to restore normal anatomy. It allows the surgeon

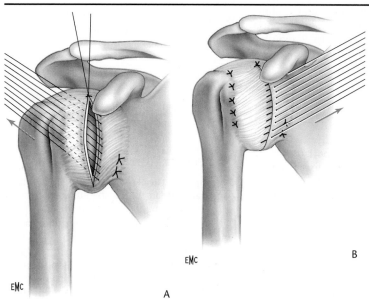

13 *A. Interval suture tied and sutures from the medial capsule.*
B. Suture of the lateral part of the capsule.

to address the spectrum of anterior instability with a high percentage of successful results. Careful preparation and adequate exposure are essential to prevent potential problems and, particularly, neurovascular complications. Errors in surgical technique can lead to an unsuccessful outcome. Treating a Bankart lesion, reducing excessive capsular laxity and closing the rotator interval are essential to success. The postoperative rehabilitation programme must be adapted and modified on an individual basis.

References

[1] Bigliani LU, Kurzweil PR, Schwartzbach CC et al. Inferior capsular shift procedure for anterior inferior shoulder instability in athletes. *Am J Sports Med* 1994 ; 22 : 578-584

[2] Flatow EL. Gleno-humeral instability. In : Post M, Flatow EL, Bigliani LU, Pollock RG eds. The shoulder. Operative technique. Baltimore : Williams and Wilkins, 1998 : 167-200

[3] Jobe FW, Gousman RE. Anterior capsulo-labral reconstruction. *Tech Orthop* 1989 ; 3 : 29-35

[4] Kvitne RS, Jobe FW, Jobe CM. Shoulder instability in overhand or throwing athletes. *Clin Sports Med* 1995 ; 14 : 917-935

[5] Leslie JT, Ryan TJ. The anterior axillary incision to approach the shoulder joint. *J Bone Joint Surg Am* 1962 ; 44 : 1193-1196

[6] Neer CS. Shoulder reconstruction. Philadelphia : WB Saunders, 1990 : 273-341

[7] Neer CS, Fithian TH, Hansen PE et al. Reinforced cruciate repair for anterior dislocations of the shoulder. *Orthop Trans* 1985 ; 9 : 44

[8] Neer CS, Foster CR. Inferior capsular shift for involuntary inferior and multidirectional instability of the shoulder. *J Bone Joint Surg Am* 1980 ; 62 : 897-908

[9] Pollock RG, Owens JM, Nicholson GP et al. Anterior inferior capsular shift procedure for anterior gleno-humeral instability: long term results. *Orthop Trans* 1993 ; 17 : 974

[10] Warner JP, Johnson D, Miller M, Caborn DN. A technique for selecting capsular lightness in repair of anterio-inferior. shoulder instability. *J Shoulder Elbow Surg* 1995 ; 5 : 352-364

[11] Wirth MA, Blatter G, Rockwood CA Jr. The capsular imbrication procedure for recurrent anterior instability of the shoulder. *J Bone Joint Surg Am* 1996 ; 78 : 246-259

Multidirectional instability of the shoulder

PP Symeonides

Abstract. – Multidirectional instability (MDI) of the shoulder is manifested by anterior posterior or inferior dislocation or subluxation. They can be voluntary or involuntary. Both these types of instability should be treated conservatively initially, for at least six months to one year. Operative treatment is indicated for patients with involuntary instability only if conservative treatment fails. Patients with voluntary instability who have psychological problems are excluded from operative treatment because it is likely to fail.

The inferior capsular shift continues to be the procedure of choice for MDI of the shoulder, aiming at the global reduction of the volume of the redundant capsule. The shifting of the inferior capsule can be performed by open and closed (arthroscopic) methods. The results of open procedures are satisfactory in over 80% of cases.

For arthroscopic shifting of the inferior capsule, more satisfactory results are being obtained as more experience is gained and these are tending to match the results of open procedures. Very recently, arthroscopic thermal shrinkage of the slack capsule has also been introduced with encouraging results.

Keywords: shoulder, multidirectional instability.

Introduction

The treatment of multidirectional instability (MDI) of the shoulder (*fig 1*) is a complex problem that has not yet been completely solved. Our knowledge on this subject continues to improve as more research is performed and as more clinical studies with long follow up are published. Until now, various specific exercise systems, as well as open and closed (arthroscopic) operative procedures have been introduced for the management of this difficult affliction.

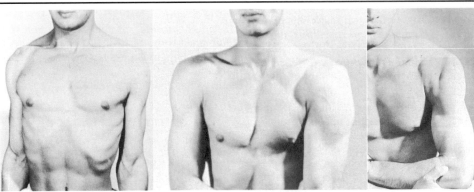

1 *Patient with MDI of the left glenohumeral joint: inferior, anterior, posterior.*

Type of instability

Before deciding to apply any treatment to a patient with glenohumeral instability, it is very important to determine whether the instability is of traumatic or atraumatic origin or if it is the result of repetitive trauma (acquired) [12]. This differentiation is based on:

– History of the patient's instability.

– Physical examination using the various tests of shoulder instability.

PP Symeonides, M.D., Professor of Orthopaedics, Orthopaedic Department, University of Thessaloniki. Former Dean of the Medical School, Aristotle University of Thessaloniki. 3 Grigoriou Palama Street, 54622 Thessaloniki, Greece.

– Radiographic findings.

– CT and MRI findings, particularly the arthro-MRI.

– Examination under general anaesthesia [13].

– Arthroscopy.

Once the surgeon is convinced that the instability is of an atraumatic MDI type, which is different from multidirectional hyperlaxity (MDH) [7], he must clarify in which of the following categories the instability belongs:

– Involuntary.

– Voluntary with an involuntary component [4].

– Voluntary without psychological disorders.

– Voluntary with psychological disorders.

The treatment of MDI is non-operative and/or surgical.

Non-operative treatment

Almost all authors agree that the treatment of atraumatic MDI should be initially non-operative, regardless of the type of instability (involuntary or voluntary) [6, 13, 16].

The non-operative treatment includes a prolonged rehabilitation programme of specific exercises which aim to strengthen both the deltoid and rotator cuff muscles as well as the scapular stabilisers. The length of this kind of treatment ranges from six months [16] to one year [13], depending on the individual case and the surgeon's preference.

Matsen et al [11] suggested that for patients with atraumatic instability, vigorous co-ordinated contractions of the rotator cuff muscles of the shoulder are of particular importance. They create a dynamic stabilising mechanism which resists humeral head displacement.

Kromberg, Brostrom and Nemeth [9], in an investigation of patients with generalised joint laxity, found significant muscular imbalance in comparison to normal controls. They therefore recommended a special training programme for muscle strengthening and co-ordination to improve the stability of the shoulder.

Burkhead and Rockwood [3] investigated 140 unstable glenohumeral joints in 115 patients who were treated using a specific system of exercises. Patients with atraumatic instability responded favourably (80%) to this exercise programme. In contrast, those with traumatic instability showed poor results (16% success rate). The authors concluded that in patients with atraumatic MDI of the shoulder, a trial of specific resistance strengthening exercises should be embarked upon before reconstruction of the shoulder is considered

For patients with atraumatic instability, Neer [12] recommends exercises with the arm below the level of the shoulder, for at least a year, to strengthen the rotators and deltoid. Many of these patients will not need surgical treatment following this course of exercises.

Although various rehabilitation systems have been described in the literature, no marked differences between them have been shown. Our 24 patients with MDI [19] underwent the Rockwood and Burkhead [16] regimen of exercises and the results were satisfactory. The exercises were most effective for patients with involuntary atraumatic posterior shoulder instability, similar to Burkhead and Rockwood's findings [3], and were less effective for patients with atraumatic anterior and inferior instability. However, the percentage of successful results in our study was inferior to those of the above mentioned authors, probably because of our limited experience in applying the system of exercises and perhaps owing to reduced patient compliance.

Surgical treatment of MDI

For patients with MDI who fail to respond to conservative management for a period of six months to one year, surgical treatment is indicated. The surgeon should closely monitor his patients during this period so as to ascertain that the conservative treatment,

which was demonstrated to them, has been appropriately carried out. At the same time the surgeon can assess the patients' motivation and maturity to cooperate in such an operation, by examining them several times. Voluntary dislocators with psychiatric disorders should be excluded from surgical treatment despite failure of any prolonged conservative treatment. However, prejudice should not exist against voluntary dislocators, because not all of them have psychiatric problems [17].

The inferior capsular shift designed by Neer and Forster in 1980 continues to be the operation of choice in the treatment of MDI. The aim of this procedure is to reduce the capsular volume of the shoulder joint by overlapping and tightening the capsule on the side of greatest instability. This leads to obliteration of the inferior capsular pouch and to tension of the posterior capsule.

The classical operative methods (Bankart, Putti-Platt, Magnuson-Stack, Bristow-Letarjet, etc.) which have proved successful in treating traumatic unidirectional shoulder instability have not been effective in treating MDI of the shoulder [12].

OPERATIVE TECHNIQUE

The shoulder in MDI is approached from the side of greatest instability. Shoulders with anterior and posterior instability are usually approached from the anterior side because all sides of the capsule may be tightened from this side. The surgeon must also be prepared to use a posterior approach if necessary. This must also be explained to the patient prior to operation.

ANTERIOR APPROACH

The patient is placed in a beach chair position. General anaesthesia or an intrascaline block is used. Although the direction of greatest instability will have been determined before the operation, on the basis of history and clinical examination using the various tests, an examination of the shoulder while the patient is under general anaesthesia is necessary to confirm the clinical impression concerning the side of greatest instability.

An incision, 7 to 8 cm long, is extended from the upper fold of the axilla towards the coracoid process *(fig 2)*. This incision gives better cosmetic results, but topographically is located medially to the deltopectoral space. For a surgeon with moderate experience, a longer incision extending from the coracoid process to 2 cm lateral and distal to the upper fold of the axilla (which follows exactly the deltopectoral interval) is preferable. The skin with its subcutaneous tissue is cut and mobilised on both sides and up to the clavicle. The deltopectoral groove which is marked by the cephalic vein comes into view. However, it is not always easy to trace the vein and the deltopectoral interval especially in obese patients. Looking

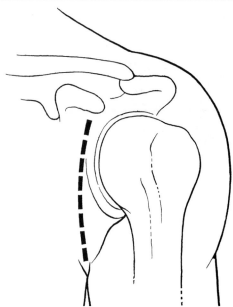

2 *The skin incision in the anterior approach to the glenohumeral joint.*

for a yellow, longitudinal line of fat after retracting the skin and subcutaneous tissue may be of some help [20]. The deep fascia is incised along this line to reveal the cephalic vein and the deltopectoral interval. The vein is retracted with the deltoid muscle laterally, and the two muscles are bluntly separated reaching the second anatomical layer that consists of the short head of the biceps and coracobrachialis. Dissection above the coracoid process should be done carefully, as the cephalic vein is at risk in the upper corner of the deltopectoral interval. The clavipectoral fascia is incised laterally to the conjoined tendon with the corresponding muscles. These are gently retracted medially, because of the vulnerability of the musculocutaneous nerve. There is no need to osteotomise the coracoid process. The arm is then externally rotated and the third anatomical layer consisting of the subscapularis tendon and muscle is brought into view. A thin layer of synovium that covers the anterior aspect of the subscupularis tendon is removed. The latter facilitates a clear definition of the boundaries of the subscapularis tendon with the arm in external rotation. The anterior circumflex vessels that run along the inferior margin of the subscapularis muscle are carefully dissected and ligated or cauterised. Cauterisation is not always effective in preventing bleeding from these vessels. Keeping the arm in external rotation eliminates the risk to the axillary nerve.

According to the classical description by Neer and Forster [13], the subscapularis tendon is divided vertically 1 cm medial to its insertion to the lesser tuberosity. The division only includes the superficial half of the thickness of the subscapularis tendon, leaving the posterior half of the tendon to reinforce the anterior capsule. If the vertical incision of the subscapularis tendon is more medial, care must be taken to leave a thin

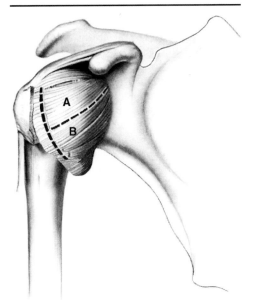

3   *T shaped incision of the anterior capsule of the glenohumeral joint. Note that the vertical limb of this incision is not made at the level of the stump of the subscapularis but 3/4 to 1 cm medially, to facilitate the suturing of the inferior and superior capsular flaps laterally.*

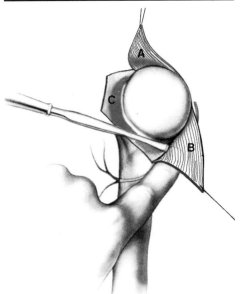

4   *The index finger is used to palpate and protect the axillary nerve during the detachment of the inferior capsular flap from the lower part of the neck of the humerus, as recommended by Neer [12].*

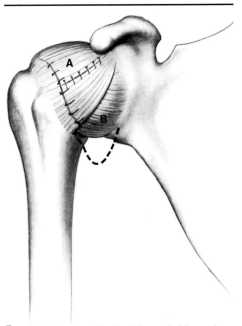

5   *The inferior capsular flap is first pulled forward, upwards and laterally and is sutured to the lateral part of the capsule, reducing the excess volume of the joint capsule and eliminating the inferior capsular pouch.*

tendinous part on the medial stump of the subscapularis because, otherwise, suturing the muscle to the tendinous lateral stump is difficult and unsafe [19].

The superficial half of the subscapularis tendon is carefully and completely separated from the posterior half and it is retracted medially. The interval between the superior and middle glenohumeral ligaments should be closed at this stage with one or two 0 non-absorbable sutures. The sutures should not be very tight because this may cause a limitation of the lateral rotation of the arm [1]. A T shaped incision is made on the anterior capsule while the arm is kept at about 30⁰ abduction and at 20⁰ external rotation *(fig 3)*. The horizontal limb of the T incision is made between the middle and inferior glenohumeral ligaments, whereas the vertical one is located laterally at the insertion of the capsule to the cut subscapularis and the neck of the humerus. Two traction sutures are used, one for the upper and one for the lower capsular flaps. Through this T opening, the humeral head and the glenoid cavity can be seen. Detachment or splitting of the labrum and capsule, although very rare, are also looked for and if detached they are sutured to the anterior glenoid rim by two 0 non-absorbable sutures. The arm is then gradually externally rotated, and the inferior glenohumeral ligament and capsule are cautiously detached from the inferior and posterior part of the neck of the humerus with a sharp periosteal elevator. The area of capsule detachment from the humeral neck is curetted and roughened to facilitate the healing of the shifted capsule to the bone. This stage is crucial because of the risk of injury to the axillary nerve. The index finger, as suggested by Neer [12], is therefore used to palpate and protect the nerve while the

detachment is carried out *(fig 4)*. The inferior capsular flap is freed completely from any adhesions to the surrounding tissues and is pulled upward and forward, so that its superolateral corner is sutured and fixed at the superior end of the vertical limb of the T incision, as well as to the lateral stump of the subscapularis and capsule using one or two 0 non-absorbable sutures. Care is taken to hold the capsular flap in contact with the roughened area of the neck of the humerus. During the upward pull of the inferior capsular flap, the elimination of the inferior capsular pouch can be checked by palpation with the little finger.

At this stage it is important that the arm be held in a neutral position (flexion-extension) and at approximately 10⁰ external rotation and 10⁰ abduction. After the completion of the suturing of the inferior capsular shift, the superior capsular flap is pulled down and sutured to the soft tissues of the neck of the humerus and to the lower part of the inferior capsular flap *(fig 5)*. The medial stump of the subscapularis tendon, with the muscle, is relocated in its original position and sutured to the lateral tendinous stump of subscapularis and capsule. The deltopectoral space is closed with three or four sutures, and a subcuticular suture is used for skin closure. The upper limb is immobilised in a spica cast or in an orthosis with the arm held in approximately 10° of abduction and 10° of external rotation for 6 weeks. During this period, the patient is seen regularly to check that the plaster spica is not moving inferiorly. Only isometric exercises of the arm and gentle elbow motion are performed, if the latter is possible. The plaster or orthosis is removed six weeks postoperatively and mild exercises of the shoulder muscles are gradually

introduced. Immobilisation of the shoulder for six weeks does not cause any loss of motion to the joint [10].

Modifications to the inferior capsular shift procedure

Since the description of the inferior capsular shift procedure by Neer and Forster [13], various modifications of capsulorrhaphy have been described for the reconstruction of MDI of the shoulder. They can be classified into four types including the original, according to the position of the vertical incision of the capsule.

A. The classical inferior capsular shift described by Neer and Forster [13] in which the vertical line of the T incision of the capsule is located at the level of the medial end of the lateral stump of the cut subscapularis tendon. The horizontal one is located between the inferior and middle glenohumeral ligaments.

B. The subscapularis tendon is cut transversely 1 cm from its insertion to the lesser humeral tuberosity. A thin layer of the deep surface of the tendon is left with the capsule, for reinforcement. The capsule is separated from the subscapularis muscle. The vertical line of the T opening is located laterally, approximately 3/4 to 1 cm medial to the cut subscapularis tendon and the insertion of the capsule into the neck of the humerus. This narrow part of capsular tissue facilitates safer suturing of the inferior capsular flap [6]. We have also used this surgical technique for the cases of MDI we have operated on.

C. The capsule is divided midway between its attachment to the humerus and to the

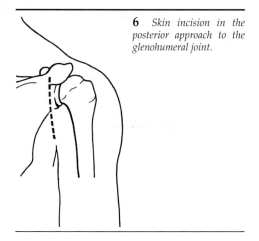

6 *Skin incision in the posterior approach to the glenohumeral joint.*

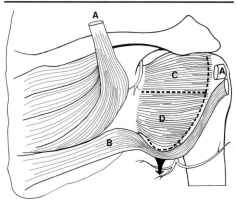

7 *Exposure of the posterior capsule by medial reflection of the cut infraspinatus and traction of the teres minor distally. A T shape incision is made on the posterior capsule.*

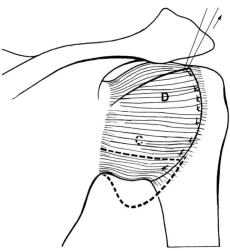

8 *The superior capsular flap (C) is first pulled downwards and laterally, and sutured to the lateral stump of the capsule. Then the inferior capsular flap (D) is shifted upwards and sutured by overlapping the superior one and eliminating the inferior pouch of the loose joint capsule.*

glenoid rim as described by Rockwood [15]. The medial flap is brought superiorly and laterally under the lateral capsular flap, which is brought, superiorly and medially, over the medial capsular flap.

D. The subscapularis is not cut transversely at its insertion to the lesser tuberosity but is divided horizontally along its fibres at the junction of its upper two-thirds and lower one-third; thus the capsule is approached. The horizontal line of the T opening of the capsule follows the direction of the split in the subscapularis, whereas the vertical one is performed parallel to the edge of the glenoid process, just medial to the labrum. The inferior capsular flap that develops is shifted superiorly and sutured onto the glenoid. The superior capsular flap is then overlapped on the inferior and is also sutured to the glenoid bone [18].

Posterior approach to the glenohumeral joint

General anaesthesia is used. The patient is placed in the lateral decubitus position lying on the normal shoulder. A vertical skin incision is performed, starting 2 cm medial to the posterolateral corner of the acromion, and extending 10 cm distally towards the posterior fold of the axilla *(fig 6)*. The deltoid muscle is split in line with its fibres for 5 cm. A stay suture is placed at the distal end of the split in the deltoid muscle to prevent its extension distally. The origin of the deltoid may be detached subperiosteally for 2 cm, one at each side of the split, to facilitate the approach to the infraspinatus. The two parts of the deltoid are then retracted gently to expose the underlying infraspinatus and the proximal portion of the teres minor. The surgeon should remember that the axillary nerve emerges distal to the teres minor muscle through the quadrangular space. The infraspinatus tendon is incised vertically 1 cm medial to its attachment to the greater tuberocity. A thin layer of the deep part of the tendon is left attached to the capsule for reinforcement. The infraspinatus is gently reflected medially, and the teres minor is retracted distally, to expose the capsule *(fig 7)*. Care is taken not to injure the suprascapular nerve that innervates the infraspinatus. A T incision is performed on the capsule, with its vertical limb 1 cm medial to its humeral neck attachment. The incision is extended inferiorly around the humeral neck as far as is needed to eliminate the capsular pouch. The index finger is used to protect the axillary nerve during this inferior capsular incision. The glenoid labrum is inspected and should it be detached, which is rare, it is reattached. The upper capsular flap is then pulled downwards and sutured to the lateral part of the capsule, and the lower capsular flap is shifted superiorly upwards and is also sutured to the lateral part of the capsule, overlapping the upper capsular flap *(fig 8)*. The infraspinatus is reattached to its anatomical position, the detached origin of the deltoid is sutured with non absorbable sutures and the skin is closed with a subcuticular suture. The upper limb is immobilised either in a light plastic brace or in a light plastic spica cast for six weeks with the arm in slight abduction and 10 to 20 degrees external rotation. After the removal of the brace or spica, the shoulder is mobilised by exercises. Mobilisation should be slow but progressive. The rotator cuff muscles and deltoid should be gently strengthened to protect the sutured capsule and ligaments. A period of 3 to 6 months is needed to complete the mobilisation of the glenohumeral joint. Patients who have been operated on should not resume their athletic activities for 9-12 months.

Other surgical procedures for the treatment of MDI

Glenoid osteotomy has been used by Nobuhara and Ikeda [14] for the treatment of MDI. The aim of the osteotomy is to change the inclination of the glenoid cavity so that it faces more superiorly. This reduces the excess volume of the capsule, establishes a new fulcrum for the shoulder musculature, and controls the tendency of the humeral head to slip inferiorly. They operated on 111 patients over a period of 14 years and have reviewed 100 with a follow up of more than a year. The results were satisfactory. In all but three patients, symptomatic instability almost completely subsided. However, the operation seems technically demanding. A larger series with a longer follow up is needed to evaluate the efficacy of the procedure.

Arthroscopic treatment and thermal capsular shrinkage of MDI

Arthroscopic treatment and thermal capsular shrinkage represent two new methods in the management of MDI of the shoulder. (For details see relevant chapter in this book.)

RESULTS

The results of the open inferior capsular shift procedure have been satisfactory in patients with atraumatic involuntary MDI of the shoulder. The successful results of these mid-term follow up studies exceeded 80% *(table I)*. Reports with longer follow up are needed to confirm the long-term efficacy of the inferior capsular shift procedure.

Conclusions

Involuntary MDI can be managed effectively using a specific system of exercises, and, if this

Table I. – Results of mid-term follow up.

Author	Year	Shoulders	% satisfactory results	Unsatisfactory results	Follow up
Neer-Forster [13]	1980	32	31 (97%)	1	1-2 years
Neer [12]	1990	100	97%	3	Not stated
Cooper-Brems [5]	1992	43	34 (79%)	9 (21%)	3.3 y
Bigliani et al [1]	1993	52	94%	6%	2-11 y
Hamada et al [8]	1999	22	86%	14%	8.3 y

fails, an open inferior capsular shift procedure can be performed. Successful results of over 80% have been reported. The arthroscopic inferior capsular shift procedure as well as arthroscopic thermal shrinkage of the redundant capsule have also produced encouraging results, but more studies are needed to determine the long term effectiveness of these procedures. Voluntary MDI remains an unresolved problem, which should be further investigated and treated accordingly.

References

[1] Bigliani LU. Recurrent anterior instability: Open surgical repair. In : Bigliani LU ed. The unstable shoulder. AAOS Monograph Series, 1996 : 59-67

[2] Bigliani LU, Pollock RG, Owens JM et al. The inferior capsular shift procedure for MDI of the shoulder. *Orthop Tran* 1993 ; 17 : 576

[3] Burkhead WZ, Rockwood CA. Treatment of instability of the shoulder with an exercise program. *J Bone Joint Surg Am* 1992 ; 74 : 890-896

[4] Cofield RH, Irving JF. Evaluation and classification of shoulder instability with special reference to examination under anaesthesia. *Clin Orthop* 1987 ; 223 : 32-43

[5] Cooper RA, Brems AA. The inferior capsular shift procedure for multidirectional instability of the shoulder. *J Bone Joint Surg Am* 1992 ; 74 : 1516-1521

[6] Flatow EL. Glenohumeral instability. In : Post M, Bigliani LU, Flatow E, Pollock RG eds. The shoulder. Operative technique. Baltimore : Williams and Wilkins, 1998 : 167-200

[7] Gerber C. Observations on the classification of instability. In : Warner P, Iannott JP, Gerber C eds. Complex and revision problems in shoulder surgery. Philadelphia : Lippincott-Raven, 1997 : 9-18

[8] Hamada K, Fukuda H, Nakajima T, Yamada N. The inferior capsular shift operation for instability of the shoulder. *J Bone Joint Surg Br* 1999 ; 81 : 218-225

[9] Kronberg M, Brostrom LA, Nemeth G. Differences in shoulder muscle activity between patients with generalized joint laxity and normal controls. *Clin Orthop* 1991 ; 269 : 181-192

[10] Mallon WJ, Speer KP. Multidirectional instability. Current concepts. *J Shoulder Elbow Surg* 1995 ; 4 : 54-64

[11] Matsen FA, Thomas SC, Rockwood CA. Anterior glenohumeral instability. In : Rockwood CA, Matsen FA eds. The shoulder. Philadelphia : WB Saunders, 1990 : 576-605

[12] Neer CS 2nd. Shoulder reconstruction. Philadelphia : WB Saunders, 1990 : 326-327

[13] Neer CS 2nd, Foster GR. Inferior capsular shift for involuntary inferior and multidirectional instability of the shoulder. *J Bone Joint Surg Am* 1980 ; 62 : 897-908

[14] Nobuhara K, Ikeda H. Glenoid osteotomy for loose shoulder. In : Watson MS ed. Surgical disorders of the shoulder. Edinburgh : Churchill Livingstone, 1991 : 44-50

[15] Rockwood CA. Approach to treatment of atraumatic and multidirectional glenohumeral instability. In : Rockwood CA, Matsen FA eds. The shoulder. Philadelphia : WB Saunders, 1990 : 608-612

[16] Rockwood CA, Burkhead WZ. Subluxation of the glenohumeral joint. Response to rehabilitative exercise. Traumatic versus atraumatic instability. Proceedings of the third international conference on surgery of the shoulder, 1986 : 293-298

[17] Rowe CR, Pierce DS, Clark JG. Voluntary dislocation of the shoulder: a preliminary report on a clinical electromyographic and psychiatric study of twenty-six patients. *J Bone Joint Surg Am* 1973 ; 55 : 445-460

[18] Rubenstein DL, Jobe FW, Glousman RE, Kvinte RS, Pink MM, Giagara CE. Anterior capsulolabral reconstruction of the shoulder in athletes. *J Shoulder Elbow Surg* 1992 ; 1 : 229-273

[19] Symeonides PP. Surgical management of the unstable shoulder. In : Watson MS ed. Practical shoulder surgery. London : Grune and Stratton, 1984 : 67-127

[20] Symeonides PP. The Putti-Platt procedure. In : Watson MS ed. Surgical disorders of the shoulder. Edinburgh : Churchill Livingstone, 1991 : 379-385

Chronic posterior dislocations of the shoulder

M Randelli
PL Gambrioli

Abstract. – Chronic posterior dislocations of the shoulder are usually the result of a missed posterior dislocation or fracture-dislocation of the humeral head, which has been reduced for not more than three weeks and is characterised by varying degrees of damage to the humeral head (the McLaughlin anterolateral humeral defect), and less often by lesions involving the posterior glenoid margin and periarticular soft tissues. Surgical treatment is principally based on the size and depth of the humeral defect.

In Type 1 chronic posterior dislocations with a humeral bone defect that involves 20% to 50% of the head profile, closed reduction has been proposed for recent lesions with humeral damage of up to 20% of the articular surface. In small head lesions, the indication is either transposition of the subscapularis tendon into the humeral impression fracture as proposed by McLaughlin, or transposition of the lesser tuberosity according to Neer's technique. In acute lesions where the articular cartilage is impacted but not destroyed, it has been suggested to reshape the humeral surface by means of joint cartilage disimpaction and cancellous bone grafting. In chronic humeral head defects approaching 50% of the articular surface, and for patients with good bone stock, the reconstruction of the humeral head surface can be attempted by means of bone allografts to avoid resorting to arthroplasty.

Type 2 is a deep and wide humeral defect covering more than 50% of the joint surface. This kind of lesion could be an indication for either non-intervention or treatment with prosthetic surgery, according to the patient's age, functional requirements and general clinical condition.

Type 3 is a fracture-dislocation of the humeral head, where a posterior bony hinge keeps the posteriorly dislocated head in continuity with the diaphysis. The articular profile of the humeral head is preserved. The surgical indication is open reduction of the dislocation, repositioning of the humeral head and interfragmentary osteosynthesis. There is a risk of delayed humeral head necrosis and this must always be communicated to the patient.

Type 4 is a multi-fragmented fracture-dislocation with the remnants of the posteriorly dislocated humeral head showing a completely altered joint profile. The only surgical indication is for hemi- or total shoulder arthroplasty.

A full evaluation must also include any glenoid lesions, even if these are very rare. If treatment choices are sufficiently adapted to the various anatomo-pathological situations and the patient's condition, the outcome is generally satisfactory.

© 2001, Editions Scientifiques et Médicales Elsevier SAS. All rights reserved.

Keywords: shoulder, chronic posterior dislocation, fracture-dislocations, classification of humeral lesions, open reduction, reconstruction of humeral head.

Definition

Chronic posterior dislocation of the shoulder is usually the result of a missed posterior dislocation or fracture-dislocation of the humeral head, which has not been reduced for more than three weeks and is characterised by varying degrees of damage to the humeral head (the McLaughlin anterolateral humeral defect), and less often by lesions involving the posterior glenoid margin and peri-articular soft tissues.

Mario Randelli, M.D., Professor.
Istituto Clinico Humanitas, Via Manzoni 56, 20089 Rozzano Milan, Italy.
Pier Luigi Gambrioli, M.D.
Istituto Ortopedico "G. Pini", Milan, Italy.

Classification and treatment choice

Among the different classifications that have been put forward [10, 13], a classification based on the extent of humeral damage and combining both posterior and fracture-dislocations can be a useful guideline for evaluating different treatment options [14].

A good evaluation of the size and depth of the humeral defect can be obtained by means of an axillary lateral X-ray view, and a computed tomography examination (CT) sometimes with a 3D reconstruction. On this basis, chronic posterior dislocations and fracture-dislocations of the shoulder can be classified into four types (fig 1).

Type 1 is a chronic posterior dislocation with a humeral bone defect that involves 20% to 50% of the articular surface. This is the most frequent kind of lesion and a broad range of treatments can be considered.

Closed reduction has been proposed in recent lesions having humeral damage of up to 20% of the articular surface. In small head lesions, the indication is either the transposition of the subscapularis tendon into the humeral impression fracture as proposed by McLaughlin, or transposition of the lesser tuberosity according to Neer's technique.

All references to this article must include: Randelli M and Gambrioli PL. Chronic posterior dislocations of the shoulder. Editions Scientifiques et Médicales Elsevier SAS (Paris). All rights reserved. Surgical Techniques in Orthopaedics and Traumatology, 55-190-B-10, 2001, 6 p.

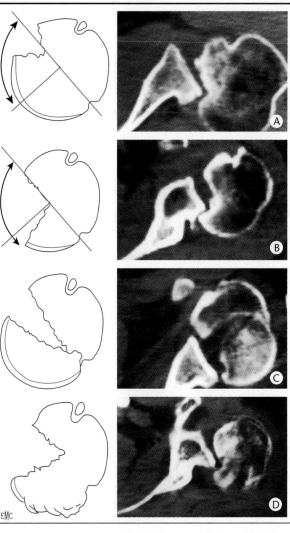

1 *Classification of the chronic posterior dislocations and fracture-dislocations.*
A. Type 1: Humeral defect of 20% to 50% of the humeral head.
B. Type 2: Humeral defect of more than 50% of the humeral head.
C. Type 3: Fracture-dislocation without damage to the humeral head.
D. Type 4: Fracture-dislocation with destruction of the humeral head.

In acute lesions where the articular cartilage is impacted but not destroyed, it has been suggested to reshape the humeral surface by means of joint cartilage disimpaction and cancellous bone grafts [4, 7].

In chronic humeral head defects approaching 50% of the articular surface, and in patients with a good bone stock, the reconstruction of the humeral head surface can be attempted by means of bone allografts to avoid resorting to arthroplasty [5, 6].

Type 2 is a deep and wide humeral defect covering more than 50% of the joint surface. This kind of lesion could be an indication for either non-intervention or treatment by prosthetic surgery, according to the patient's age, functional requirements and general clinical condition.

Type 3 is a fracture-dislocation of the humeral head, where a posterior bony hinge keeps the posteriorly dislocated head in continuity with the diaphysis. The fracture may be at the level of the anatomical neck or involve part of the diaphysis medially. The articular profile of the humeral head is preserved. The surgical indication is open reduction of the dislocation, repositioning of the humeral head and interfragmentary osteosynthesis. There is a risk of delayed humeral head necrosis and this must always be communicated to the patient.

Type 4 is a multi-fragmented fracture-dislocation with the remnants of the posteriorly dislocated humeral head showing a completely altered joint profile. The only surgical indication is hemi- or total shoulder arthroplasty.

A full evaluation must also include any glenoid lesions, even if these are very rare. Only fractures that involve at least a third of the glenoid surface and make the humeral head unstable posteriorly require corrective surgery, usually by means of allografts. Where there is both serious glenoid and humeral damage, the indication is for a total arthroplasty.

Selecting the most appropriate treatment cannot be based solely on the size of the humeral head or glenoid defect, but should also consider clinical aspects (severe limitations in daily living activities and pain), the patient's age, functional needs and compliance to the rehabilitation programme, time since the dislocation, the state of the articular cartilage and the quality of the humeral head bone stock.

Non-operative treatment

This is based on abstaining from any attempt to reduce the dislocation, and initiating gradual rehabilitation to lead to

limited movement recovery, mainly in active forward elevation. The choice of a treatment based on purposeful non-intervention usually concerns elderly patients with limited functional requirements and little pain, patients with severe humeral lesions that offer no guarantee of a good surgical outcome, and subjects with major general contraindications to surgery or who refuse surgical treatment.

Closed reduction for small humeral defects

This may be applied with reasonable success in patients who consult within two to three weeks for Type I posterior dislocations with a humeral defect involving around 20% of the humeral head profile.

Even if some recent posterior dislocations with minor osseous damage can be reduced without anaesthesia, more extensive and older lesions usually require a reduction under scalene block or general anaesthesia, always bearing in mind the risk of an intraoperative humeral fracture.

The reduction procedure is performed with traction in line with the axis of the arm along with a de-coaptation manoeuvre that disengages the humeral head impression fracture from the posterior glenoid rim. At this moment, gradual external rotation of the arm should result in repositioning the humeral head in front of the glenoid. Following the reduction, the limb should be immobilised in an orthosis or prefabricated splint with arm abduction at 45° and external rotation of 20° for three to four weeks.

If the reduction fails or the humeral head remains posteriorly unstable, an open reduction and stabilisation using an appropriate technique should be considered.

Open reduction

Surgical reduction of a locked posterior dislocation is indicated if the dislocation is more than 3 weeks old, in Type 1 lesions with a humeral defect that involves over 20% of the articular surface and in Type 3 inveterate posterior fracture-dislocations.

Historically, different surgical approaches have been proposed: anterior [10, 13], posterior [3], superior [15, 16], or else a combined anterior and posterior approach [1]. Each one of these procedures has its advantages and drawbacks.

The most frequently used access is currently the standard deltopectoral approach because the anterior exposure permits a good anterior capsular release, easy transfer of the subscapularis, and optimal exposure for repair of the humeral head defects by bone grafts or, when necessary, for arthroplasty. A posterior access can only occasionally be associated, when there might be reduction difficulties or the need to repair a posterior glenoid bone lesion. The patient is in an half-sitting position with the arm free and the shoulder out from the table, accessible both anteriorly and posteriorly to allow manual manoeuvres on the head posteriorly, or the performance of a posterior access by gently turning the patient onto the opposite side. The iliac crest is also prepared if an autoplastic bone graft is planned.

The anterior approach is the classic deltopectoral one. The anterior humeral circumflex artery must be identified and preserved in all procedures where the humeral head is to be conserved.

The subscapularis tendon is vertically sectioned 1 cm from its insertion if a simple open reduction is planned, or near its insertion if subscapularis transpositioning according to McLaughlin's procedure is to be performed. If the humeral head defect is more extensive, an osteotomy of the lesser tuberosity with the tendon inserted, as described in Neer's technique, is performed.

An ample vertical capsular section is fundamental for performing the reduction, avoiding further trauma and damage to an osteoporotic humeral head. Sometimes in capsular sectioning, it has to be pushed far down and therefore attention must be paid to the axillary nerve. Before the reduction, the impression fracture is freed of all scar tissue.

The difficulty of reducing a posteriorly dislocated humeral head is directly related to the depth of the humeral impression fracture. The reduction can be obtained in different ways: by manual de-coaptation with lateral traction on the arm and/or by introducing a blunt Hohmann-type retractor between the posterior glenoid border and the humeral head in order to lever the humeral head. If the reduction is especially difficult, a laminar spreader may be used to enlarge the space between the glenoid posterior edge and the head impression fracture, disengaging with a simple manoeuvre the McLauglin lesion from the posterior glenoid border. When the intact edge of the humeral head appears at the posterior glenoid border, manual posterior pressure on the humeral head and gentle external rotation of the arm allow the reduction to be completed.

Open repair and stabilisation of the humeral head

Once the joint is reduced, an evaluation of the humeral head lesions is made to determine the extent of the McLaughlin's humeral impression fracture, the state of the articular cartilage and any localised or general softening or collapse of the humeral head structure.

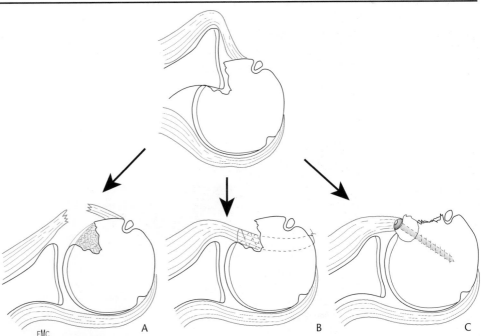

2 *Surgical treatments in Type 1 chronic dislocations with a humeral defect of up to 20% of the articular profile.*
A. Reshaping of the humeral surface by means of local cancellous bone grafts.
B. McLaughlin's subscapularis transfer.
C. Neer's lesser tuberosity transfer.

If the humeral head reveals good bone stock, stabilisation can be obtained by different techniques. We mention in passing the seldom used external rotation osteotomy of the proximal humerus, proposed by Keppler et al [9].

The most currently used techniques are listed below.

RESHAPING THE HUMERAL SURFACE BY MEANS OF LOCAL CANCELLOUS BONE GRAFTS

This technique is applicable to recent lesions where the cartilage has been impacted but not destroyed in young patients or elderly people with adequate humeral bone stock (fig 2A).

A bone window is made in the greater tuberosity just on the opposite site to the cartilage defect. The local spongiosa and/or cancellous bone chips obtained from the iliac crest are pushed below the area of the cartilage impaction, raising the chondral surface until the normal articular contour is regained. If there are loose cartilage fragments, these may be kept in place by suturing their edges with reabsorbable threads or by fixing them with bio-absorbable K-wires through the humeral surface. Two parallel screws may be positioned below the graft zone in order to support the cancellous bone fragments. The capsula is not usually surgically addressed at the end of the operation. The subscapularis is mobilised from its origin to the scapular neck, sectioning the capsule along the anterior glenoid border and detaching the muscle from its scapular insertion. The subscapularis is also freed from all adherences and finally sutured into the normal insertion site on the lesser tuberosity.

Post-operatively, the shoulder is positioned in a brace with the arm in slight abduction and neutral rotation. Movements that bring the humeral grafted area into contact with the glenoid are avoided for at least six weeks.

TRANSFER OF THE SUBSCAPULARIS

The transfer of the subscapularis muscle, as described by McLaughlin (fig 2B), is best applied in small humeral defects (less than 25% of the humeral head profile) in patients having good bone stock and humeral head cartilage preservation.

Through an anterior deltopectoral approach, the subscapularis tendon is detached from its insertion at the lesser tuberosity. The humeral head is reduced and the humeral defect cleared of cartilage residue and scar tissue so that a fresh bed of cancellous bone can be prepared for insertion of the subscapularis tendon. The tendon, freed from any adherences, is tightly reinserted by means of transosseous sutures within the humeral head defect. Shoulder stability is controlled in internal rotation. If the shoulder shows a tendency to posterior subluxation, the humeral head can be temporarily fixed in front of the glenoid with two percutaneous and transarticular Kirschner wires in a position of 45° abduction and 20° external rotation. After having stabilised the joint, the transosseous sutures are tied and the wound closed. The arm will be kept in position with a splint or a plaster spica cast for 4 weeks. Following this, both the immobilisation and percutaneous Kirschner wires are removed and a gradual rehabilitation programme is started.

TRANSFER OF THE LESSER TUBEROSITY

Hawkins and Neer [8] have suggested transferring the lesser tuberosity with its attached subscapularis tendon in cases where the bone defect involves 20%-45% of the humeral head's articular profile. The advantages of this technique are better bone filling of the humeral defect and more secure reinsertion of the subscapularis (fig 2C).

Osteotomy of the lesser tuberosity should be performed obliquely, starting from the medial edge of the bicipital groove, avoiding destabilisation of the long head of the biceps tendon within the groove. The lesser tuberosity osteotomy is limited distally at the anterior humeral circumflex vessels. The lesser tuberosity fragment is fixed into the defect with one, or occasionally two, cancellous lag screws anchored into the cancellous bone of the humeral head. If the shoulder is stable, immobilisation is undergone for 4 weeks as described for McLaughlin's operation. Should the humeral defect be too large to be filled with a lesser tuberosity graft, a humeral head reconstruction by means of an autogenous bone graft or an allograft must be considered.

AUTOGENOUS OR ALLOGENIC BONE GRAFT RECONSTRUCTION

Autogenous massive bone grafts from the iliac crest or allogenic bone grafts obtained from conserved humeral or femoral heads are more and more widely used to reconstruct the humeral surface even in defects of limited width, whereas in the past, subscapularis or lesser tuberosity transfer techniques were used (fig 3).

Allograft technique outcomes were published by Gerber in 1996 [6]. Classical indications for this procedure concern either young or elderly patients having good bone stock and a large humeral lesion involving up to 50% of the articular surface.

The most suitable grafts are those obtained from a size-matched, fresh-frozen humeral head. Should this source not be available, a fresh-frozen femoral head may be used.

The anterior deltopectoral access involves the detachment of the subscapularis insertion from the lesser tuberosity, reduction of the dislocation and careful preparation of the humeral defect, whose walls should be prepared with a bed of well-vascularised spongy bone.

It should be checked that the bone graft has an outline that will adapt to the diameter of the humeral head. An allograft is prepared with dimensions about 2 mm wider than the humeral defect in order to obtain a press-fitting of the bone graft into the defect. No fixation is needed if the graft is perfectly stable, but in most cases it is better to perform fixation with one or two lag screws or Herbert screws, avoiding conflict of the heads of the screws with the glenoid articular surface. Rigid fixation seems to

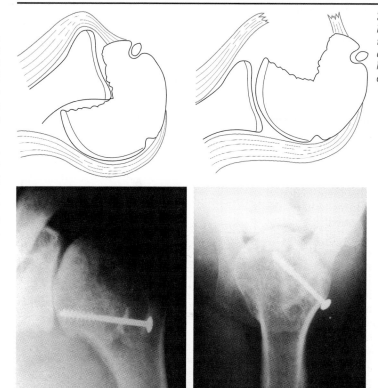

3 *Reconstruction of the humeral head by means of massive allografts in a Type 1 chronic dislocation with a humeral defect of up to 50% of the articular profile.*
A. Humeral defect approaching 50%.
B. Reduction of the dislocation.
C. Reconstruction of the head by means of an autogenous or allogeneic massive bone graft fixed with screws.

favour graft rehabilitation, encouraging a creeping vascular substitution mechanism.

Reduction and fixation of Type 3 chronic posterior fracture-dislocations

A Type 3 chronic posterior fracture-dislocation is usually due to a two-part anatomical neck fracture where the humeral head is luxated posteriorly but has preserved its articular surface intact and is joined to the greater tuberosity by a bony bridge.

Although the risk of delayed necrosis is significant, the indication, especially in younger subjects, is for a repositioning of the humeral head and its fixation using lag screws (fig 4).

Reducing the dislocation through an anterior deltopectoral approach can be difficult because the impression fracture deriving from the fracture is often wide and deep, almost as much as the humeral head diameter. Sometimes, the posterior bony bridge has to be interrupted between the humeral head and greater tuberosity by repositioning the humeral head onto the tuberosities and obtaining the reduction of the dislocation with a leverage manoeuvre using a blunt Hohmann retractor between the humeral head and the posterior edge of the glenoid. These are difficult movements which must be carried out in the most gradual and atraumatic way possible, to avoid damaging the humeral head cartilage. When the dislocation is reduced, the scar tissue is removed from within the defect between the humeral head and the tuberosity. The humeral head is then repositioned in its anatomical location and fixed with two cancellous lag screws.

Arthroplasty in chronic posterior dislocations

A shoulder hemi- or total arthoplasty is indicated in Type 2 dislocations with a

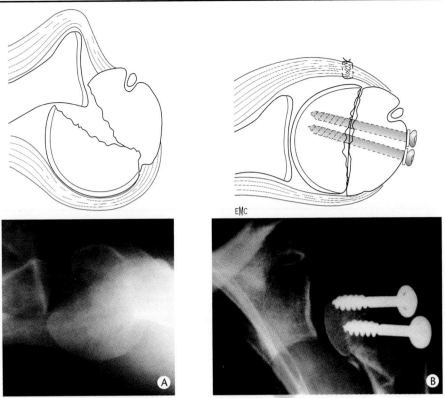

4 *Surgical treatment of a Type 3 chronic posterior shoulder fracture-dislocation.*
A. Fracture-dislocation without damage of the humeral head.
B. Humeral head reduction and fixation with two cancellous lag screws.

humeral defect wider than 50% of the articular profile and in Type 4 fracture-dislocations with complete destruction of the articular segment. Other indications are the collapse of the humeral head, severe damage to the humeral cartilage and irreparable glenoid injuries.

Compared to the usual humeral prosthesis implantation technique, some procedural details must be considered.

If the reduction manoeuvres for the dislocated humeral head are difficult, the head fragments may be removed piecemeal, but care must be taken during this manoeuvre not to alter the support section of the prosthetic head.

The humeral head retrotorsion angle has to be chosen intra-operatively, checking the shoulder's passive stability with various orientations of the prosthetic head, but preferring the normal retroversion angle presented by the patient when it offers good stability.

It is better to use a prosthetic head diameter equal to that of the patient's anatomical one; this facilitates passive motion and

reinsertion of the subscapularis tendon without excessive tension.

Sometimes a capsular plicature or a temporary posterior capsular retensioning can be carried out, as described by Mestdagh, Boileau and Walch [12], where two large absorbable sutures are passed in the posterior capsule before prosthesis insertion and tied over the subscapularis tendon before suturing it. Any excessive retensioning that could create an anterior subluxation must be avoided.

The choice between hemi-arthroplasty and total shoulder arthroplasty depends on the condition of the glenoid cartilage. A hemi-arthroplasty is to be preferred in younger subjects and where glenoid cartilage is preserved. Resurfacing of the glenoid is indicated in cases of serious cartilage wear or grave glenoid bone lesions that require reconstruction with bone grafts.

The arm is usually held in a splint in neutral rotation, and rehabilitation must avoid any internal rotation of the arm for a period of about 40 days.

Glenoid lesions and periarticular soft tissue repair

It is a rare to have to resort to a repair of the posterior glenoid bone structure in a chronic posterior dislocation or fracture-dislocation. Small splits in the posterior glenoid rim do not usually require treatment since they do not influence post-reduction articular stability. In the very rare situations when the dislocation reduction is unstable due to a glenoid rim fracture, a posterior access and reconstruction of the glenoid surface can be considered by repositioning the glenoid bone fragment or by reconstructing the glenoid with an iliac crest graft or an allograft. When the glenoid is extensively damaged, the usual indication is a total shoulder arthroplasty.

Posterior capsulolabral detachments or a posterior capsular redundancy are commonly seen in this condition. In most cases they do not require any surgical treatment and heal up during the postoperative period, when the arm is maintained in a position of slight external-rotation. A posterior capsular plicature, sometimes used in shoulder prosthesis, is rarely performed. The subscapularis and the long head of the biceps can occasionally be disrupted, mainly in elderly subjects and in posterior dislocations deriving from electric shock or convulsions. Such lesions are easily treatable by an anterior approach at the same time as the reduction and repair of the humeral head.

Conclusion

If the treatment choices are sufficiently adapted to the various anatomo-pathological situations and the patient's condition, the outcome of the techniques described above are generally satisfactory.

Although the subscapularis transfers according to the procedures of McLaughlin and Neer have provided good results, the more frequent current tendency is to reconstruct the humeral surface using bone allografts, and to maintain the anatomical insertion of the subscapularis tendon.

Clinical results can be compromised because of complications such as stiffness, pain, residual posterior instability or humeral head collapse. Humeral head necrosis and progressive damage to the articular cartilage may be satisfactorily treated by shoulder arthroplasty.

References ➤

References

[1] Augereau B, Leyder P, Apoil A. Traitement des luxations postérieures invétérées de l'épaule par double abord et butée osseuse rétro-glénoidiénne. *Rev Chir Orthop* 1983 ; 69 (suppl II) : 289-290

[2] Checchia SL, Santos PD, Miyazaki AN. Surgical treatment of acute and chronic posterior fracture-dislocation of the shoulder. *J Shoulder Elbow Surg* 1998 ; 7 : 53-64

[3] Dubousset J. Luxations postérieures de l'épaule. *Rev Chir Orthop* 1967 ; 53 : 65-85

[4] Gerber C. L'instabilité posteriéure de l'épaule. In : Cahiers d'énseignement de la SOFCOT n° 40. Paris : Expansion Scientifique Francaise, 1991 : 223

[5] Gerber C. Chronic, locked anterior and posterior dislocations. In : Warner JJ, Iannotti JP, Gerber Ceds. Complex and revision problems in shoulder surgery. Philadelphia : Lippincott-Raven, 1997 : 99-113

[6] Gerber C, Lambert SM. Allograft reconstruction of segmental defects of the humeral head for the treatment of chronic locked posterior dislocation of the shoulder. *J Bone Joint Surg Am* 1996 ; 78 : 376-382

[7] Griggs SM, Holloway GB, Williams GR, Iannotti JP. Treatment of locked anterior and posterior dislocation of the shoulder. In : Iannotti JP, Williams GReds. Disorders of the shoulder. Philadelphia : Lippincott-William and Wilkins, 1999 : 335-359

[8] Hawkins RJ, Neer CS, Mendoza FX. Locked posterior dislocation of the shoulder. *J Bone Joint Surg Am* 1987 ; 69 : 9-18

[9] Keppler P, Holz U, Thielemann FW, Meinig R. Locked posterior dislocation of the shoulder: treatment using rotational osteotomy of the humerus. *J Orthop Trauma* 1994 ; 8 : 286-292

[10] McLaughlin HL. Posterior dislocation of the shoulder. *J Bone Joint Surg Am* 1952 ; 34 : 584-590

[11] McLaughlin HL. Posterior dislocation of the shoulder. *J Bone Joint Surg Am* 1962 ; 44 : 1477

[12] Mestdagh H, Boileau P, Walch G. Intra- and postoperative complications of the shoulder arthroplasty. In : Walch G, Boileau P eds. Shoulder arthroplasty. Berlin : Springer-Verlag, 1999 : 414

[13] Neer CS 2nd. Fractures. In : Neer CS 2nded. Shoulder reconstruction. Philadelphia : WB Saunders, 1990 : 394

[14] Randelli M. La fracture-luxation postérieure de l'épaule : nouveaux éléments de classification et thérapeutiques. Abstract 2e congrés de la Société européenne de chirurgie de l'épaule et du coude, Berne, 1 Octobre1988

[15] Rowe CR, Zarins B. Chronic unreduced dislocation of the shoulder*J Bone Joint Surg Am* 1982 ; 64 : 494-505

[16] Stableforth PG, Sarangi PP. Posterior fracture-dislocation of the shoulder*J Bone Joint Surg Br* 1992 ; 74 : 579-584

[17] Walch G, Boileau P, Martin B, Dejour H. Luxations et fracture-luxations postérieures invétérées de l'épaule. À propos de 30 cas. *Rev Chir Orthop* 1990 ; 76 : 546-558

Arthroscopic subacromial decompression (ASAD)

U Jonsson-Lillkrona
B Salomonsson

Abstract. – *The clinical outcome after arthroscopic subacromial decompression is comparable to that after open acromioplasty. The learning curve for this procedure is long, but severe complications are rare. A posterior portal is generally used for the scope, while a lateral one is used as the working portal. It is important to have a complete picture of the anatomy before resection is started. After the bursal tissue and periosteum have been resected, approximately 5 mm of bone is resected along 2 cm of the undersurface of the anterior acromion.*

Keywords: shoulder, arthroscopy, subacromial decompression, impingement syndrome, arthroscopic acromioplasty.

Introduction

It is widely believed that contact between the greater tuberosity, the rotator cuff tendons and the coraco-acromial arch in certain shoulders can lead to the painful impingement syndrome. It has also been shown in cadaver examinations that increased contact occurs between these structures in Hawkin's test and Neer's test for impingement [30]. The arthroscopic equivalent of open anterior acromioplasty was first described in 1987 by Ellman [8].

Indications for surgery

The symptoms caused by impingement syndrome are pain at night and pain in connection with activity. Arthroscopic acromioplasty is indicated if these symptoms are present for more than one year despite conservative treatment during at least six months. The treatment prior to surgery should be physical therapy, primarily involving rotator muscle strengthening, steroid injections and possibly non-steroid anti-inflammatory medication (NSAID) [20]. A positive impingement sign and a positive injection test must also be present before a decision is made to perform surgery.

Ulf Jonsson-Lillkrona, M.D., Associate Professor and Head.
Björn Salomonsson, M.D.
Division of Orthopaedics, Karolinska Institutet, Danderyd Hospital, S-182 88 Danderyd, Sweden.

Secondary impingement due to a multidirectional instability must be excluded. Other relevant causes of pain must be considered, such as osteoarthrosis of the acromioclavicular or glenohumeral joints. In addition, patients with partial thickness tears and small full-thickness tears can be treated by arthroscopic acromioplasty without any additional surgery [15].

The surgical treatment options in cases of complete cuff rupture must be evaluated separately.

Pathological changes in the supraspinatus muscle as revealed by MRI are not more frequent among patients with impingement syndrome than among age-matched controls [12] and great caution should be shown when using the MRI findings as a contribution to the decision to perform surgical treatment for impingement.

Before making the decision to perform an acromioplasty, an X-ray examination of the shoulder joint should be carried out. This must include 2 perpendicular views of the humeroscapular joint. If two anteroposterior views of the humerus are made, with the arm in internal and external rotation, there is a high chance of identifying any calcific deposits in the rotator cuff. Signs of osteoarthritic changes in this joint will also be shown, as well as signs of skeletal malformations, for example unfused acromial epiphyses (os acromiale), which should sometimes be treated specifically. It is also important to perform a radiographic examination of the acromioclavicular joint. If there are isolated inferior osteophytes or

osteoarthritic joint changes, these must be considered before surgery. The lateral view can be an axillary or a true scapulolateral projection. The scapular outlet view is especially suited to visualise the undersurface of the acromion at the outlet of the supraspinatus tendon. The patient is positioned as for the true scapulolateral X-ray and the tube is angled anterocaudal 5-10 degrees. An MRI may provide supplementary information, especially concerning the integrity of the rotator cuff, but this examination is seldom mandatory before an ASAD. Ultrasonography can also be very informative for the surgeon if the radiologist has special experience with shoulders.

The morphology of the acromion has been assessed in various ways by a number of investigators to determine if there are situations which increase the risk for rotator cuff tears and impingement. The acromion has been identified as being of three different types: flat (I), curved (II) and hooked (III) [5] (*fig 1*). Although the three morphological classes of the acromion have been shown to have different incidences of rotator cuff tears [5], it is not known whether there is any study demonstrating their relationship to impingement syndrome.

Technical overview

Surgery can be performed with the patient in either the lateral decubitus position or the beach chair position. One advantage of the

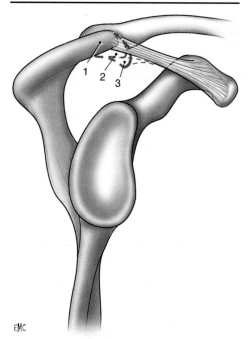

1 *The three configurations of the acromion: 1 (Type I: flat), 2 (Type II: curved) and 3 (Type III: hooked).*

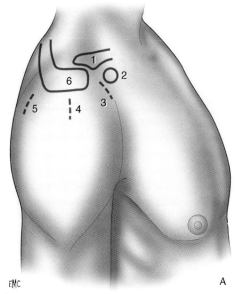

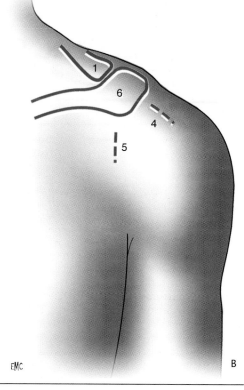

2 *The bony landmarks of the acromion (6), lateral clavicle (1) and the processus coracoideus (2) are marked with a pen, then the anterior (3) and lateral (4) portals are identified. The posterior (5) portal is found 2 cm medial and 2 cm inferior of the posterior corner of the acromion.*
A. Lateral view.
B. Posterior view.

lateral position is that it is easier to suspend the arm with continued traction. Esch has recommended that the traction be 5-7 Kp [9]. In the beach chair position, the assistant may have to pull the arm downwards during certain moments of the procedure.

The ASAD procedure is technically demanding and the learning curve is long. Before starting to perform ASAD, the surgeon should have arthroscopic experience (for example, he should have already performed arthroscopic meniscectomies). There is at least one virtual training system available, which will probably speed up the learning process [25].

It is advisable to use an arthroscopic infusion pump with a pressure sensor. The pressure should be kept between 40 and 100 mm/Hg [9]. Morrison [22] has shown that a fluid pressure in the subacromial bursa of 49 mm/Hg below the systolic pressure reduces the bleeding from the acromion undersurface in most cases; however, there are still situations in which the pressure needs to be increased still further. Sperber and Wredmark [28] found no harmful effects in the deltoid muscle with a bursal pressure of 150 mm/Hg for 25 minutes. To stop bleeding, it is acceptable to raise the pressure towards 150 mm/Hg for a few minutes.

Surgical techniques

During the learning period, it is advisable to outline the margins of the acromion and the lateral clavicle with a pen, and also to mark the coracoid process and the recommended portals. Start with two free hands to localise the posterior soft spot between the infraspinatus and the teres minor. This point

is approximately 2 cm medial of the posterior corner of the acromion and 2 cm inferior of the rim. Use the thumb, for example, to palpate this spot, and move the humeral head anteriorly and posteriorly with the other hand to identify the position of the joint space. The axillary nerve is underneath the teres minor, and branches from the suprascapular nerve to the infraspinatus muscle are more than 1.5 cm medial of this portal (*fig 2*).

Make small incisions and preferably use a conical obturator so as not to injure the joint structures. Direct the obturator approximately 45 degrees medially towards to collum scapulae area and allow the conical tip to slide laterally on the scapula until you feel the joint line. Repeat this "scapular glide" technique until you feel confident. Verify that you can move the humeral head forwards with the obturator when its tip is lateral to the supposed joint line. Then introduce the obturator with a fair degree of force through the capsule in the direction of the coracoid.

The shoulder joint can be inspected by either 40 cc of air (with a 20 cc syringe) or water, if necessary with an anterior portal with a cannula lateral to the coracoid. After the glenohumeral joint has been inspected, change to the obturator once again and withdraw it from the joint, then redirect it from the same dorsal portal superiorly and anteriorly towards the anterior margin of the acromion. If the surgeon allows the tip to slide tightly against the undersurface of the acromion, it may be possible to enter superior to the bursa. Identification of the bursal space may be difficult, as normally it is fairly narrow. When entering the bursa, a

small change in tissue resistance is felt. Sweep the tip from medial to lateral several times in the bursa just posterior to the anterior border of the acromion and recognise the sensations from the tip when it is sliding with light contact on the undersurface of the acromion. Thereafter, start the infusion pump and fill the bursa.

The skin incision for the lateral portal will be about 3 cm lateral to the lateral acromial border and 1 cm posterior to the anterior border. Push a wide cannula with an obturator inside it into the bursa and localise the outlet cannula from the arthroscope or try to establish contact between the two tips. In most cases, an adequate view can be obtained with the 30° arthroscope directed towards the supraspinatus. Try to identify the margins of the acromion, especially anteriorly and laterally. There is a pad of fat under the acromioclavicular joint which can also be localised by pushing the lateral clavicle. A soft tissue shaver is used and in most cases some of the bursal tissue has to be removed before a good overview is gained. Electrocautery may be used for soft tissue resection, together with laser techniques, radiofrequency and other thermal devices.

However, "blind resection" should be avoided. Do not start resecting tissue before the shaver is localised and some anatomical landmarks have been localised. The localisation of the acromioclavicular (AC) joint and the anterolateral corner can be facilitated by introducing small needles from superior to inferior at these positions. Confirmation of an impingement situation can be seen in many patients as an erosion at the bursal side of the rotator cuff or at the insertion of the coraco-acromial ligament. The size and the extension of this bursa – the largest in the human body – varies a lot. Although it often extends several cm lateral and anterior of the acromion, it can generally be fully inspected from the dorsal portal. As there is no evidence that the bursal tissue is insignificant in relation to the pain in impingement situations, it is advisable to resect as much bursal tissue as possible. Continue to remove the periosteum and the extension of the coraco-acromial ligament on the undersurface of the acromion over an area of at least 2 x 2 cm, i.e. from the anterior border, and 2 cm posterior and all the way from the lateral border towards the AC joint.

When the bursa is cleared from all soft tissue and the acromial periosteum has been resected, change to an acromioniser or burr with a diameter of 4-5.5 mm. According to Bigliani et al [4], in most cases it is sufficient to resect an amount of bone equivalent to 5 mm at the anterior acromion. This resection decreases successively in height posteriorly and ends approximately 2 cm posterior to the anterior rim. One way of helping to estimate the amount of bone that has been resected is to start by establishing a groove 1 cm behind the anterior rim and to make this groove almost as deep as the acromioniser *(fig 3, 4)*. This groove is then levelled off posteriorly and 5 mm is resected anterior to the groove.

Some surgeons also prefer to abrade 5 mm of the anterior tip of the acromion so that it does not protrude anterior to the lateral clavicle [11, 25]. This technique transforms a type II acromion (curved) and type III acromion (hooked) to a type I (flat). In some shoulders with impingement, the acromion is a type I which is transformed to an inverted type II by this technique. Do not forget to resect the undersurface of the anterior lateral corner of the acromion.

The procedure is finished by inspecting the entire undersurface of the acromion to ensure that there are no troublesome spurs or other irregularities remaining. The insertion of the coraco-acromial ligament is resected *(fig 5, 6)*.

If the procedure is not performed under plexus anaesthesia, it is advisable to administer about 10 ml local anaesthesia, possibly mixed with 5 mg of morphine, to reduce postoperative pain. The incisions can be sutured since the shoulder is usually fairly swollen from the water leakage. This swelling will reduce in a few hours.

Rehabilitation

The postoperative regimen includes passive pendulum exercises each day. During the first two weeks, a sling can be used. After two weeks, active training can be started, and strength exercises with rubber bands can start after six weeks. Full physical activity should not be begun until after

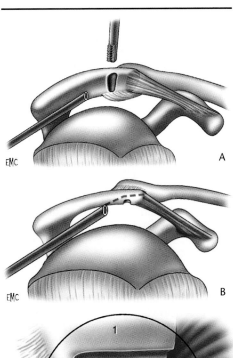

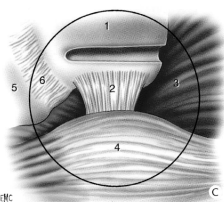

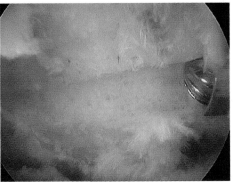

3 A. Lateral view: scope from posterior, burr from lateral portal, 5 mm groove in the undersurface of the acromion.
B. Lateral view: schematic drawing of planned resection.
C. Arthroscopic view from posterior portal, showing a 5 mm groove in the undersurface of the acromion (1). The coraco-acromial ligament (2) is intact and the lateral clavicle (5) is medial to the AC joint (6). The deltoid muscle (3) and supraspinatus part (4) of the rotator cuff are also seen.

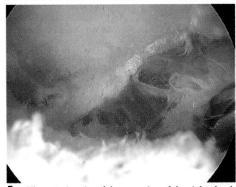

5 The anterior rim of the acromion of the right shoulder is being resected. Some fibres of the deltoid muscle are seen in front.

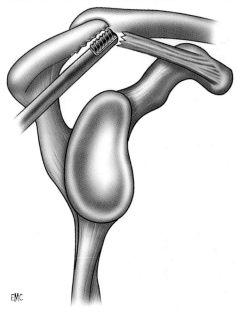

6 With the arthroscope in the lateral portal, the burr can be introduced in the posterior portal and held flat against the undersurface of the acromion during resection.

Special considerations

Many surgeons prefer to interchange the positions of the arthroscope and the burr at the end of the procedure. This technique ensures that the acromion is flat after the resection. It also makes it easier to resect the anterolateral corner of the acromion *(fig 6)*. In some patients, it can be advantageous to resect some part of the bursa or acromion with the arthroscope in a strict anterior portal.

Electrocautery and other thermal devices can be used to stop bleeding, especially in situations where it seems unwise to reduce the patient's blood pressure significantly. Murphy et al did not find less bleeding (or any other benefit) when using Holmium laser compared to electrocautery in ASAD [23].

There are studies which indicate that resection of the inferior AC capsule may induce minor instability of the joint as well as tenderness [7]. There is also a suspicion that this will cause future pain in the AC

4 Subacromial space of the right shoulder with the burr in a lateral portal. The groove in the acromion has been resected. Some patches of remaining periosteum are seen.

3 months. If the patient is carefully instructed after the procedure and given written instructions, there appears to be no advantage in scheduling a regular consultation with the patient [2].

joint upon activity [17]. Although Snyder et al [6] have shown that resection of inferior AC joint osteophytes during ASAD is safe, it is probably wiser not to resect a symptom-free AC joint even if there are osteoarthritic changes. If the patient has tenderness in the AC joint, a positive cross-body test and a positive injection test, then a concomitant ASAD and resection of the AC joint should be performed. If necessary the AC joint resection can be performed from an anterior portal (in line with the AC joint).

There are findings to indicate that calcific deposits in the supraspinatus tendon do not need to be resected at surgery. Loew et al [19] have furthermore shown that there is no correlation between calcifying tendonitis and other MRI findings associated with subacromial impingement. Tillander and Norlin [29] have shown that significant calcific deposits in the supraspinatus tendon decrease or disappear within two years after ASAD.

Lasares et al [18] have shown that the incidence of postoperative calcific deposits is higher after arthroscopic subacromial decompression than after the open procedure. Berg and Ciullo [3] have shown

that postoperative heterotopic ossification after acromioplasty or distal clavicle resection may be symptomatic. The incidence appeared to be higher among patients with pulmonary diseases. They suggest that these patients at risk should be given prophylactic treatment for heterotopic ossification when ASAD is planned.

Symptoms from an os acromiale (unfused anterior acromion) have been associated with symptoms from impingement [26]. ASAD with complete or near-complete resection of the unstable os acromiale has shown good early results. The technique is basically the same, except that the lateral portal is positioned in line with the fibrous nonunion, which is 1-2 cm posterior to the normal lateral portal.

If a patient has persistent symptoms after an ASAD and re-operation is planned due to a suspicion of inadequate bone resection, an open procedure is generally preferred [14].

Results

Many surgeons have presented functional results of the shoulders with 85-90 percent

rated as good or excellent [8, 13, 16, 24, 25, 27]. These results are of the same order as those after open procedures. The failures are generally attributed to inadequate diagnosis [14]. Full recovery does not generally occur until some months after the procedure [1].

Complications

The most frequent complication is extravasion of fluid into adjacent tissues. This is seldom deleterious, but it makes the procedure more difficult. Leakage is controlled by having the joint tissue tight around the cannulas, by keeping the pressure moderate and by avoiding prolonged operation times. Several different types of nerve lesions have been described [21]. In many cases it has been difficult to clarify whether these lesions are caused by the interscalene block or by the surgical procedure itself. One case with mid-clavicular resection is described as an example where the surgeon did not control the anatomy [10]. A bone resection which is too vigorous can of course result in a fracture of the acromion.

References

[1] Altchek DW, Warren RF, Wickiewicz TL, Skyhar MJ, Ortiz G, Schwartz E. Arthroscopic acromioplasty. Technique and results. *J Bone Joint Surg Am* 1990 ; 72 : 1198-2007

[2] Andersen NH, Sojbjerg JO, Johannsen HV, Sneppen O. Self-training versus physiotherapist-supervised rehabilitation of the shoulder in patients treated with arthroscopic subacromial decompression: A clinical randomized study. *J Shoulder Elbow Surg* 1999 ; 8 : 99-101

[3] Berg EE, Ciullo JV. Heterotopic ossification after acromioplasty and distal clavicle resection. *J Shoulder Elbow Surg* 1995 ; 4 : 188-193

[4] Bigliani LU, Colman WW, Kelkar R, Flatow EL, Pollock RG, Soslowsky LJ et al. The effect of anterior acromioplasty on rotator cuff contact: An experimental and computer simulation. Proceedings of the American Shoulder and Elbow Society, Orlando, 1995

[5] Bigliani LU, Morrison DS, April EW. The morphology of the acromion and its relationship to rotator cuff tears. [abstract]. *Orthop Trans* 1986 ; 10 : 228

[6] Buford D, Mologne T, McGrath S, Heinen G, Snyder S. Midterm results of arthroscopic co-planing of the acromioclaviculat joint. *J Shoulder Elbow Surg* 2000 ; 9 : 498-501

[7] Checchia SL, Doneu PS, Miyazaki AH, Funchel LF, Pinheiro JA. Proceedings of the 7th International Congress on Surgery of the Shoulder, Sydney, 1998

[8] Ellman H. Arthroscopic subacromial decompression: Analysis of one- to three-year results. *Arthroscopy* 1987 ; 3 : 173-181

[9] Esch JC. Operating room environment. In : Esch JC, Baker CL, Whipple TL eds. Arthroscopic surgery: the shoulder and elbow. Philadelphia : JB Lippincott, 1993 : 49-62

[10] Esch JC. The subacromial space and rotator cuff lesions. In : Esch JC, Baker CL, Whipple TL eds. Arthroscopic surgery: the shoulder and elbow. Philadelphia : JB Lippincott, 1993 : 365-405

[11] Flugstad D, Matsen FA, Larry I, Jackins SE. Failed acromioplasty and the treatment of the impingement syndrome. Paper presented at ASES 2nd open meeting, New Orleans, 1986

[12] Frost P, Andersen JH, Lundor E. Is supraspinatus pathology as defined by magnetic resonance imaging associated with clinical signs of shoulder impingement? *J Shoulder Elbow Surg* 1999 ; 8 : 565-568

[13] Hartig A, Rojczyk M. Arthroscopic subacromial decompression. Comments on indications and surgical technique. *Unfallchirurg* 1993 ; 96 : 109-115

[14] Hawkins RJ, Chris T, Bokor D, Kiefer G. Failed anterior acromioplasty. A review of 51 cases. *Clin Orthop* 1989 ; 243 : 106-111

[15] Hoe-Hansen CE, Palm L, Norlin L. The influence of cuff pathology on shoulder function after arthroscopic subacromial decompression: A 3- and 6-year follow-up study. *J Shoulder Elbow Surg* 1999 ; 8 : 585-589

[16] Jerosch J, Strauss JM, Schneider T. Arthroscopic decompression. 1-3 year results. *Z Orthop Ihre Grenzgeb* 1992 ; 130 : 406-412

[17] Kuster MS, Hales PF, Davis SJ. The effects of arthroscopic acromioplasty on the acromioclavicular joint. *J Shoulder Elbow Surg* 1998 ; 7 : 140-143

[18] Lazarus MD, Chansk HA, Misra S, Williams GR, Iannotti JP. Comparison of open and arthroscopic subacromial decompression. *J Shoulder Elbow Surg* 1994 ; 3 : 1-11

[19] Loew M, Sabo D, Wehrle M, Mau M. Relationship between calcifying tendinitis and subacromial impingement: A prospective radiography and magnetic resonance imaging study. *J Shoulder Elbow Surg* 1996 ; 5 : 314-319

[20] Matsen FA, Arntz CT. Subacromial impingemnt. In : The shoulder. Philadelphia : WB Saunders, 1990 : 623-646

[21] Mohammad KD, Hayes MG, Saies AD. Unusual complications of shoulder surgery. *J Shoulder Elbow Surg* 2000 ; 9 : 350-353

[22] Morrison D. The relationship between subacromial space pressure, blood pressure and visual clarity during arthroscopic subacromial decompression. *Arthroscopy* 1995 ; 11 : 557-560

[23] Murphy MA, Noelle MM, Boyd JL, Donald CQ, Buss DD. Cost-benefit comparison: Holmium laser versus electrocautery in arthroscopic acromioplasty. *J Shoulder Elbow Surg* 1999 ; 8 : 275-278

[24] Nielsen KD, Wester JU, Lorentsen A. The shoulder impingement syndrome: The results of surgical decompression. *J Shoulder Elbow Surg* 1994 ; 3 : 12-16

[25] Norlin R, Tillander B, Grund-Pedersen J. Virtual shoulder arthroscopy - An excellent tool in training and education. Proceedings of the 10th congress of the European Society for Surgery of the Shoulder and the Elbow. Salzburg, 1997

[26] Ortiguera CJ, Freehill MQ, Buss DB. Arthroscopic treatment of the unstable mesoacromion. *Tech Shoulder Elbow Surg* 2001 ; 3 : 219-224

[27] Speer KP, Lohnes J, Garrett WE. Arthroscopic subacromial decompression: results in advanced impingement syndrome. *Arthroscopy* 1991 ; 7 : 291-296

[28] Sperber A, Wredmark T. Intramuscular pressure and fluid absorption during arthroscopic acromioplasty. *J Shoulder Elbow Surg* 1999 ; 8 : 414-418

[29] Tillander BM, Norlin RO. Change of calcification after arthroscopic subacromial decompression. *J Shoulder Elbow Surg* 1998 ; 7 : 213-217

[30] Valadie AL III, Jobe CM, Pink MM, Ekman EF, Jobe FW. Anatomy of provocative test for impingement of the shoulder. *J Shoulder Elbow Surg* 2000 ; 9 : 36-46

Open anterior acromioplasty

F Postacchini
S Gumina

Abstract. – The skin incision runs from the lateral end of the anterior margin of the acromion to the lateral aspect of the coracoid process. In the presence of a pure subacromial impingement syndrome, the skin incision may be 4-5 cm in length. Alternatively, a saber-cut incision can be carried out. The deltoid can be sectioned transversely at a distance of 5 mm from the anterior border of the acromion or, preferably, detached with a needle-tip electrocautery from the bone. We section the coraco-acromial ligament and then remove its lateral portion, attached to the acromion, while performing the acromioplasty. The latter is carried out with an osteotome directed obliquely downwards and backwards to remove the antero-inferior portion of the acromion for approximately one-third of its sagittal length. The subacromial bursa is removed as extensively as possible, particularly when it is thickened. Areas of erosion of the bursal side of the cuff are excised and the resulting defect is then closed. Full-thickness cuff tears, when present, are repaired. Great care is taken to suture the edges of the deltoid, or to reattach the muscle to the acromial border with transosseous sutures.

Keywords: shoulder, impingement syndrome, open acromioplasty.

Introduction

Neer [7] first used the term "subacromial impingement" to indicate a condition characterised by different degrees of pathological change of the subacromial bursa and rotator cuff tendons, as a result of an abnormal narrowness of the coraco-acromial space. He described the clinical symptoms caused by the impingement, and the indication for surgical treatment, consisting of an oblique anterior acromioplasty.

Many authors have reported their experience with the open subacromial decompression, usually obtaining a high proportion of good results [5, 8, 10, 11]. In 1985, Ellman [4] reported satisfactory results with the use of arthroscopy. This study raised the question of which type of surgical treatment should be preferred in patients with subacromial impingement syndrome. Although this is still a current debate, it should be remembered that Lazarus et al [6] found that open surgical decompression gave a lower rate of unsatisfactory clinical

results and symptomatic postoperative calcifications, than arthroscopic surgery, independently of the learning curve of the latter.

Indications for surgery

Open subacromial decompression is indicated in patients presenting the typical clinical signs and symptoms of chronic subacromial impingement syndrome, when no improvement has been obtained by conservative management for at least 6 months. The main problem in recommending the operative treatment, is the lack of diagnostic investigations capable of irrefutably demonstrating that the patient's pain is caused by a subacromial impingement. The latter can be suspected when the radiographs (true AP view and 30° caudal tilt view) show a type III acromion [1], an abnormal thickness of the anterior aspect of the acromion and/or a gross proliferation of the latter extending beyond the anterior border of the clavicle, or marked degenerative hypertrophy of the AC joint. Shoulder arthrography is negative, unless a rotator cuff tear is present. MRI may show degenerative changes of the rotator cuff and inflammatory changes of the subacromial bursa. However, the most reliable diagnostic tool is the so-called

impingement test, which consists of injecting 5-10 ml of a local anaesthetic into the subacromial space. Results of surgery are significantly better in patients experiencing a considerable decrease or disappearance of shoulder pain, compared to those with little or no improvement in pain following the impingement test [9].

Patient positioning and preparation of surgical field

Either general anaesthesia or an interscalene block of the brachial plexus can be performed. The patient is placed in a modified beach chair position with the trunk angled at 50°- 60° to the horizontal plane with the head displaced and rotated towards the non-affected shoulder. A sand bag or towel is placed under the scapula to elevate it from the plane of the bed. A short arm board is connected to the operating table to support the forearm during the operation. The whole upper limb and the axilla, the shoulder, the supraclavicular region and the ipsilateral hemithorax are painted with antiseptic solution. The arm is draped free to permit shoulder movements during the operation. The inner sheets should be placed medially to the coracoid process to allow for

Franco Postacchini, M. D.
S Gumina, M. D.
Orthopaedic Department, University "La Sapienza", Piazzale Aldo Moro, 5, I-00185 Rome, Italy.

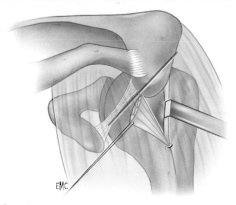

1 *The skin incision (continuous line) runs from the lateral end of the anterior margin of the acromion down to the lateral aspect of the coracoid process. The deltoid is cut transversely at a distance of 5 mm from the acromial border and the muscle bundles are split vertically.*

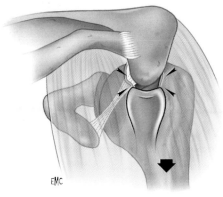

2 *The deltoid is sectioned just along the anterior border of the acromion, starting from the anterolateral corner of the bone and proceeding medially. Traction is applied to the arm distally (arrow) to obtain a better view of the subacromial space (arrowheads).*

palpation of the tip of the process, which is an important anatomical landmark, together with the anterior and lateral border of the acromion and the AC joint. To decrease bleeding, an epinephrine solution may be injected in the skin and subcutaneuos tissue along the skin incision. The surgeon is placed anterolaterally to the shoulder, and the first assistant cranially to him. The second assistant, placed at the level of the elbow, applies traction caudally and moves the arm, when necessary, during the operation.

Surgical approach

The skin incision runs in the line extending from the lateral end of the anterior margin of the acromion down to the lateral aspect of the coracoid process (fig 1). The length of the incision ranges from 4 to 10 cm depending on the patient's age and sex and, particularly, on whether a rotator cuff tear is present. In the absence of a cuff tear, a small skin incision, centred over the anterior border of the acromion, allows for an adequate subacromial decompression to be performed with little or no cosmetic defect.

An alternative approach is through a saber-cut incision, which starts from the superior surface of the acromion and extends to the anterolateral aspect of the shoulder, passing just lateral to the AC joint.

The incision is deepened to the subcutaneous tissue, thus exposing the anterior acromial edge and the superficial fascia of the deltoid.

The anterolateral border of the acromion and the subacromial space can be exposed in two ways:

1) The muscle bundles of the deltoid are split, starting at the level of the middle portion of the anterior border of the acromion, for a distance not exceeding 4 cm (fig 1). A suture is placed at the distal end of the split to avoid further separation of the muscle bundles, and possible injury to the axillary nerve. The muscle is then sectioned

transversely, at a distance of 5 mm from the acromial border (fig 1), leaving a lamina of muscle tissue to make the suture of the deltoid easier at the end of the operation. The drawback of this method is that the anterior border of the acromion may be poorly visible, thus making the acromioplasty more difficult.

2) The deltoid is sectioned with a needle-tip electrocautery just along the anterior border of the acromion, starting from the anterolateral corner of the bone and proceeding medially (fig 2). The incision is extended over the acromion, following a posteromedial direction, just lateral to the AC joint. To locate the anterior border of the acromion better, the surgeon can palpate the edge of the bone with a finger, while the second assistant applies traction to the arm distally to increase the acromion humeral space. The length of the deltoid detachment depends on the length of the skin incision and on whether the pathological condition is only a subacromial impingement or a cuff tear and, in the latter instance, on the size of the tear. For a simple subacromial decompression, it may be sufficient to detach only 3 to 5 cm of muscle from the acromion. A short deltoid detachment makes the acromial osteotomy more difficult, but has the advantage of facilitating the postoperative rehabilitation and speeding-up the functional recovery of the shoulder. This is related, to a large extent, to the length of the deltoid origin which has been left intact. When using this method, the deltoid may or may not be split longitudinally. The advantages of detaching the deltoid from the acromion are to obtain better exposure of the acromial edge and subacromial space, and to perform a more secure deltoid repair at the end of the operation.

In patients with a subacromial impingement, the anterior border of the acromion often appears thicker than normal, or its anterior border shows a more or less prominent spur, which is easily exposed when the deltoid is detached from the acromial edge. These findings, as well as a very narrow

subacromial space, are usually good prognostic elements for the result of surgery. If a large or massive cuff tear is present, this is clearly visible as soon as the subacromial space is exposed. Small tears can often be identified only after the acromioplasty.

Subacromial decompression

The coraco-acromial ligament is easily visible under the deep fascia of the deltoid, lateral to the AC joint. When the deltoid has been detached for a short distance only, the ligament can be felt with a finger as a fibrous band inserting into the inner portion of the undersurface of the acromion. The ligament can be sectioned at the level of its middle portion, or removed for about 1 cm, halfway between the coracoid and the acromion. In the presence of a massive cuff tear, an alternative is to detach the ligament from the acromion and to reattach it to the undersurface of the bone, to limit the upward migration of the humeral head [2]. The coraco-acromial ligament is simply cut after cauterisation of the acromial branch of the thoraco-acromial artery, which crosses the superficial portion of the ligament. The lateral portion, attached to the acromion, together with the caudal portion of the bone, are then removed during acromioplasty.

While distally retracting the portion of the deltoid detached from the acromion with its superficial and deep fascia, a periosteal elevator is used to detach the adhesions between the undersurface of the acromion and the bursal side of the cuff. The periosteal elevator or, alternatively, an osteotome, is placed under the acromion to protect the cuff and simultaneously depress the humeral head. The acromioplasty is performed with an osteotome 1 to 2 cm in width. The cutting edge of the osteotome is placed just below the anterosuperior border of the acromion, and the instrument is directed obliquely downwards and backwards to remove a wedge of bone whose base corresponds to the anterior aspect of the acromion (fig 3). The thickness of the base depends on the height of the anterior aspect of the acromion; usually 5 to 7 mm of bone are removed. Since the thickness of the acromion varies considerably in different individuals, great care should be taken not to remove too much bone and risk a fracture of the acromion. In the sagittal direction, approximately the anterior one-third of the acromion is removed, whilst in the transverse direction the osteotomy should involve the entire anterior aspect of the bone. A rongeur is then used to smooth the undersurface of the acromion and remove any remaining ridge of bone. The adequacy of bone removal is tested by flexing and abducting the arm. When enough bone has been excised, no impingement is detected while flexing the arm in neutral, internal and external rotation, whilst a residual

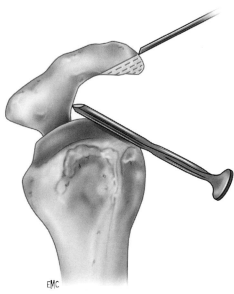

3 *An oblique anterior acromioplasty. An osteotome, or any flat instrument, is used to gently push the rotator cuff and humeral head down to expose the anterior border of the acromion better.*

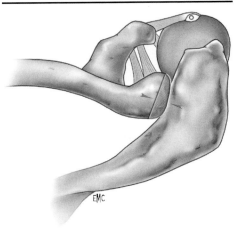

4 *The superior view of the right shoulder. Arrowheads indicate the clavicular portion that must be removed in the rare cases in which degenerative changes of the articular facets of the clavicle contribute to, or are responsible for, subacromial impingement. Not more than 1 cm of bone should be removed.*

impingement may be observed during abduction. This can occur when the most lateral part of the acromion has not been removed with the osteotome. In this instance, the undersurface of the lateral acromion should be removed with the osteotome, or a rongeur if the deltoid has not been detached from the lateral portion of the bone.

In approximately 10%-20% of cases, the undersurface of the AC joint contributes to, or is responsible for, subacromial impingement. When this condition is found, the caudal prominent part of the acromion and of the lateral end of the clavicle should be excised using an osteotome, a rongeur, or a burr *(fig 4)*. Rarely, a greater portion of clavicle needs to be removed. In this case, it has been suggested excising more bone inferiorly than superiorly, and more bone posteriorly than anteriorly, to preserve the superior AC joint ligament, deltoid origin and trapezius insertion [3].

In the presence of an unfused acromial epiphyses, it should be determined whether the unfused portion is a pre-acromion or a mesacromion before and/or during surgery. The former should be excised, whilst the latter should not only be preserved, but grafting and fixation may be necessary, particularly if the superior AC joint ligaments and trapezius fascia, which provide acromion stability, have been sectioned.

Bursectomy can be avoided when the bursa is normal in appearance. However, this may

be a poor prognostic sign, since in the presence of a true subacromial impingement, the subacromial bursa is almost consistently thickened, due to chronic inflammation. When this is the case, the bursa is removed as extensively as possible by grasping and cutting it with the scissors. The arm is then moved in all directions to detect small full thickness cuff tears or partial tears of the bursal side of the cuff. The latter are usually repaired by removing the area of partial tear and closing the cuff defect with slowly absorbable sutures.

Closure

Usually, no suction drain is used. The deltoid is reattached to the acromion with three or four transosseous non absorbable number 2 sutures. For the transosseous reattachment of the muscle, it is easier to insert the needle from the inferior rather than the superior aspect of the acromion, because after the acromioplasty, the trabecular bone of the inferior aspect is more easily perforated than the cortical bone of the superior aspect.

Injection of 20-30 ml of 0.25% bupivacaine into the subcutaneous tissue decreases the immediate postoperative pain. The deep subcutaneous tissue is closed with absorbable sutures; the superficial fatty layer with thin 3-0 catgut, and the skin, with running subcutaneous 2-0 proline stitches.

Postoperative care

Patients with subacromial impingement only, or an associate partial tear of the bursal side of the rotator cuff, wear a sling all day

for 2 to 4 days following surgery. They are then encouraged to carry out active pendulum movements of the operated arm several times a day. Five to seven days after surgery, passive shoulder exercises are started, both with the help of a physiotherapist and autonomously. In this phase, the use of a pulley is extremely helpful for performing passive flexion exercises of the operated shoulder, which is raised by the opposite arm. The sling is usually worn for at least several hours a day and during the night until the surgical wound has healed. Active shoulder movements are initiated 3 to 4 weeks after the operation, depending on the length of deltoid disinsertion from the acromion. A too early and energetic rehabilitation programme runs the risk of delayed reattachment of the deltoid to the acromion, and may result in shoulder pain and the appearance of a sulcus just below the anterior border of the acromion. This is more likely to occur when the length of the deltoid detachment exceeds 5 cm. A full range of active shoulder motion is usually obtained 4 to 6 weeks after surgery. Exercises of muscle strengthening are then begun and continued for 2 or more weeks.

References

[1] Bigliani LU, Morrison D, April EW. The morphology of the acromion and its relationships to rotator cuff tears. *Orthop Trans* 1986 ; 10 : 228

[2] Bigliani LU, Rodosky MW. Techniques of repair of large rotator cuff tears. *Tech Orthop* 1994 ; 9 : 133-140

[3] Craig EV. Open anterior acromioplasty for full-thickness rotator cuff tears. In : Craig EV ed. The shoulder. New York : Raven Press, 1995 : 3-33

[4] Ellman H. Arthroscopic subacromial decompression: a preliminary report. *Orthop Trans* 1985 ; 9 : 49

[5] Hawkins RJ, Brock RM, Abrams JS, Hobeika P. Acromioplasty for impingement with an intact rotator cuff. *J Bone Joint Surg Br* 1988 ; 70 : 795-797

[6] Lazarus MD, Chansky HA, Misra S, Williams GR, Iannotti JP. Comparison of open and arthroscopic subacromial decompression. *J Shoulder Elbow Surg* 1994 ; 3 : 1-11

[7] Neer CS 2nd. Anterior acromioplasty for the chronic impingement syndrome in the shoulder. A preliminary report. *J Bone Joint Surg Am* 1972 ; 54 : 41-50

[8] Post M, Cohen J. Impingement syndrome. A review of late stage II and early stage III lesions. *Clin Orthop* 1986 ; 207 : 126-132

[9] Postacchini F. Coracoacromial attrition syndrome. Anatomy, clinical aspects and surgical treatment. *Ital J Orthop Traumatol* 1989 ; 15 : 15-24

[10] Rockwood CA Jr, Lyons FR. Shoulder impingement syndrome: diagnosis, radiographic evaluation, and treatment with a modified Neer acromioplasty. *J Bone Joint Surg Am* 1993 ; 75 : 409-424

[11] Thorling J, Hakan B, Gunnar H, Hovelius L, Olle H. Acromioplasty for impingement syndrome. *Acta Orthop Scand* 1985 ; 56 : 147-148

Rotator cuff tears: the arthroscopic techniques

JF Kempf
F Bonnomet

Abstract. – Endoscopic sutures are without a doubt an interesting development, as they combine the recognised advantages of arthroscopic surgery with preservation of the deltoid. Arthroscopy may be performed in either the lateral or the beach chair position. A thorough assessment of the joint is a mandatory first step, to confirm the preoperative radiological aspect of the lesion as well as to evaluate its location, extension and tendon trophicity. The second step is analysis by buroscopy of supraspinatus tendon trophicity, thickness and reducibility into the tuberculum major, as well as the potential presence of an associated split. An acromioplasty is performed: the coracoacromial ligament is cut by electrocatutery. Suture insertion can be done as a one-step or two-step technique. In the first, the screw is preloaded with non-absorbable suture and passed through the tendon, then screwed into the bone. In the two-step technique, the anchoring systems require pre-insertion of the suture in the tendon with the help of a suture punch or a suture needle. If possible, the knot should be a sliding knot (for example, a fisherman's knot).

The best indication is a distal and isolated tear of the supraspinatus. In this anatomical situation, high rates of healing and good results can be achieved.

Keywords: shoulder, rotator cuff, tears, arthroscopy.

Introduction

At its beginning, the technique of shoulder arthroscopy improved our knowledge of the anatomy of the glenohumeral joint and subacromial region, as well as that of shoulder pathology.

Further development of reinsertion devices and sutures have improved the arthroscopic procedures for shoulder stabilisation and reinsertion of rotator cuff tears.

Johnson [20] surely opened the way with using metallic staples for reinsertion of the cuff onto the tuberculum major, as described in his first book published in 1986. Kempf et al [17] were the first in France to develop an interest in arthroscopic reinsertion of cuff tears, having used these staples between 1987 and 1991.

Then, several devices appeared which allowed suture anchorage into the bone (fig 1) and stitching without impairing the metallic structures left in the subacromial bursa [29, 32].

Jean-François Kempf, Professeur des Universités - Praticien Hospitalier.
François Bonnomet, Praticien Hospitalier.
Service d'Orthopédie, Hôpital de Hautepierre, 1, avenue Molière, 67098 Strasbourg cedex, France.

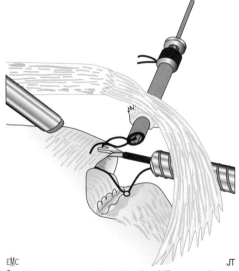

1 *Supraspinatus reinsertion by different anchor or screw devices.*

Suture techniques continue to improve with the development of increasingly better-performing anchors, and varied and clever autosuture devices. Some of the latter even avoid using knots, which are always a challenge in arthroscopic treatment.

Endoscopic sutures are without any doubt an interesting development, because they combine the recognised advantages of arthroscopic surgery (low morbidity, day surgery, no scar, less infection risk) with preservation of the deltoid. This point is important: every shoulder surgeon fears a failure of the reinsertion of the deltoid onto the acromial process in open rotator cuff surgery, as this usually leads to disaster.

Nevertheless, numerous problems need to be pointed out. Arthroscopic surgery is indeed a difficult and sometimes troublesome technique. Good preoperative radiological assessment is highly advisable, as evaluation of the rupture and the degree of retraction may paradoxically be difficult.

The therapeutic procedure itself is not free from pitfalls: correct positioning of the stitches for the anchoring device and tight knotting are not always an easy task.

We will discuss the various pitfalls of this technique later, with the aim of avoiding them.

Techniques

A complete joint assessment should be the first step. This should be followed by an acromioplasty, debridement of the tear margins, burring of the tuberculum major, and finally, by tendon reinsertion onto the bone.

JOINT ASSESSMENT

Arthroscopy may be performed either in the lateral position with the arm abducted 45° and under traction by a 5 kg weight, or in a semi-seated position (the so-called beach chair position).

A thorough joint assessment is a mandatory first step, in order to confirm the preoperative radiological aspect of the lesion and to estimate its location, extension and tendon trophicity.

The second step is an analysis by bursoscopy of the supraspinatus tendon trophicity, thickness, and reducibility onto the tuberculum major, as well as the potential presence of an associated split.

ACROMIOPLASTY

A preliminary thorough cleaning of the bursa will facilitate analysis of the supraspinatus tear.

At least two portals will be needed: a posterior portal for the scope and a lateral portal for the instruments. A third anterolateral portal is sometimes performed, lateral to the acromiocoracoid ligament, for efficient pump-aided washout.

After identification, the acromiocoracoid ligament is cut by electrocautery. The fibrous tissue covering the inferior side of the acromion is then carefully trimmed. Burring is started only after good exposure of the anterior and lateral corners of the acromion. A 8 mm large bone chisel is introduced by an anterolateral portal, as described for instance by Gazielly [14, 15]. In this way, resection of the anteroinferior corner, which is very aggressive towards the underlying tendons, may be performed. The authors trim the acromion with a motorised burr, aiming for the level of the inferior side of the posterior part of the acromion.

Others [13] use only motorised burrs for a complete acromioplasty, thus obtaining a perfectly flat acromion.

In fact, when repair criteria for a rotator cuff tear cannot be fulfilled, this type of acromioplasty may well be the only treatment possibility [3, 9, 13, 19, 20, 21, 25, 26, 28, 31].

DEBRIDEMENT OF TEAR MARGINS

Tear margins should be thoroughly trimmed with a rongeur until sound tissue is discovered. Only at this stage can tear repair criteria be assessed in a definitive way. Good tendon reduction onto the tuberculum major as well as muscle trophicity (already studied by preoperative CT scan: see "Indications" below) need to be assessed.

In case of retraction, a paraglenoid capsulotomy with a scalpel will debride the deep side of the supraspinatus; the superficial side can be debrided with a periosteum elevator.

In case of tensionless reduction, the arthroscopic procedure can be continued. If

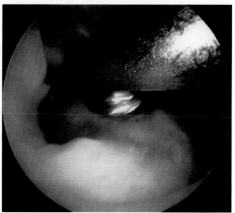

2 *Burring of the tuberculum major.*

not, it is advisable to convert the operation to a mini-open procedure, using a short longitudinal incision parallel to the medius deltoid fibres and landing on the tear. This allows performance of a conventional transosseous reinsertion onto the tuberculum major [1, 14, 16, 19, 25, 31].

MINI-OPEN TECHNIQUE

This relatively easy technique may follow an arthroscopic acromioplasty and acromiocoracoid ligament section. After a short lateral transdeltoid approach without any muscle detachment (a positive point of this technique), the tuberculum major is burred and the tendinous stump of the supraspinatus is refixed onto it [11, 23].

ARTHROSCOPIC REINSERTION OF THE ROTATOR CUFF

The initial step prepares the tuberculum major by burring until bleeding subchondral bone is seen (fig 2); nevertheless, the cut should not be too deep, so as not to compromise the solidity of the anchoring device which will be implanted.

The surgeon may now choose between two options: some devices such as the Corkscrew® (Arthrex) and Harpoon® (Biomet) are anchors passed through the tendon; alternatively, anchoring systems such as Mitek® (G2), Revoscrew® (Linvatec) and Statak® (Zimmer) require the pre-insertion of a suture in the tendon.

■ *One-step suture insertion technique*

The most commonly used technique was developed by Burkhart [11]. The anchoring device consists of a 2 mm core Corkscrew® (Arthrex); its small diameter allows an atraumatic intratendinous passage before screwing into the bone.

In this ready-to-use system, each screw is preloaded with two non-absorbable sutures (fig 3, 4). The Corkscrew® offers good resistance to avulsion from cancellous bone, and may be unscrewed in case of an operative incident. Nevertheless, visualisation of the screw position in the

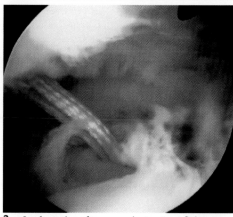

3 *Implantation of a supraspinatus transfixing screw with two sutures.*

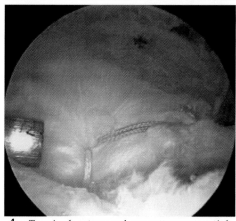

4 *Two simple sutures and one mattress suture tied.*

bone is much more difficult due to impairment of the visual field by the tendon margins.

■ *Two-step suture insertion technique*

Wolf [32] uses the Mitek® (G2) anchoring device. The first step leads the suture into the tendon margin with the help of a specially-designed tool, such as the suture punch developed by Caspari [7] or the Hauwkeye Suture Needle® (Linvatec).

The use of two cannulas, anterolateral and lateral, is mandatory. The definitive suture is passed through the tendon by means of a shuttle relay suture. The two suture arms are hooked by a crochet hook or a special grasper introduced into a cannula. One of the arms is then slid through the anchor or screw eyelet and positioned in the bone under direct view. Depending on the anchor or screw used, it may be necessary to predrill a hole in the tuberculum major.

Whatever the anchoring system chosen, two or three such devices must be implanted.

■ *Which stitch?*

The two classical stitches, at present the only two possible under arthroscopy (i.e. simple and mattress stitches) are not considered the best solutions by Gerber [16]. He has shown that the modified Mason-Allen stitch offers

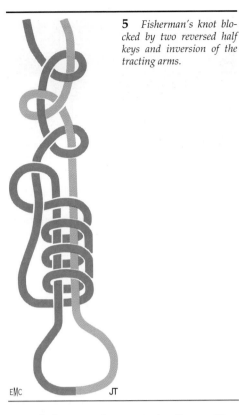

5 *Fisherman's knot blocked by two reversed half keys and inversion of the tracting arms.*

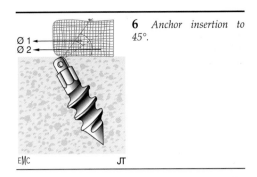

6 *Anchor insertion to 45°.*

a much better resistance to loading, with a rupture point reaching 359 N as compared to 184 N for the simple stitch and 269 N for the mattress stitch. Thus, it seems more advisable to perform mattress stitches than simple ones in arthroscopy, and even to double them.

■ *Knots*

Practically speaking, the surgeon may be confronted with two situations: either the suture slides in the anchor eyelet or it does not.

When the suture slides: D. Harryman and T. Loutzenheiser showed in 1995 [19] that the first knot has to be either a simple flat key or better a sailor's knot *(fig 5)*. This sailor's knot will be possible only if the sutures slide freely without tension; if not, they may break. For the following knots, the half keys must be inverted and the tracting arm as well, in order to ensure that the knot is blocked.

When the suture does not slide: it is not possible to use a sailor's knot. Two half keys in the same direction start the procedure, maintaining the traction on one arm and avoiding any pulling force on the second arm, until an inverted third half key is made to block the two previous ones. The next five or six half keys will be carried out, insuring their inversion and the tracting arm inversion.

■ *Which suture?*

Arthroscopic surgery imposes the use of long-lasting (six to eight weeks at least) and resistant sutures. Thus, only non-absorbable or slowly-absorbable material, such as PDS®, should be used.

C. Gerber [16] demonstrated that the best results regarding elongation and rupture tests are given by non-absorbable braided sutures, Ethibond® for instance. He reported good results for absorbable braided sutures such as Vicryl®, but their absorption is too quick, with an average duration of satisfactory strength varying between 12 and 30 days. Furthermore, PDS® type absorbable monofilament sutures offer not only good resistance but also high elongation under stress.

In practical terms, if an absorbable suture is desired, it is best to use a suture which is slow to resorb, such as PDS®; this is the suture we prefer for intra-articular surgery.

However, for highly stressed stitches, it seems wiser to use a non-absorbable braided suture such as Ethibond®. Although tying is harder to perform, the result is very solid. This is a very resistant and less-deformable material, and especially indicated for rotator cuff surgery.

■ *Pitfalls*

The inexperienced arthroscopist may encounter some problems:

Problems with suture insertion

Whichever technique is used, two large diameter cannulas are mandatory, generally lateral and anterolateral. Also, pre-insertion of a traction suture will be most helpful, especially in cases of large tears.

A wire-loop suture passer, such as the Caspar suture punch, will be placed at a right angle to the tear margin, and a shuttle-relay device used. The insertion of a crochet hook, the Linvatec® for instance, needs a much more tangential access to the tendon in order to transfix it easily. Here again, a shuttle-relay may be very useful, but it is also possible to use a wire-loop suture passer with a provisional no. 3 PDS® passed through the tendon, and then to insert a definitive suture.

Anchorage quality and tolerance

Arthroscopic reinsertion devices may lead to problems of tolerance and reliability.

As far as tolerance is concerned, the relatively easily performed stapling quite often imposes a revision operation for removal of an impairing metallic element. The recently developed stitches do not present this disadvantage.

Barber [2] has tested almost all available reinsertion devices, without comparing them to traditional transosseous sutures. He studied them in pork bone at different levels of the diaphyseal cortex, metaphyseal cortex and cancellous bone.

Schematically, all screwed systems and especially the larger ones come first in performance: the best performances were recorded for 5 or 5.2 mm Stratak®. A lesser resistance was offered by Mitek® anchors, Revoscrew® and Statak® 3.5 screwed systems, Tag Wedge Style® and Harpoon®.

The avulsion resistance of the various devices available reaches 100 to 200 N, comparable to the values for transosseous stitches. Nevertheless, the extreme variability of bony density in the proximal humerus, according to age and sex, needs to be pointed out. The most avulsion-resistant systems are also the largest ones, and their arthroscopic management is therefore more difficult.

These systems can be used in certain situations; we would not mind inserting them in rotator cuff tears without retraction and where the tension on the reinserted zone is expected to be low.

Positioning the anchor

This procedure is easier in two-step systems; the chosen anchor will be placed at a 45° angle to the tuberculum major plane *(fig 6)* to offer the best resistance to traction, as described by Burkhart [4]. If a one-step system is preferred, a tendon and bone transfixing screw (Corkscrew® for instance) may be used. The correct position of the material after insertion will be checked by lifting up the tendon margins *(fig 4)*.

Knots

Efficient knot tying imposes the avoidance of any twisting or mixing of the various sutures involved; thus, we recommend placing only one suture with its two arms into the cannula where the knot will be tied, the other cannula protecting the other sutures.

Results

MINI-OPEN REINSERTION

Flynn [11] records 100% success in his 10 cases. Liu [23] has performed this technique 44 times and reports 84% good and excellent results after an average 4.2 year follow-up.

ARTHROSCOPIC STITCHES

Only a few series have been published on this recent technique. Johnson [20], a pioneer of the method, reports in his book the results of 31 reinsertions with staples. 67% of the patients now have a pain-free shoulder and the best score is for distal tears. When performing a systematic removal of staples, he noted 7 cases of non-healing and a persistent continuity solution in 3 cases (partial healing).

Kempf et al [17] reported an experience of 20 patients with an average 18 month follow-up. The Constant score was 76 points at revision. Anatomically, 17 controls were performed either by an arthro-CT or by revision arthroscopy when staple removal was indicated. Healing was confirmed to be complete in 7 cases, partial in 5 other cases and missing in 5 patients. As a result, these authors have now abandoned this technique, because of the staple's aggressivity for the subacromial space, and small tears due to stitches.

Snyders [29] published in 1994 a preliminary series of 30 patients repaired with a Revoscrew® technique. He reported good results without giving any details encouraging this procedure.

Wolf [32] reported his 54 first endoscopic repairs using Mitek® anchors with resorbable no. 0 PDS® sutures. According to the UCLA score, his outcomes were excellent in 52%, good in 33%, medium in 7.5% and poor in 7.5% of the patients. An arthroscopic control of the repair was possible in 23 of his 43 patients, showing complete healing in 16 patients (70%), who claimed 80% excellent and good functional results, as well as incomplete healing in 7 patients who obtained only 71% excellent and good outcomes.

Gazielly [14] gave preliminary results of 15 supraspinatus isolated distal tears reinserted according to Snyder (Revoscrew®) between 1993 and 1995, with an average 17.7 months follow-up. He used an Ethibond® no. 1 type non-resorbable suture. The Constant score reached 87.6 points on an average. Results were excellent in 73% and good in 27% of the cases. An arthro-CT or ultrasound control showed cuff healing in 93.3%. He did not note any specific complications due to the technique, but there was one postoperative infection and one case of stiffness requiring manipulation under anaesthesia three months postoperatively.

Indications

The two conditions necessary for arthroscopic surgical repair of a rotator cuff tear to be indicated are:

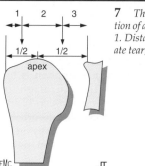

7 *Three grade classification of a supraspinatus tear: 1. Distal tear; 2. intermediate tear; 3. retracted tear.*

Clinically, the patient must be relatively young (less than 60-65 years old), voluntary and motivated. Chronic complaints, the importance of functional disability, and compensations for work accidents and insurance benefits should be taken into account as well.

Radiologically, an arthro-CT or MRI will indicate the severity of the tear, i.e. the amount of torn tendons: isolated supraspinatus, supraspinatus with a posterior extension towards the infraspinatus or supraspinatus with anterior extension towards the subscapularis.

The degree of tear retraction will be estimated in the frontal plane; we use Patte and Bernageau's classification [27]. This classification distinguishes between distal tears with a tendon stump staying close to the tuberculum major, medium tears where the stump retracts towards the apex of the humeral head, and finally, tears in the glenoid area *(fig 7)*. The position and state of the tendon of the long head of the biceps is also an important criterion.

The quality of the tendon stump may be estimated by its thickness, and the quality of the muscle by its fatty degeneration, as described by Goutailler and Bernageau [18]. This fatty degeneration seems to be a very important prognostic factor.

The subacromial space provides a good indication of the tear width. As shown by Walch [31], good clinical results after repair may be obtained only when the remaining subacromial space is larger than 7 mm. This is always the case when dealing with an isolated and distal supraspinatus tear.

Arthroscopic repair criteria must be respected. Our indication for this kind of procedure is the distal isolated supraspinatus tear *(fig 8)*. Any posterior or anterior extension will lead us towards conventional surgery, arthroscopic operations being extremely difficult in such cases.

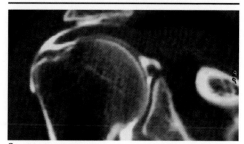

8 *Ideal indication for arthroscopic repair of a distal isolated supraspinatus tear.*

Long biceps viability is another important factor: a tenotomy or tenodesis will be performed if the long biceps is degenerated or unstable.

Perspectives

For the time being, we perform arthroscopic repair of rotator cuff tears only in patients less than 60 years old, who have good tendinous and muscular trophicity (fatty degeneration inferior or equal to 2), and only on isolated and distal supraspinatus tears, exclusive of any posterior or anterior extension.

Nevertheless, improvement of these techniques will probably lead to increasing indications, especially regarding the severity of cuff retraction. Whereas a posterior extension towards the infraspinatus should no longer be a contraindication, we regard an anterior extension towards the subscapularis as a limitation of the technique. Indeed, arthroscopic treatment of these superior lesions of the subscapularis, although theoretically possible, is a major challenge. The main pitfall is an underestimation of the lesions.

Second, an important intratendinous extension is very difficult to assess and to treat arthroscopically. We still regard this lesion as a contraindication.

We have already underlined the difficulty of tying tight and resistant knots. New systems are being proposed, which hopefully will no longer require knot tying. On the other hand, automatic stitching forceps such as Acufex® or Arthrotek® suture punches could help perform mattress or even Mason - Allen stitches, shown by Gerber [16] to have the best grip.

Although surgeons need to pay attention to new techniques proposed by manufacturers, we cannot forget that a good conventional surgical repair is always more rewarding than a brilliant but somewhat uncertain arthroscopic procedure.

References

[1] Adamson GJ, Tibone JE. Ten years assessment of primary rotator cuff repairs. *J Shoulder Elbow Surg* 1993 ; 2 : 57-63

[2] Barber AF, Herbert MA, Click JN. The ultimate strength of suture anchors. *Arthroscopy* 1995 ; 11 : 21-28

[3] Bartolozzi A, Andreychik D, Ahmad S. Determinants of outcome in the treatment of rotator cuff disease. *Clin Orthop* 1994 ; 308 : 90-97

[4] Burkhart SS. Arthroscopic rotator cuff repair: Corkscrew™ suture anchor technique. Oral communication at speciality day of Arthroscopy Association of North America. San Francisco. 16 February 1997 : 80-98

[5] Burkhart SS. Reconcilling the paradox of rotator cuff repair versus debridement: A unified biomechanical rationale for the treatment of rotator cuff tears. *Arthroscopy* 1994 ; 10 : 4-19

[6] Carpenter JE, Fisch DN, Huston LJ, Goldstein SA. Pull-out strength of five suture anchors. *Arthroscopy* 1993 ; 9 : 109-113

[7] Caspari RB, Thal R. A technique for arthroscopic subacromial decompression. *Arthroscopy* 1992 ; 8 : 23-30

[8] Ellman H, Kay SP, Wirth M. Arthroscopic treatment of full-thickness rotator cuff tears: midterm follow-up. *Arthroscopy* 1992 ; 8 : 403

[9] Ellman H, Kay SP, Wirth M. Arthroscopic treatment of full-thickness rotator cuff tears: 2 to 7 years follow-up study. *Arthroscopy* 1993 ; 9 : 195-200

[10] Fischer SP. Tying good knots arthroscopically. Oral communication at speciality day of Arthroscopy Association of North America. San Francisco. 16 February 1997 : 55-60

[11] Flynn IM. Arthroscopically assisted rotator cuff repair with Mitek anchor. *Am J Arthrosc* 1994 ; 1 : 15-18

[12] France PE, Paulos LE, Harner CD. Straight biomechanical, evaluation of rotator cuff fixation methods. *Am J Sports Med* 1989 ; 17 : 173-181

[13] Gartsman GM. Arthroscopic treatment of rotator cuff disease. *J Shoulder Elbow Surg* 1995 ; 4 : 228-241

[14] Gazielly DF, Gleyze P, Montagnon C. Functional and anatomical results after rotator cuff repair. *Clin Orthop* 1994 ; 304 : 43-53

[15] Gazielly DF, Gleyze P, Montagnon C, Thomas T. Arthroscopic repair of distal supraspinatus tears with Revoscrew™ and permanent mattress sutures. A preliminary report. *J Shoulder Elbow Surg* 1997 ; 6 : 199-200, 229-230

[16] Gerber C, Schneeberger AG, Beck M, Schlegel W. Mechanical strength of repairs of the rotator cuff. *J Bone Joint Surg Br* 1994 ; 76 : 371-380

[17] Gleyze P, Kempf JF. Résultats cliniques et anatomiques d'une série de ruptures de la coiffe des rotateurs réparées par agrafage endoscopique. *Acta Orthop Belg* 1995 ; 61 : 32-36

[18] Goutallier D, Postel JM, Bernageau J, Lavau L, Voisin MC. Fatty muscle degeneration in cuff ruptures: pre- and postoperative evaluation by CT scan. *Clin Orthop* 1994 ; 304 : 78-83

[19] Harryman DT, Mack L, Wang K, Jackins S, Richardson M, Matsen FA. Repairs of the rotator cuff: correlation of functional results with integrity of the cuff. *J Bone Joint Surg Am* 1991 ; 73 : 982-989

[20] Johnson LL. Diagnostic and surgical arthroscopy. St Louis : CV Mosby, 1993

[21] Kempf JF, Gleyze P, Bonnomet F, Nerisson D. Ruptures de la coiffe des rotateurs. Traitement symptomatique par acromioplastie sous arthroscopie. Résultats et analyse des 31 premiers cas. *Rev Chir Orthop* 1994 ; 80 (suppl I) : 194

[22] Kuhn JE, Hawkins RJ. Arthroscopically assisted techniques in diagnosis and treatment of rotator cuff tendinopathy. *Sports Med Arthrosc Rev* 1995 ; 3 : 60-67

[23] Liu S. Arthroscopically assisted rotator cuff repair. *J Bone Joint Surg Br* 1994 ; 76 : 592-595

[24] Loutzenheiser TD, Harryman DT 2nd, Yung SW, France MP, Sidles JA. Optimizing arthroscopic knots. *Arthroscopy* 1995 ; 11 : 199-206

[25] Montgomery TJ, Yerger B, Savoie SH. Management of rotator cuff tears : A comparison of arthroscopic debridement and surgical repair. *J Shoulder Elbow Surg* 1994 ; 3 : 70-78

[26] Neer CS. Anterior acromioplasty for the chronic impingement syndrome in the shoulder. *J Bone Joint Surg Am* 1972 ; 54 : 41-50

[27] Patte D. Classification of rotator cuff lesions. *Clin Orthop* 1990 ; 254 : 81-86

[28] Rockwood CA, Williams GR, Burkhead WZ. Debridement of degenerative, irreparable lesions of the rotator cuff. *J Bone Joint Surg Am* 1995 ; 77 : 857-868

[29] Snyder SJ, Heath DD. Arthroscopic repair of rotator cuff tears with miniature suture screw anchors and permanent mattress sutures. *Arthroscopy* 1994 ; 10 : 345-346

[30] Walch G, Marechal E, Maupas J, Liotard JP. Traitement chirurgical des ruptures de la coiffe des rotateurs. Facteurs pronostiques. *Rev Chir Orthop* 1992 ; 78 : 379-388

[31] Walch G, Nove-Josserand L, Levigne C, Renaud E. Tears of the supraspinatus tendon associated with "hidden" lesions of the rotator interval. *J Shoulder Elbow Surg* 1994 ; 3 : 353-360

[32] Wolf EM. Arthroscopic rotator cuff repair. Oral communication at speciality day of Arthroscopy Association of North America. San Francisco. 16 February 1997 : 71-74

Rotator cuff tears: the open technique

D Gazielly

Abstract. – The indications for open surgery of full-thickness rotator cuff tears are based on precise criteria for muscle-tendon anatomical lesions and depend upon the patient's ability to carry out postoperative rehabilitation. In all cases, preoperative imaging must provide the surgeon with as much information as possible about the tear, and preoperative rehabilitation must, within an ideal period of three months, be used to prepare, educate and better understand the patient. Under specific conditions concerning the indications, operative technique and rehabilitation, open surgical repair of reparable full-thickness cuff tears can be safely recommended, with or without a cuff reinforcement device, to motivated patients.

Keywords: *shoulder, rotator cuff, full-thickness tear, repair.*

Introduction

A rotator cuff tear is one of the most frequent causes of shoulder pain and is currently a frequent reason for orthopaedic consultation by an increasingly older population. However, full-thickness rotator cuff tears – partial tears are excluded from this chapter – do not all require surgery. The preoperative period is precisely an indispensable opportunity to identify those tears which can be repaired, basing selection first on muscle-tendon anatomical criteria and second on the patient's motivation and physical ability to carry out postoperative rehabilitation, which has been shown to account for one-half of final functional results [4]. When the decision for surgical treatment has been made on the basis of precise selection criteria, surgical treatment requires not only properly adapted technique but also, and just as important, postoperative rehabilitation which must be organised with extreme care, in order to avoid the well-known complications of this type of surgery.

Open surgery of "reparable" cuff tears

A rotator cuff tear is said to be "reparable" if the torn tendon or tendons have maintained

Dominique F Gazielly, M.D., Shoulder Unit, Institut de la Main, Clinique Jouvenet, 6, Square Jouvenet, 75016 Paris, France.

sufficient resilience and thickness to allow their tension-free reattachment, with the arm to the side, to the anatomical site of insertion on the humerus, and if fatty degeneration of one or more cuff muscles has not reached a stage where it could be responsible for poor functional results and/or recurrent postoperative tear [10]. It is mandatory that these anatomical lesions be identified and assessed by quality preoperative imaging before the patient is offered the opportunity of surgical cuff repair.

PREOPERATIVE PERIOD

The preoperative period has a twofold purpose: 1) to provide the surgeon with full information about the tear and surrounding cuff muscle status, and 2) to prepare and educate the patient through specific rehabilitation which will enable the surgeon and physiotherapist to better understand the patient's motivation [4].

■ *Preoperative imaging*

The objective of preoperative imaging is to assess the size and possible repair of the tear, completing the important picture provided by clinical examination concerning passive and active range of motion, and to identify the site of the tear, its anteroposterior extension (supraspinatus test, lift-off test, resistance to external rotation) and its muscle environment (possible atrophy of the supra- and/or infraspinatus fossae).

The preoperative imaging of choice is CT scan or MRI which should always be

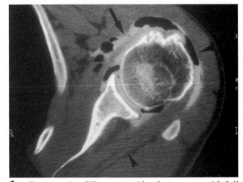

1 *Preoperative CT scan provides the surgeon with full information on the tear to be repaired.*

preceded by standard radiography to document indirect signs of cuff tear and any subacromial impingement, demonstrating the shape and thickness of the anterior acromion to be taken into account for anterior acromioplasty.

The surgeon should obtain as much data as possible *(fig 1)*. The retraction of the torn tendon(s) must not extend further than the upper part of the head for a tear to be considered amenable to tension-free repair. The tear may involve only the supraspinatus tendon or it may extend forwards to the subscapularis (anterosuperior tear) or backwards to the infraspinatus (posterosuperior tear), which will make surgical repair more difficult. Cuff status also enters into a difficult surgical prognosis: for example, a thinned tendon end or tendon lamination will add to the actual size of the tear. The stage of fatty muscle degeneration is

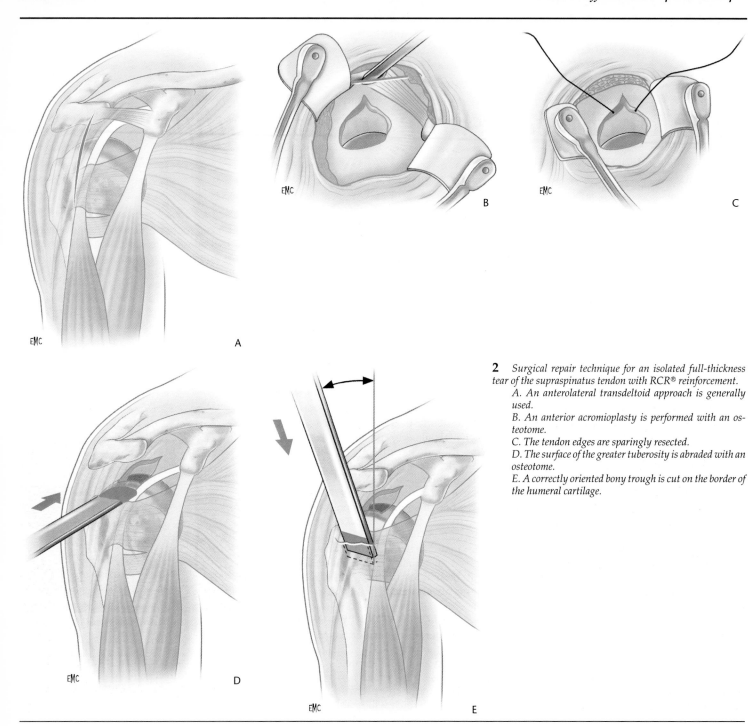

2 *Surgical repair technique for an isolated full-thickness tear of the supraspinatus tendon with RCR® reinforcement.*
A. An anterolateral transdeltoid approach is generally used.
B. An anterior acromioplasty is performed with an osteotome.
C. The tendon edges are sparingly resected.
D. The surface of the greater tuberosity is abraded with an osteotome.
E. A correctly oriented bony trough is cut on the border of the humeral cartilage.

proportional to the age of the corresponding tendon tear, with the exception of the infraspinatus, whose degeneration may not necessarily be associated with a tear of its tendon and which represents a risk factor for postoperative recurrent tear [10].

■ *Preoperative rehabilitation: to prepare, educate and better understand the patient*

The objective of rehabilitation is to overcome shoulder stiffness, especially in flexion and internal rotation. Any reduction in passive range of motion is a formal contraindication for surgery, as it always leads to postoperative stiffness [5]. The rehabilitation exercises learned by the patient are identical to those that will be carried out regularly

after surgery, with 3 to 4 daily sessions [6]. It is during this preoperative rehabilitation phase that the surgeon and therapist will learn to better know the patient's personality, his or her family and occupational environment, and his physical and intellectual ability to carry out rehabilitation exercises. We have shown that the optimal period for this preoperative phase is 3 months [7]. The study of a series of 671 patients for a Symposium held in 1998 by the Société Française de Chirurgie Orthopédique et Traumatologique (SOFCOT) confirmed that the ideal period between the indication for open surgical repair and the actual surgery is 3 months, which gives time to conduct imaging of the lesions and to rehabilitate a stiff shoulder.

This 3 month period is an apparently favourable predictive factor [1].

SURGICAL TECHNIQUES

Surgery can be performed under general or regional anaesthesia, whichever is customarily used by the surgical team.

The patient is seated in a beach chair position. The entire upper limb is prepared and draped. An anterolateral transdeltoid approach is generally used, avoiding unnecessary detachment of the deltoid *(fig 2A)*. A transacromial approach may be used to permit better exposure of the posterior superior cuff [11].

Anterior acromioplasty should preferably be performed with an osteotome and not with a motorised burr *(fig 2B)* [1]. The resection of the anterior part of the acromion must be sufficient to avoid any contact with the repaired, and possibly reinforced, tendon. The coraco-acromial ligament must be resected in its entirety to avoid any impingement with the cuff. The acromioclavicular joint is excised on its under-surface if inferior osteophytes are found. Resection of the lateral centimetre of the clavicle need not be systematic.

The subacromial bursa is only sparingly resected to expose the tear, as its vascular supply will make a valuable contribution to healing.

The technique used for surgical repair will depend on whether the tear is:

– restricted to the upper supraspinatus,

– an anterosuperior tear extending towards the subscapularis tendon, or

– a posterosuperior tear involving the infraspinatus tendon.

■ Repair of an isolated tear of the supraspinatus tendon

The tendon edges are sparingly resected (fig 2C). It is important to check that the torn tendon is mobile and can be reattached to the upper end of the greater tuberosity without being pulled taut. Coracoid detachment of the coracohumeral ligament and posterior superior capsulotomy will facilitate reattachment of the tendon to the greater tuberosity with minimal tension. Any lamination is sutured with nonabsorbable sutures. The long head of the biceps is systematically inspected for subluxation. The current trend is to perform tenodesis of the long head of the biceps in the event of subluxation or severe degenerative change. Tenodesis techniques vary: single suture to the rotator cuff, embedding in the bicipital groove, or use of metal anchors [13].

An osteotome is used to abrade the surface of the greater tuberosity, removing cortical bone to promote tendon healing in contact with bleeding cancellous bone (fig 2D).

A bony trough is made on the border between the humeral cartilage and the abraded greater tuberosity to permit insertion of the implant base; the trough must be directed towards the centre of the humeral head to avoid weakening the greater tuberosity (fig 2E).

The edges of the torn tendon are reattached with non-absorbable sutures through the bone of the greater tuberosity in the deep part of the trough. On the basis of the work conducted by the SOFCOT Symposium in 1998 [1], which focused particularly on the intactness of the repaired cuff at control imaging two years after surgery, it would appear that the suture technique had a statistically significant influence on the rate of recurrent tear. These rates were: 20% in the case of reattachment with U-shaped sutures which cross through a bony trough;

36% with U-shaped juxtaposed sutures in the bony trough; and 59% after use of simple sutures on Mitek® anchors with no bony trough ($P = 0.004$).

■ Repair of an anterosuperior cuff tear

The tear of the supraspinatus tendon may extend forwards in the direction of the rotator interval, laying bare the long head of the biceps in its intra-articular portion. These are difficult tears to repair, as the torn coracohumeral ligament is fragile and often difficult to suture, which may leave the long head of the biceps uncovered, a source of incapacitating postoperative pain.

The tear of the supraspinatus tendon may be associated with a reparable tear of the upper subscapularis tendon. The long head of the biceps may be in position in its groove with an intact superior glenohumeral ligament (fig 3A). If it is dislocated inwards, we prefer to perform a tenodesis rather than to attempt its re-positioning with the risk of incapacitating postoperative pain [8].

Reattachment of the subscapularis tendon is performed with nonabsorbable sutures mounted on 2 to 3 suture anchors positioned on the abraded lesser tuberosity (fig 3B), giving an anatomical repair (fig 3C).

■ Repair of a posterosuperior cuff tear

The tear of the supraspinatus tendon may extend backwards in the direction of the infraspinatus tendon. In this type of moderately retracted tear, the upper portion of the humeral head is entirely laid bare. It is necessary to assess whether it is possible to return the torn tendons to their anatomical point of insertion without undue tension, holding the arm to the side. Tendon retraction may require section of the coracohumeral ligament on the lateral edge of the coracoid process and a periglenoid capsulotomy so that the tendon may freely reach the greater tuberosity.

■ Technical variant: repair with a rotator cuff reinforcement device (RCR®)

In the vast majority of cases, the torn tendon is thinned and degenerate. It is known that there is a non-negligible risk of tear recurrence if a fragile tendon is reattached [1, 7, 12]. For this reason, since 1989, we have been using a cuff reinforcement device of polypropylene, RCR® (Biomet-Merck), to protect the reattached tendon and allow its safe healing with no risk of tear recurrence, especially during the first 45 postoperative days, during which range of motion must be recovered through early repetitive passive mobilisation [9].

The bony trough must be sufficiently deep and wide to house the implant base without having to bend the implant (fig 4A).

To avoid collapse of the 1 cm bone bridge when tightening the knot, if the bone of the

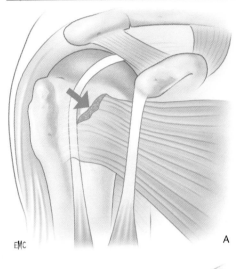

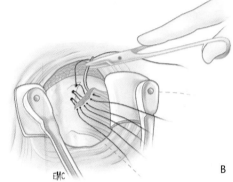

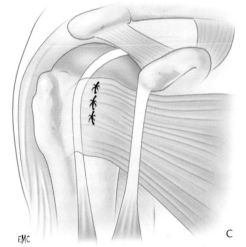

3 *Surgical repair technique for detachment of the upper two thirds of the subscapularis tendon.*
A. The long head of the biceps remains in position in the groove.
B. The subscapularis tendon is reattached with anchored sutures.
C. Anatomical repair of the subscapularis tendon.

greater tuberosity is fragile, it is possible to add support with two small plates of metal or bioabsorbable material (fig 4B). The tendon of the supraspinatus is now reattached to the greater tuberosity. The vertical side of the triangular tear is sutured with interrupted sutures which are pulled tight over the implant. Finally, the two branches of the RCR® are sutured to the supraspinatus tendon. The size of reinforcement is chosen such that the distal ends of each branch can, like the entire peripheral edge of the implant, be sutured

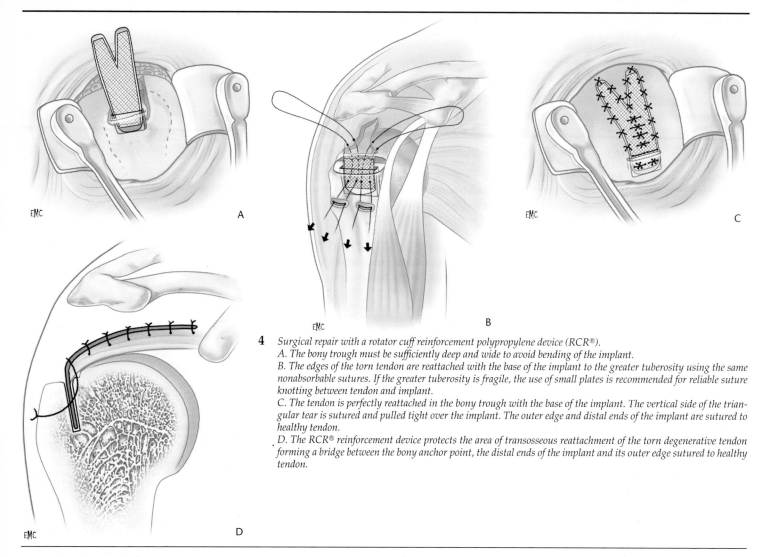

4 *Surgical repair with a rotator cuff reinforcement polypropylene device (RCR®).*
A. The bony trough must be sufficiently deep and wide to avoid bending of the implant.
B. The edges of the torn tendon are reattached with the base of the implant to the greater tuberosity using the same nonabsorbable sutures. If the greater tuberosity is fragile, the use of small plates is recommended for reliable suture knotting between tendon and implant.
C. The tendon is perfectly reattached in the bony trough with the base of the implant. The vertical side of the triangular tear is sutured and pulled tight over the implant. The outer edge and distal ends of the implant are sutured to healthy tendon.
D. The RCR® reinforcement device protects the area of transosseous reattachment of the torn degenerative tendon forming a bridge between the bony anchor point, the distal ends of the implant and its outer edge sutured to healthy tendon.

to healthy tendon and not to muscle, taking advantage of the elastic properties of the polypropylene braid *(fig 4C)*. Thus positioned, the RCR® reinforcement will protect the sutures used to reattach the degenerate tendon by bridging the reattachment area between the base of the implant, firmly anchored in the bony trough, and the two ends and outer edge of the implant sutured to healthy tendon. The RCR® is designed to reinforce the cuff and not to substitute for it *(fig 4D)*.

For repair of an anterosuperior tear, if a reinforcement of RCR® type is used, the anterior branch can be sutured to the coracohumeral ligament. In our experience, a tenodesis of the long head of the biceps should be performed whenever it shows degenerative lesions and cannot be properly covered at the time of repair.

The risk of re-rupture is very high in a posterior superior cuff tear [7], and the author feels it is necessary to protect the tendon reattachment with a rotator cuff reinforcement as previously described.

POSTOPERATIVE REHABILITATION

This must started the day after surgery with warm-up pendulum exercises and passive mobilisation, under continuous cryotherapy or adequate analgesia such as an interscalene block. Recovery of passive flexion must be given the utmost attention by the therapist and surgeon, as postoperative stiffening may be of sudden onset, causing pain and a subsequent vicious circle (pain and stiffness), especially if more than 3 months were required to overcome preoperative shoulder stiffness. It is essential at this stage to emphasise the contribution that the patient must make towards final functional results by regularly carrying out self-rehabilitation exercises at home. One of the advantages of the cuff reinforcement is that it eliminates the need for wearing an abduction brace and enables immediate passive mobilisation without limitation, in all ranges of motion, with no risk of early tear recurrence. In general, active exercising will be allowed only when passive joint motion has been fully recovered. Afterwards, deltoid muscle and humeral head depressor strengthening will restore a functional shoulder at the third postoperative month, and a "useful" or "sports" shoulder at the sixth postoperative month.

Results and indications

The results achieved after repair of full-thickness rotator cuff tears by open surgery can be analysed: first, in relation to the restored function of the operated shoulder, and second, by the anatomical results obtained on the repaired cuff. In order to use these results to guide a logical treatment strategy, patient review must be based on the same functional scoring system, and radiological analysis must be based on reproducible imaging of the repaired cuff. The follow-up period must be at least two years. Numerous authors have published results on the surgical treatment of full-thickness cuff tears [5], but the results of these different series are difficult to compare, because the functional scoring systems used are not the same, and often no imaging is performed to ascertain the anatomical results of repaired cuffs. However, these results do tally on one essential point: repair of a torn cuff must not be delayed too long and must be performed before the tear has become too extensive or fatty degeneration of the cuff muscles has become too advanced.

We refer to two multicentre studies which had the advantage of using both Constant's score system [2] and investigating anatomical results using ultrasound CT scanning or MRI: the European Symposium on the Rotator Cuff [8] and the Symposium organised by the Société Française de Chirurgie Orthopédique et Traumatologique [1], both of which entailed a series of more than 600 patient files.

The indications for open surgery of cuff tears relate to several criteria [3]:

– size of the tendon tear,

– extent of fatty degeneration, in particular of the infraspinatus and subscapularis muscles,

– whether or not the humeral head is properly positioned in relation to the glenoid,

– physiological age.

Indications also depend upon the factors below, some of which may indicate a poor prognosis [1]:

– age over 55 years,

– drinking or smoking habits,

– industrial injury,

– extended preoperative sick leave,

– medical treatment lasting more than 6 months,

– atrophy of the supra- and infraspinatus fossae,

– highly positive supra- and infraspinatus tests,

– limited passive forward elevation,

– preoperative Constant score of less than 40/100 points,

– subacromial distance of less than 6 mm,

– osteoarthritis beyond Samilson's stage 2,

– fatty degeneration of cuff muscles greater than stage 2 in Goutallier's classification,

– atrophy of more than 2/3 of muscle volume on the Y-view at preoperative MRI.

Indications depend upon these numerous criteria and predictive factors, and vary according to type of lesion: reparable or irreparable tears. In reparable tears of the rotator cuff, open surgery is indicated before the age of 55. Between 55 and 65, the indication for open surgery is determined by a favourable socio-professional environment, and fatty muscle degeneration must not be greater than stage 2. Open surgery of subscapularis tears should be performed at an early stage in order to guarantee good functional results and should entail tenodesis of the long head of biceps if there is tendinopathy.

Under these conditions for indications, which take into consideration a certain number of precise criteria and which exclude systematic surgical repair for all cuff tears, the particular complications of this type of surgery can be limited:

– Postoperative stiffness will be avoided if passive range of motion is restored preoperatively through a rehabilitation programme lasting an optimum period of 3 months, and if postoperative rehabilitation is started immediately and properly managed.

– Recurrent tears will be less frequent if open surgery is properly performed, step by step. The work achieved by the two symposiums referred to above demonstrates that the use of a cuff reinforcement improves the quality of anatomical results in supraspinatus and infraspinatus tendon tears, and that for both these tendons, reattachment in a bony trough is more reliable than fixation by suture anchors.

Overall, open surgical repair of rotator cuff repairs should not inspire apprehension, and will be all the more effective the earlier it is performed.

References

[1] Augereau B, Gazielly DF. Les ruptures transfixiantes de la coiffe des rotateurs, subscapularis inclus. Symposium SOFCOT, novembre 1998. *Rev Chir Orthop* 1999 ; 85 (suppl II) : 87-139

[2] Constant CR, Murley AM. A clinical method of functional assessment of the shoulder. *Clin Orthop* 1987 ; 214 : 160-164

[3] Coudane H, Goutallier D. Pathologie de la coiffe des rotateurs. *Encycl Méd Chir* (Éditions Scientifiques et Médicales Elsevier SAS, Paris), Appareil locomoteur, 14-350-A-10, 1997 : 1-12

[4] Gazielly DF. A model of rehabilitation for repair of the rotator cuff. In : Vastamäki M, Jolovaara P eds. Surgery of the shoulder. Amsterdam : Elsevier Science BV, 1995 : 455-467

[5] Gazielly DF. La rupture de la coiffe des rotateurs. In : Cahiers d'enseignement de la SOFCOT. Conférences d'enseignement. Paris : Expansion scientifique française, 1997 : 165-185

[6] Gazielly DF. L'épaule au quotidien. Montpellier : Sauramps Médical, 1999 : 1-252

[7] Gazielly DF, Gleyze P, Montagnon C. Functional and anatomical results after rotator cuff repair. *Clin Orthop* 1994 ; 214 : 160-164

[8] Gazielly DF, Gleyze P, Thomas T. The cuff. Paris : Elsevier, 1997 : 165-185

[9] Gazielly DF, Montagnon C, Constant CR, Jully JL. The use of a reinforcement of the cuff in surgical repair: a preliminary report. *J Shoulder Elbow Surg* 1994 ; 3 : [abstract 41]

[10] Goutallier D, Postel JM, Bernageau J, Lavau L, Voisin MC. Fatty muscle degeneration in cuff ruptures: pre- and postoperative evaluation by CT scan. *Clin Orthop* 1994 ; 304 : 78-83

[11] Goutallier D, Postel JM, Leguilloux P. Fermeture chirurgicale des coiffes non réparables par suture simple. *Encycl Méd Chir* (Éditions Scientifiques et Médicales Elsevier SAS, Paris), Techniques chirurgicales - Orthopédie-Traumatologie, 44-285, 2000 : 1-14

[12] Harryman DT, Mack LA, Wang KY, Jackins SC, Matsen FA. Repairs of the rotator cuff. Correlation of functional results with the integrity of the cuff. *J Bone Joint Surg Am* 1991 ; 73 : 982-989

[13] Molé D, Sirveaux F. Principes de technique chirurgicale. In : Les ruptures transfixiantes de la coiffe des rotateurs, subscapularis inclus. Symposium SOFCOT, novembre 1998. *Rev Chir Orthop* 1999 ; 85 (suppl II) : 100-104

Rheumatoid arthritis of the shoulder

JF Loehr
N Gschwend

Abstract. – As an initial manifestation of the disease, rheumatoid arthritis will affect the shoulder joint in approximately 10% of patients. However, in the general course of this illness, about 58% will develop shoulder symptoms. Since not only the articulating surfaces but also the soft tissues of the joint are in most cases affected, particular attention should be focused on the rotator cuff tendons early on. If medical and conservative measures have failed in restoring joint function and relieving pain, the surgical options are (after a possible early synovectomy): restoration of the rotator cuff and (if the joint has been destroyed) shoulder arthroplasty.

As constrained or linked devices have given poor results due to early loosening, a non-linked prosthesis will be employed in most cases. The decision to use a glenoid implant is based on the bone stock available and the function of the rotator cuff. In rheumatoid patients, the bone may be osteopenic making anchoring of the implants difficult at the glenoid side of the joint. In contrast to osteoarthritis, the wear pattern of this arthrosis is in many cases a progressive central erosion of the glenoid bone. In cases with advanced destruction and loss of the rotator cuff, a bipolar or reversed prosthesis might be considered to restore some function and to provide pain relief. Only in a few cases will arthrodesis become an option in the rheumatoid patient. Since rheumatoid arthritis is a systemic disease, careful assessment of the function and status of other joints is necessary to co-ordinate any other therapy required.

Keywords: shoulder arthroplasty, rheumatoid arthritis, rotator cuff, synovectomy, arthrodesis.

Introduction

In rheumatoid arthritis (RA), joint deterioration proceeds from synovitis to local pannus and subchondral erosions, and finally to progressive loss of the cartilaginous surfaces, leading to complete destruction of the joint [9].

In the lower extremity, any functional disorder of the joints will soon disturb the ability of the patient to move about, thereby reducing his or her personal freedom. Unfortunately, this is not the case in the upper extremity, since a functional loss can be compensated for a long period before the patient is finally forced to seek medical attention.

In rheumatoid disease of the shoulder, it is necessary to be aware of the involvement of the soft tissues in the process, and in particular, the rotator cuff. Therapeutic

Joachim F Loehr, M.D., FRCSC, ENDO-Klinic, Holstenstr. 2, 22767 Hamburg, Germany.
Norbert Gschwend, Prof. Dr. med., Former head of Clinic Schulthess, Lengghalde 2, CH-8008 Zurich, Switzerland.

decisions must be made early, since synovectomy may still be indicated or local therapy such as steroid injections may help with a subacromial bursitis. Thorough clinical examination is important, since radiographs can tell only a little about the status of the shoulder muscles and their tendinous attachments.

Once the rotator cuff has been lost or severe joint destruction has set in, few options are left, and arthroplasty must be considered for pain relief and restoration of function. Obviously, shoulder function depends on the presence of the shoulder muscles; therefore, once the cuff has become irreparable, other therapeutic means are required, such as a bipolar prosthesis [50] or the reversed prosthesis as initially presented by Grammont [15].

Incidence of shoulder involvement

The incidence of shoulder joint involvement in RA has been reported as 57% to 96% [19]. In a review of 300 rheumatoid arthritis patients [18], the figure was found to be 58%.

Table I. – Incidence of rheumatoid arthritis by joint (n=300) [18].

Shoulder	58%
Elbow	53%
Wrist	66.6%
Finger joints	95%
Hip joints	17%
Knee joints	74.3%
Ankle and midfoot joints	52%
Forefoot	79.3%

All of these patients had an average 10-year history of onset of RA before the relevant shoulder problems became obvious (*table I*).

Rheumatoid arthritis in the shoulder joint will be the initial manifestation of the disease in less than 10% of patients [17]. As one might expect, pain is often the first symptom, followed by functional disability, in particular for elevation or rotation against resistance or loads. When the rotator cuff tendons have been torn for a longer period, muscle atrophy might present at clinical inspection, with a loss of the physiological shoulder/neck contour, particularly in the supraspinatus fossae [27]. In rare cases, a localised swelling resembles a ganglion of

Table II. – Cumulative incidence for the onset of shoulder, elbow and wrist symptoms in RA [19].

Years after onset	Shoulder (%)*	Elbow (%)*	Wrist (%)*
0-2	48.7	33.3	67.5
3-4	58.7	38.3	70.9
5-6	66.7	52.5	84.2
7-8	71.4	55.0	90.0
9-10	77.4	63.3	90.8
11-12	82.0	65.0	95.0
13-14	83.3	65.9	95.0
15-16	83.3	66.7	95.0
17+	83.3	66.7	95.0

* mean involvement rate of right and left extremities

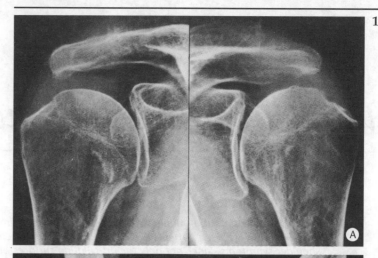
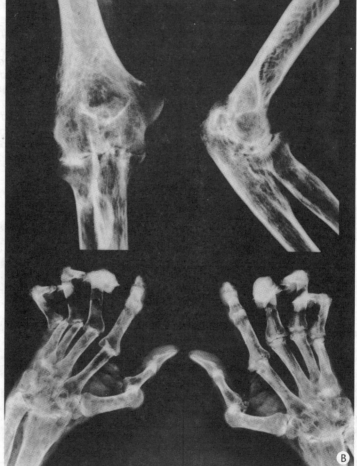

1 *A. Symmetrical early involvement of the shoulder articulations in a patient.*
B. Concurrent destruction of the elbow, wrist and finger joints in the same patient.

the AC joint; most frequently this will point to an active bursitis. Advanced involvement of the rotator cuff may be suspected in cases of spontaneous rupture of the long head of the biceps tendon [47].

Hämäläinen [19] has summarised the incidence of onset of rheumatoid arthritis in the upper extremity *(table II)*.

Pre-operative planning

PHYSICAL EXAMINATION AND CLINICAL SIGNS

As for all patients, but particularly in the RA patient, a careful examination of the cervical spine should be included in the physical examination to rule out secondary compression of cervical nerve roots or possible upper motor neuron signs with pseudobasilar impression [17].

Active and passive range of motion of the shoulder joint should be assessed, as well as muscular function. In most rheumatoid patients, many other joints will be involved, so the full chain of articulations must be assessed for the involved arm *(fig 1)*. Bilateral disease should be suspected, as well as further joint involvement of the lower extremities, which may make the use of crutches necessary in the future. This would create an additional burden on the shoulder joints and challenge any rehabilitation after shoulder surgery [14].

RADIOLOGICAL EXAMINATION

■ Classifications

Plain radiographs are needed before any intervention is undertaken [8]. Two AP views in 45° of internal and external rotation and an axillary view should be obtained *(fig 2)*. Neer [35] described three types of radiographic stages for rheumatoid arthritis:

– the wet type with periarticular erosions;

– the dry type similar to an osteoarthrosis but with less osteophytes;

– the resorptive type, with advanced bone loss, erosions and local cysts.

Since this classification assessed only the humeral head changes, Levigne [29] tried to co-ordinate the radiographic types for humeral head destruction with those of the glenoid, as well as the spatial relationship of the humeral head and the corresponding glenoid.

For the humeral head, he distinguished between three grades:

– grade I - subchondral bone intact;

– grade II - local cysts at the minor tubercle;

– grade III - loss of the spherical configuration of the humeral head.

For the glenoid:

– grade I - subchondral bone normal;

– grade II - migration of the glenoid face to the level of the coracoid base;

– grade III - glenoid bone loss medial to the coracoid base.

In an attempt to qualify also the state of the soft tissues involved, he distinguished between:

– an ascending type of deformity, where the humeral head migrates superiorly;

– a central form where the humeral head goes to the centre of the glenoid, often associated with stiffness; and

– the destroyed form.

Obviously, all classifications since the original description of the six grades by Larsen, Dahle and Eeck [26] have limitations

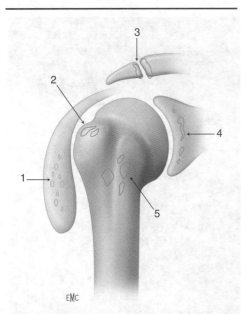

2 *Radiographic signs of rheumatoid arthritis. 1. Synovitis and rice bodies; 2. erosions and crypts; 3. A-C arthrosis and thinning of the acromion; 4. central cavity deformity with little osteophyte formation; 5. cysts.*

in providing proper staging of the state of the soft tissues related to the bony destruction *(fig 3)*.

■ **Incidence of radiological changes**

In a radiological analysis of 73 RA patients with 144 shoulder joints (2 joints which had been arthrodesed were excluded) entering the hospital for any orthopaedic surgical intervention except on the shoulder joint, a symmetrical and almost equal involvement of both shoulders was found [18]. The functional handicap of 2 groups of patients was compared. In group 1, both shoulders were radiologically staged Larsen grade 5; in group 2 both shoulders were unaffected (Larsen stage 0). It was found that all patients in group 1 belonged to the ARA (American Rheumatoid Association) Steinbrocker-Functional classes 3 and 4 (severe handicap), while those of group 2 belonged to classes 1 and 2 (no or slight handicap) *(table III)*.

■ **Rotator cuff assessment**

The functional impairment resulting from shoulder involvement in rheumatoid arthritis depends only partly on the integrity of the joint surfaces. Equal importance must be attributed to the state of the rotator cuff muscles [43]. Pathological changes within these muscle groups (fatty degeneration, thinning, or more or less extensive tears) may cause, in the earlier stages, pain due to a subacromial impingement syndrome (painful arc between 70-120°) and, in the more advanced stages, weakness and loss of function (pseudoparalysis). The site and size of the tear will determine which movements will be altered or become impossible [39]. Ultrasonography and MRI allow detection of the pathological changes in the rotator cuff [8].

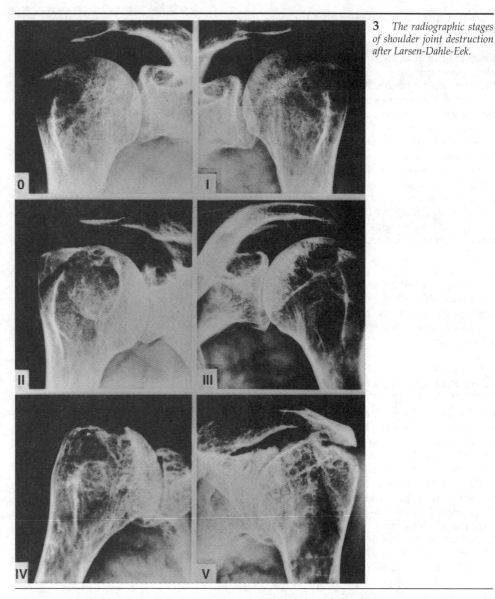

3 *The radiographic stages of shoulder joint destruction after Larsen-Dahle-Eek.*

Table III. – Radiographic signs in rheumatoid arthritis of the shoulder joint [18].

1. Decalcification, osteopenia, rounded structural changes	27-50%
2. Fissuring at the anatomical neck, subchondral erosions, ankylosing spondylitis, caries sicca, habitual shoulder disolocation	38-40%
3. Loss of joint space, subchondral bone destruction, bony ankylosis	16%
4. Erosion of subcondral bone	} 18%
5. Subchondral cysts with infection of the joint surfaces	
6. Osteosclerosis: particularly at the major tuberculum, mix of subchondral sclerosis with osteopenia, osteophyte formation	10%
7. Head deformation, osteolysis, secondary osteonecrosis	up to 20%
8. Increased subacromial space due to large bursitis	over 6%
9. AC-joint changes due to erosion, osteolysis, subluxation, diastasis, subluxation/luxation of the humeral head	up to 28%
10. Cranial migration with formation of a humeral acromial neo-arthrosis	11%
11. Fossa destruction	4%

Conservative treatment

The main goal in treating the rheumatoid patient will be directed towards the systemic disease by means of various medications (e.g. NSAIDs (non-steroidal anti-inflammatory drugs), gold, methotrexate) [9]. Physical measures and physiotherapy for the involved extremity attempt to retain joint mobility and to strengthen muscles, thereby centralising the shoulder joint after the inflammatory parameters have regressed [45].

A rheumatologist or a rehabilitation specialist with an interest in this particular disease should monitor such patients.

In the initial inflammatory phase, implementation of assisted range of motion (ROM) exercises will be limited, so as to avoid development of an adhesive capsulitis. Anterior elevation and external rotation are the main planes of interest at this stage. This will be accompanied by initial cryotherapy, in addition to medication with NSAIDs, and optional subacromial infiltration with a local anaesthetic. Local injection of an additional steroid depends on the state of the tissues and on exclusion of a possible infection [44]. Once the inflammatory phase has subsided, electrotherapy and paracervical thermal therapy will be begun. At this point, active assisted ROM exercises are started, focusing on isometric-concentric exercises of the humeral head against the glenoid. Attention must be paid to the scapulothoracic rhythm, with stabilisation of the scapula against the upper back to allow a glenohumeral motion without functional impingement [23]. Once pain-free motion has been obtained, eccentric exercises may be added, as well as training against weights. This should be co-ordinated with proprioceptive training of the arm [2].

It is obvious that one should not proceed with any conservative measures, and in particular physiotherapy, when the joint is destroyed or when the rotator cuff tear has advanced to such a degree as to render the joint unstable.

Operative options

Obviously, surgery should be given the preference if it can halt further joint destruction. One option in the early stages of the disease (Larsen stages 1 and 2) would be a synovectomy (radiosynoviorthesis and/or arthroscopic or open synovectomy) [16]. It is essential to be aware that there may be quite a difference between functional loss and the radiographic appearance of the joint; the treating physician and surgeon should suspect a possible loss of function in the rotator cuff, despite joint surfaces which still appear radiographically adequate. Hence, prevention of progressive rotator cuff tearing or reconstruction of the cuff has a high priority in the rheumatoid patient.

SYNOVECTOMY AND REPAIR OF ROTATOR CUFF TEAR

Considering the pathogenesis of the disease, it seems possible that the removal of all inflammatory tissue within the joint would lead to a partial abatement of further destruction, improved function and reduced pain [33]. Success seems to be related to the joints involved, the state of the soft tissues and the amount of synovitis present.

In addition to the clinical evaluation, ultrasonography and MRI will help to determine the state of the soft tissue involvement, and whether an early arthroscopic synovectomy is still of value [28].

The effectiveness of radiosynovectomy depends on the intra-articular situation. Here, the thickness of the synovial "carpet" will determine the effectiveness of penetration of the isotopes. Therefore, it seems sensible to perform an arthroscopic synovectomy 6 to 8 weeks before radiosynoviorthesis, so as to reduce the

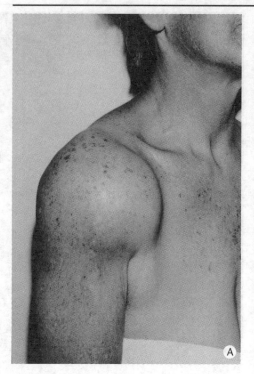
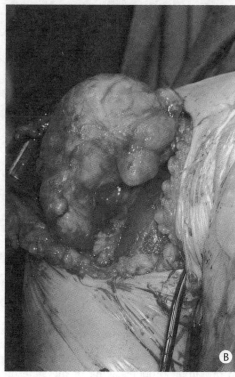

4   *A. Massive swelling of a shoulder joint due to extensive bursitis.*
   B. Peroperative situation with massive synovitis and rice bodies within the joint cavity and subacromial/subdeltoid space.

thickness of the synovial surfaces and give the radioisotopes a better chance to act upon the remaining tissues. At the same time, an arthroscopic synovectomy will reduce the load of joint-destructive enzymes and fibrin within the joint. It will also allow visual assessment of the joint surfaces and the state of the rotator cuff tendons, with the option of repair through a "mini-open" approach [28].

In the presence of larger rotator cuff tears, one can still proceed with a synovectomy, preferably carried out at the same time as cuff repair (fig 4A, B). The usual operative approaches and techniques for mobilisation and bony fixation of the cuff should be used [11]. In all cases, the coraco-acromial ligament should be preserved in order to prevent later cranioventral subluxation of the humeral head [32].

Rehabilitation after a radiosynovectomy will depend on any additional procedure performed. If the rotator cuff has been repaired, application of an abduction brace is suggested for approximately 6 weeks, with limited passive assisted exercises, going on to active assisted exercises after this period.

The results of arthroscopic synovectomy have been reported in only a few studies [9, 16, 33], and no long-term results have been presented. In two-thirds of the cases, pain and residual effusion can be reduced for a longer period, but the radiographic progression of joint disease can be prevented in only a few cases. This is one of the reasons why it is necessary to ensure close follow-up of the shoulder joint in patients

with rheumatoid arthritis, as not to miss the point of rupture or deterioration of the rotator cuff.

SHOULDER ARTHROPLASTY *(fig 5)*

Shoulder arthroplasty has become a reliable way to treat the rheumatoid patient with a painful destroyed joint and severe functional impairment [24]. An intact rotator cuff is the best prerequisite for a good functional result. A difficult aspect is the degree of bony destruction present in the glenoid, where central erosion (as is common in rheumatoid arthritis in contrast to the posterior erosion in osteoarthritic patients) may lead to a complete loss of the subchondral bone [29, 32]. This can create difficulties in finding adequate bone support to anchor a glenoid component.

Obvious contraindications for implantation of a shoulder joint prosthesis will be the presence or suspicion of active infection, or a mutilating type of rheumatoid arthritis (fig 6) with complete loss of the bony structures and extensive changes involving the acromion and AC joint [37].

Shoulder arthroplasty can be divided into linked-constrained prostheses or unconstrained prostheses. As the linked prosthesis has gone out of favour due to the high rate of early loosening [51, 52], unlinked prosthetic components are employed in most cases. Here, the options are: only to resurface the humeral head (such as in a hemiarthroplasty [11]) or to perform a total arthroplasty in which the glenoid is replaced as well [42]. In addition to "bipolar" arthroplasty [49], more recently the "reverse"

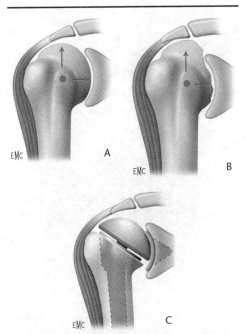

5 *A. Normal shoulder joint. Note the relationship of the rotator cuff to the humeral head and that of the centre of the head towards the centre of the glenoid.*
B. With rheumatoid destruction, medialisation of the joint occurs with loss of the rotator cuff and high riding of the head cranially.
C. Arthroplasty attempts to restore the anatomical configuration of the joint for the centre of rotation as well as the distance between the humeral head and the acromion.

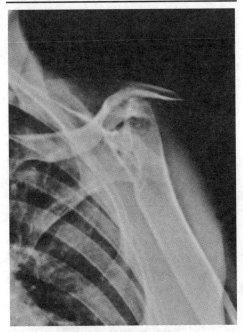

6 *Advanced rheumatoid disease of the mutilating type with complete loss of the rotator cuff.*

prosthesis has been introduced in an attempt to restore shoulder function despite the complete loss of the rotator cuff [3, 15].

Most commonly, a total shoulder arthroplasty will be indicated in rheumatoid patients when the articulating surfaces of the humeral head and the glenoid are destroyed but a proper soft tissue envelope is still present [24, 25].

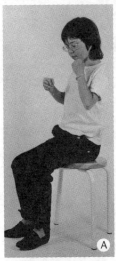
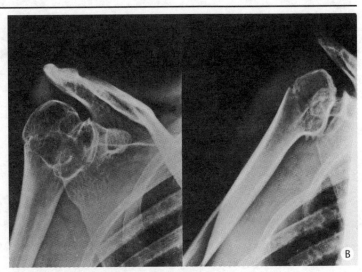

7 *A. Patient with juvenile arthritis: destroyed and painful, partially stiff shoulder joints.*
B. Shoulder joints of the same patient, not suitable for any resurfacing procedure.

Since the early success of the Neer I / Neer II prosthesis [34, 35], other devices have been introduced, reflecting in their modifications our increased knowledge of the biomechanics of joint function (Boileau and Walch [5, 46], Gerber [13]). These devices allow a much more anatomical reconstruction, giving a joint configuration which will resemble the patient's original physiological and anatomical situation.

In the rheumatoid patient, assessment of the available bone stock is a preoperative necessity. After plain radiographs, a CT examination will most likely show best any erosions and osteophytes, and delineate the version of the head versus the glenoid surface. Examination of the opposite shoulder joint for comparison may be helpful if orientation is difficult. Then, a decision can be made as to whether a glenoid reconstruction can be attempted and whether bone graft is necessary (this can easily be obtained from the resected humeral head). The other preoperative requirement is assessment of the soft tissues [21]. If the examiner has sufficient personal experience with this technique, it can easily be done through ultrasonography or MRI (magnetic resonance imaging). Since MRI is not necessarily the best tool to assess the bony situation, one might wish to compromise with an Arthro-CT (computer tomography) in some cases.

In the rheumatoid patient, most of the implants will be cemented; evidence is still missing as to whether an uncemented device might give similar success [6, 30]. Consideration must also be given to the possible need for an exchange operation at a later stage, with the option of removing an implant without destruction of the humeral shaft [48]. Rydholm [41] and others [1, 7, 22] have described cup arthroplasty. This procedure does not require the same head-neck resection as for a standard prosthesis and has in most cases replaced the indication for a resection-interposition arthroplasty [10]. It may be an option in the juvenile rheumatoid

patient, but not necessarily in the older patient where in many cases the bone stock is not suitable to support the cup (fig 7A, B). Prior to any procedure, it is important to have a clinical and radiographic assessment of the cervical spine, as positioning of the patient on the table and intubation may lead to secondary strain on the cervical column.

Surgical technique

APPROACH

The surgical technique follows the same principles as any other total shoulder or hemiarthroplasty. Usually, the deltopectoral approach will be used, retracting the cephalic vein medially. This will allow good access to the glenoid. In almost all cases, the conjoined tendon can be preserved in its origin from the coracoid process and this will protect the musclocutaneous nerve from possible injury.

In case of excessive contraction deformity, an extended exposure can be obtained by incising the proximal part of the distal deltoid insertion, or in rare cases, by developing the deltoid from the anterior acromion. Here, a periosteal sleeve should be retained to allow for later secure reattachment. Care should be taken when retracting the deltoid muscle, because it may be easily injured in the rheumatoid patient, and the acromial bone itself may be so frail as to fracture. The subacromial space is then freed with a Cobb elevator or by digital manipulation. A thickened bursa may be removed with a rongeur, with care not to injure the rotator cuff. In many cases, the long head of the biceps tendon will be rather prominent through a synovial fluid-filled sac in the intertubercular groove. Care should be taken to inspect the tendon (extra- and intra-articular) so as not to miss any fraying and possible eminent rupture. A tenodesis is then recommended.

The subscapularis tendon is elevated approximately 1/2 cm from its insertion;

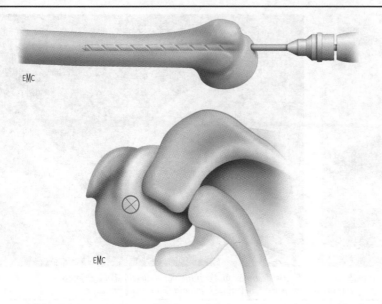

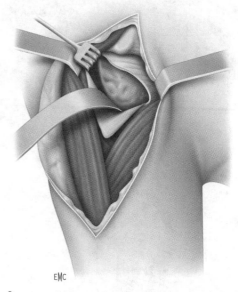

8 *It is important to find the isometric centre of the humeral shaft in relation to the humeral head. Only then will alignment of the various jigs supplied with the implants become possible.*

9 *View of a destroyed ebonised glenoid. Note the central erosion and sharp ventral/dorsal osteophytes.*

however, if it is thinned, it might be better to take it with a thin bony sliver from the lesser tubercle to allow for later reattachment. The axillary nerve should be visualised to permit later mobilisation of the capsule-tendon unit without possible nerve injury. In many cases, developing the plane between the subscapularis muscle and the capsule is impossible due to the intimate attachment and secondary fibrosis of the structures caused by the disease. Therefore, the capsule is incised along the glenoid rim and the humeral head can in most cases then be easily delivered. Should there be any resistance due to a tight inferior capsule or a dorsal subluxation, care should be taken not to attempt to dislocate the humeral head with force; in osteopenic bone this may cause fracture of the humeral shaft.

ORIENTATION OF IMPLANTS

Once the proper rotation of the humerus has been found *(fig 8)* and the head has been resected, the posterior capsule is liberated but not necessarily taken off the humeral head, so as to prevent later dorsal subluxation. The glenoid might very well have very sharp bony spicules instead of the more plump osteophytes found in osteoarthritic bone, and these should be removed.

Once the direction of the glenoid centre has been identified, a pin may be placed centrally, and digital palpation anteriorly may help to identify the ventral or anterior wall of the scapular neck, to prevent later penetration. The humeral head should be protected at this point, since the soft bone can easily be squashed when heavily retracted to obtain good visualisation of the glenoid bone. Once the decision has been made that a glenoid implant is feasible, the bone is prepared, attempting to maintain as much subchondral plate as possible [12], since this will give the best support for anchoring the glenoid component *(fig 9)*. Proper orientation is necessary, and usually one will find a central erosion, which does not necessarily require any bone graft. If the glenoid bone is destroyed down towards the coracoid base, one might consider building up the glenoid with a bone graft, but fixation may fail in the short term due to the poor bone stock available *(fig 10)*.

Once the humeral component has been set into place, a trial reduction will be done. Care must be taken not to overstuff the joint with too big a head *(fig 11)*. Proper orientation of the glenoid as well as the correct corresponding rotation of the humeral head can prevent dorsal subluxation. Ventral subluxation might require further release of the capsule dorsally and, again, proper orientation of the two components will have to be checked. In any case, the coraco-acromial arch should be preserved, so as to have some checkrein for a possible ventral-superior dislocation should the subscapularis fixation fail at one point [31].

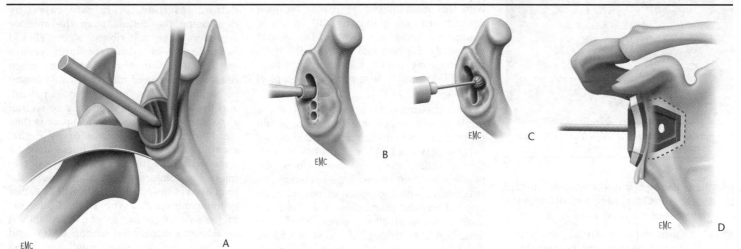

10 *A. It is important to find the correct centre of the glenoid for positioning of the glenoid component; palpation of the anterior wall may be helpful for orientation after removal of the osteophytes.*
B. Removal of the bone with a burr drill or the provided reamers should be done to
bleeding bone, without removal of the subchondral bone plate in order to maintain medial-lateral stability.
C, D. Seating of a cemented glenoid should be done in the proper depths. In particular, cement needs to be removed inferiorly and cranially in order to avoid secondary impingement.

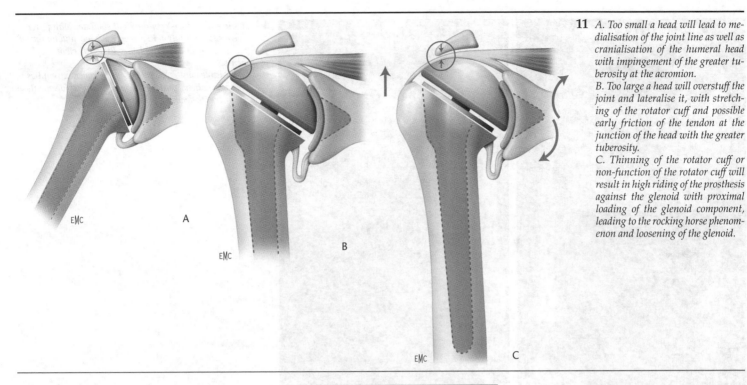

11 *A. Too small a head will lead to me-dialisation of the joint line as well as cranialisation of the humeral head with impingement of the greater tuberosity at the acromion.*
B. Too large a head will overstuff the joint and lateralise it, with stretching of the rotator cuff and possible early friction of the tendon at the junction of the head with the greater tuberosity.
C. Thinning of the rotator cuff or non-function of the rotator cuff will result in high riding of the prosthesis against the glenoid with proximal loading of the glenoid component, leading to the rocking horse phenomenon and loosening of the glenoid.

If subscapularis muscle lengthening is needed, one should take care not to "over pull" the tendon, to avoid injury to the subscapular nerve. Preparation for the sutures through the osteopenic bone should be done prior to cementing the humeral component, in order to obtain solid fixation with non-absorbable sutures.

ROTATOR CUFF REPAIR AND ALTERNATIVE IMPLANTS

If a rotator cuff tear is present at the time of surgery, it seems advantageous to attempt a repair to improve function and to cover the joint in the subacromial space [39]. If this not possible, a decision will have been made during the initial approach as to whether a bipolar prosthesis would better suit the patient's needs. A reverse prosthesis can be utilised as well [38], but one should be aware that the loads on the glenoid (metaglen) are quite high and therefore excellent fixation of the glenoid component into the bonestock seems to be a prerequisite to secure fixation against these forces [12].

Closure is performed in the usual way, the subscapularis being reattached with the arm in approximately 40 degrees external rotation. An abduction external rotation test is performed to avoid a spontaneous subluxation *(fig 12).*

Postoperative management

The general rehabilitation procedures after total shoulder arthroplasty have been described in detail elsewhere [4, 36]. For the rheumatoid patient, it is important to assess the function of the other joints of the upper extremity as well *(fig 13)*. Elbow stiffness can

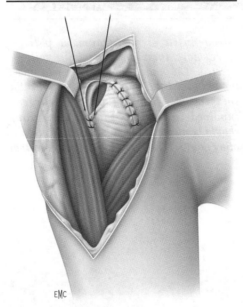

12 *Closure might require mobilisation of the subscapu-laris to allow appropriate external rotation; in a few cases an interval gap might prevail.*

easily develop if a sling is applied for a too long a period without early implementation of exercises for this joint. Care must also be taken concerning the skin, as many patients have taken steroid medication for long periods, leading to a particularly delicate skin which is prone to abrasion or subcutaneous haematoma.

Arthrodesis of the shoulder

Prior to the advent of shoulder arthroplasty, arthrodesis was a much more common procedure to treat the painful arthritic shoulder joint. As one-third of shoulder

motion is gained through the scapulotho-racic joint, the shoulder and arm might still be quite functional when fused. Obviously, the demands of the patient and the functional state of the opposite and adjoining articulations will all be factors to consider prior to shoulder fusion.

One indication for shoulder arthrodesis is complete destruction of the joint with a possible but subacute infection or paralysis after a plexus lesion. Another indication might be post-traumatic arthrosis in a very young patient. The patient's ability to attend to his personal hygiene and to feed himself will have to be considered prior to the procedure.

The technique is described in detail elsewhere [40] and the decision as to whether an arthrodesis should be done (either by screw osteosynthesis or with a pre-templated compression plate) depends on the fixation one can obtain in the bony situation found. Supplementation by bone graft might become necessary to ensure union. For postoperative rehabilitation, an abduction brace might be needed for 2-3 months, to allow fusion to progress without development of a non-union.

The generally suggested positioning of the arm is abduction of 20-30° between the lateral rim of the scapula and the medial ridge of the humeral shaft. A flexion of 30° and approximately 40-45° internal rotation will facilitate most daily activities.

Huber and Gschwend [20] reported on 22 shoulder arthrodeses, with an average follow-up of approximately 5.4 years. Although the patients subjectively stated a good result, the functional results were still inferior to any joint reconstruction.

Arthrodesis of the shoulder will be indicated in the rheumatoid patient only in a few

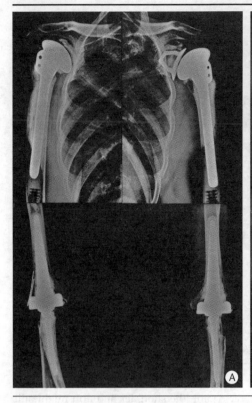

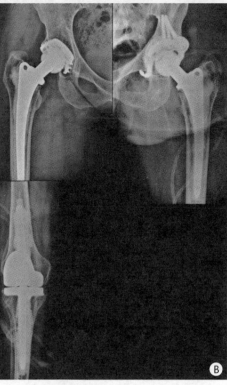

13 *A. Hemiarthroplasty of the right shoulder with progressive medial migration in osteopenic bone, and on the left side a total joint arthroplasty. Bilateral elbow replacements.*
B. Multiple joint replacements of the lower extremities in the same patient, putting the upper joint replacements at risk if crutch-walking becomes necessary.

cases, and seems to be reserved as a salvage procedure, or for the younger patient.

Conclusion

In the rheumatoid patient, the indications for shoulder surgery differ from those of the osteoarthritic or post-traumatic patient, since more than just one joint will be affected. The underlying disease will affect not only the bone and cartilage, but also the soft tissues. The orthopaedic surgeon involved in treating this patient group should be aware of the possible implication of other joints. Thus, it is a prerequisite that strategic planning be done for reconstruction of the various joints as they become involved. The success of shoulder surgery is in many ways dependent on the patient's motivation as well as on the skills of physiotherapists experienced in dealing with this patient group. A combined effort by all is necessary for a successful outcome.

References

[1] Alund M, Hoe-Hansen C, Tillander B, Heden BA, Norlin R. Outcome after cup hemiarthroplasty in the rheumatoid shoulder: a retrospective evaluation of 39 patients followed for 2-6 years. *Acta Orthop Scand* 2000 ; 71 : 180-184

[2] Aydin I. Die propriozeptive Fähigkeit der normalen und der instabilen Schulter. *Dtsch Z Sportmed* 2000 ; 51 : 336-340

[3] Baulot E, Chabernaud D, Grammont PM. Results of Grammont's inverted prosthesis in omarthritis associated with major cuff destruction. A propos of 16 cases. *Acta Orthop Belg* 1995 ; 61 (suppl 1) : 112-119

[4] Boardman ND, Cofield RH, Bengtson KA, Little R, Jones MC, Rowland CM. Rehabilitation after total shoulder arthroplasty. *J Arthroplasty* 2001 ; 16 : 483-486

[5] Boileau P, Walch G. Prosthetic adaptability: A new concept in shoulder arthroplasty. In : Walch G, Boileau P eds. Shoulder arthroplasty. Berlin : Springer-Verlag, 1999 : 83-85

[6] Cofield RH. Uncemented total shoulder arthroplasty: A review. *Clin Orthop* 1994 ; 307 : 86-93

[7] Copeland SA. Surface replacement arthroplasty of the shoulder. In : Copeland SA ed. Shoulder surgery. Philadelphia : WB Saunders, 1997 : 290-299

[8] Dijkstra J, Dijkstra PF, VdKlundert W. Rheumatoid arthritis of the shoulder. Description and standard radiographs. *ROFO Fortschr Geb Roentgenstr Nuklearmed* 1985 ; 142 : 179-185

[9] Fehr K. Systemische entzündliche Gelenk- und Wirbelsäulenerkrankungen. Rheumatoide Arthritis-Ätiologie und Pathogenese. In : Miehle M, Fehr K, Schattenkircher M, Tillmanmn K eds. Rheumatologie in Praxis und Klinik. Stuttgart : Thieme-Verlag, 2000 : 425-475

[10] Fink B, Sallen V, Guderian H, Tillmann K, Ruther W. Resection interposition arthroplasty of the shoulder affected by inflammatory arthritis. *J Shoulder Elbow Surg* 2001 ; 10 : 365-371

[11] Frank C. Ligament healing: current knowledge and clinical applications. *J Am Orthop Surg* 1996 ; 4 : 74-83

[12] Frich LH, Odgaard A, Dalstra M. Glenoid bone architecture. *J Shoulder Elbow Surg* 1998 ; 7 : 356-361

[13] Gerber CH. The treatment of the rheumatoid shoulder. In : Rheumatoid arthritis. Stuttgart : Thieme-Verlag, 1994 : 186-197

[14] Gill DR, Cofield RH, Morrey BF. Ipsilateral total shoulder and elbow arthroplasties in patients who have rheumatoid arthritis. *J Bone Joint Surg Am* 1999 ; 81 : 1128-1137

[15] Grammont PM, Baulot E. Delta shoulder prosthesis for rotator cuff rupture. *Orthopedics* 1993 ; 16 : 65-68

[16] Gschwend N. Synovectomy. Textbook of rheumatology, Philadelphia : WB Saunders, 1980

[17] Gschwend N. Surgical treatment of rheumatoid arthritis. Stuttgart : Thieme-Verlag, 1980

[18] Gschwend N, Kentsch A. Surgery of the rheumatoid shoulder. In : Bateman J, Welsh P eds. Surgery of the shoulder. St Louis : CV Mosby, 1984 : 269-280

[19] Hämäläinen M. Epidemiology of upper limb joint affections. In : Rheumatoid arthritis. Stuttgart : Thieme-Verlag, 1995 : 158-161

[20] Huber HM, Gschwend N. Schulterarthrodese. *Z Orthop Ihre Grenzgeb* 1993 ; 131 : 18-21

[21] Ibarra C, Craig EV. Soft-tissue balancing in total shoulder arthroplasty. *Orthop Clin North Am* 1998 ; 29 : 415-422

[22] Johnsson E, Egund N, Kelly I, Rydholm U, Lidgren L. Cup arthroplasty of the rheumatoid shoulder. *Acta Orthop Scand* 1986 ; 57 : 542-546

[23] Kelley M. Shoulder rehabilitation. In : Ianotti J ed. Disorders of the shoulder. Baltimore : Williams and Wilkins, 1999 : 979-1019

[24] Kelly IG. Unconstrained shoulder arthroplasty in rheumatoid arthritis. *Clin Orthop* 1994 ; 307 : 94-102

[25] Koorevar RC, Merkies ND, De Waal Malefijt MC, Teeuwen M, van den Hoogen FH. Shoulder hemiarthroplasty in rheumatoid arthritis. 19 cases re-examined after 1-17 years. *Acta Orthop Scand* 1997 ; 68 : 243-245

[26] Larsen A, Dahle K, Eek M. Radiographic evaluation of rheumatoid arthritis and related conditions by standard reference films. *Acta Radiol Diagn* 1977 ; 18 : 481-491

[27] Lehtinen JT, Belt EA, Kauppi MJ, Kaarela K, Kuusela PP, Kautiainen HJ et al. Bone destruction, upward migration, and medialisation of rheumatoid shoulder: a 15 year follow-up study. *Ann Rheum Dis* 2001 ; 60 : 322-326

[28] Lehtinen JT, Kaarela K, Belt EA, Kautiainen HJ, Kauppi MJ, Lehto MU. Relation of glenohumeral and acromioclavicular joint destruction in rheumatoid shoulder: a 15 year follow-up study. *Ann Rheum Dis* 2000 ; 59 : 158-160

[29] Lévigne C, Franceschi JP. Rheumatoid arthritis of the shoulder: presentation and results of arthroplasty. In : Walch G, Boileau P eds. Shoulder arthroplasty. Berlin : Springer-Verlag, 1999 : 221-230

[30] Levy O, Copeland SA. Cementless surface replacement arthroplasty of the shoulder. *J Bone Joint Surg Br* 2001 ; 83 : 213-221

[31] Loehr JF, Flören M, Schwyzer HK, Simmen BR, Gschwend N. Schulterinstabilität nach primärem Schultergelenkersatz. *Orthopäde* 1998 ; 27 : 571-575

[32] McCoy SR, Warren RF, Bade HA, Ranawat CS, Inglis AE. Total shoulder arthroplasty in rheumatoid arthritis. *J Arthroplasty* 1989 ; 4 : 105-113

[33] Mohing W. Zur Synovektomie des Schultergelenks. *Orthopäde* 1973 ; 2 : 84-87

[34] Neer CS 2nd. Articular replacement for the humeral head. *J Bone Joint Surg Am* 1955 ; 37 : 215-228

[35] Neer CS 2nd. Shoulder reconstruction. Philadelphia : WB Saunders, 1990

[36] Neer CS 2nd. Shoulder rehabilitation. In : Neer CS 2nd ed. Shoulder reconstruction. Philadelphia : WB Saunders, 1990 : 487-533

[37] Neer CS 2nd, Craig EV, Fukuda H. Cuff tear arthropathy. *J Bone Joint Surg Am* 1983 ; 65 : 1232-1244

[38] Rittmeister M, Kerschbaumer F. Grammont reverse total shoulder arthroplasty in patients with rheumatoid arthritis and nonreconstructible rotator cuff lesions. *J Shoulder Elbow Surg* 2001 ; 10 : 17-22

[39] Rozing PM, Brand R. Rotator cuff repair during shoulder arthroplasty in rheumatoid arthritis. *J Arthroplasty* 1998 ; 13 : 311-319

[40] Rybka V, Raunio P, Vainio K. Arthrodesis of the shoulder in rheumatoid arthritis. *J Bone Joint Surg Br* 1979 ; 61 : 155-158

[41] Rydholm U, Sjögren J. Surface replacement of the humeral head in the rheumatoid shoulder. *J Shoulder Elbow Surg* 1993 ; 2 : 286-295

[42] Smith KL, Matsen FA. Total shoulder arthroplasty versus hemiarthroplasty. Current trends. *Orthop Clin North Am* 1998 ; 29 : 491-506

[43] Sojberg JO, Frich LH, Johannsen HV, Sneppen O. Late results of total shoulder replacement in patients with rheumatoid arthritis. *Clin Orthop* 1999 ; 366 : 39-45

[44] van der Windt DA, Koes BW, Deville W, Boeke AJ, de Jong BA, Bouter LM. Effectiveness of corticosteroid injections versus physiotherapy for treatment of painful stiff shoulder in primary care: randomised trial. *Br Med J* 1998 ; 317 : 1292-1296

[45] van der Windt DA, van der Heijden GJ, van den Berg SG, ter Riet G, de Winter AF, Bouter LM. Ultrasound therapy for musculoskeletal disorders: a systematic review. *Pain* 1999 ; 81 : 257-271

[46] Walch G, Boileau P. Prosthetic adaptability: a new concept for shoulder arthroplasty. *J Shoulder Elbow Surg* 1999 ; 8 : 443-451

[47] Waldmann BJ, Figgie MP. Indications, technique, and results of total shoulder arthroplasty in rheumatoid arthritis. *Orthop Clin North Am* 1998 ; 29 : 435-444

[48] Wirth MA, Rockwood CA. Complications of total shoulder replacement arthroplasty. *J Bone Joint Surg Am* 1996 ; 78 : 603-616

[49] Worland RL, Arredondo J. Bipolar shoulder arthroplasty for painful conditions of the shoulder. *J Arthroplasty* 1998 ; 13 : 631-637

[50] Worland RL, Jessup DE, Arredondo J, Barburton KJ. Bipolar shoulder arthroplasty for rotator cuff arthropathy. *J Shoulder Elbow Surg* 1997 ; 6 : 512-515

[51] Wretenberg PF, Wallensten R. The Kessel total shoulder arthroplasty. A 13- to 16-year retrospective follow up. *Clin Orthop* 1999 ; 365 : 100-103

[52] Zippel J. Vollständiger Schultergelenkersatz aus Kunststoff und Metall. *Biomed Tech* 1972 ; 17 : 87-92

Massive rotator cuff tears: the musculo-tendinous transfer

AG Schneeberger
C Gerber

Abstract. — *Rotator cuff tears with cranial subluxation of the humeral head, an acromiohumeral distance below 5 mm, and advanced degeneration and atrophy of the involved muscles are considered irreparable. Attempted repairs of such tears usually result in re-tears, or function is not restored due to the quality of the muscles. Shoulder function and strength with irreparable tears can be restored by tendon transfer.*
The subscapularis can be replaced by the pectoralis major. Our personal experience using the pectoralis transfer is good to fair. Repair of the subscapularis should always be attempted, as no muscle can really replace it.
The supraspinatus can be substituted by transfer of the trapezius or lateral deltoid. In our experience, however, both tendon transfers do not restore abduction strength sufficiently.
Two muscles, the latissimus dorsi and the teres major, can be successfully used to substitute for the infraspinatus and restore external rotation strength. Wide experience is available for the latissimus dorsi transfer. Patients who have a complete loss of functional external rotation, and who can still elevate their arm but only by internally rotating it, are good candidates for the latissimus dorsi transfer. It is, however, contraindicated for subscapularis insufficiency, deltoid deficiency, and complete pseudoparalysis.

Keywords: *shoulder, rotator cuff tears, tendon transfers.*

Introduction

Certain massive tears of the rotator cuff cannot be successfully repaired due to the size of the defect, the poor quality of the tendon and irreversible severe atrophy, degeneration and retraction of the torn muscles, so that even a healed repair is of limited functional value. An established method of restoring shoulder function is replacement of the irreparable rotator cuff by musculo-tendinous transfer.

Indications for tendon transfers in rotator cuff deficiency

The indications for tendon transfers are not well established. They should be considered in a symptomatic rotator cuff defect which is beyond successful repair. Reparability depends on the size of the tear and on two parameters which define whether or not a repair will lead to a successful functional outcome.

Alberto G Schneeberger, M.D.
Christian Gerber, M.D., Department of Orthopaedic Surgery, University of Zurich, Balgrist, Forchstrasse 340, 8008 Zurich, Switzerland.

One parameter is subluxation of the humeral head. If the acromiohumeral distance on an AP view in neutral rotation is below 7 mm, the potential for successful repair is severely compromised. If the distance is below 5 mm, successful repair is generally impossible.

The second parameter is degeneration and atrophy of the muscles of the rotator cuff, as demonstrated on MRI scans or advanced fatty degeneration, as demonstrated on CT-scans [15, 16]. This is the most important indicator for tendon transfer.

The reason for tendon transfers in shoulders with irreparable rotator cuff tears is to restore shoulder function and strength. For elderly patients with few functional demands, cuff debridement should be considered instead. Three muscles of the rotator cuff, the subscapularis, the supraspinatus and the infraspinatus muscle, can all be replaced by musculo-tendinous transfers.

The subscapularis muscle

The subscapularis is an internal rotator and head depressor. It pulls the head posteriorly and with its tendinous insertion situated high on the humeral head, it also abducts the humerus.

To substitute for the subscapularis, the acromial part of the trapezius and the pectoralis major have been proposed.

TRAPEZIUS TRANSFER

Although too weak and of somewhat short amplitude [17], the trapezius has been tried as a substitute for the subscapularis. Its tendon is released from the acromion. The lateral clavicle is resected. The tendon is then brought through the enlarged acromioclavicular joint and fixed to the lesser tuberosity. The pull of the transferred muscle is backward but unfortunately also upward. Nonetheless, the early results of Goutallier et al [14] of 25 cases with subscapularis deficiency treated with transfer of the trapezius were good to excellent for pain relief, and acceptable for function in cases where the subscapularis and the supraspinatus were replaced. The authors feel that this transfer probably prevents superior migration of the head, but that it does not recentre a cranially-migrated head.

PECTORALIS MAJOR TRANSFER

The pectoralis major is much better suited in terms of strength and amplitude to replace the subscapularis, but it runs anterior to the chest and therefore does not pull the humeral head backward. Our preferred technique is to release and transfer the entire pectoralis major tendon. Other authors transfer only the superior half of the tendon [23] *(fig 1)*. The tendon must be freed

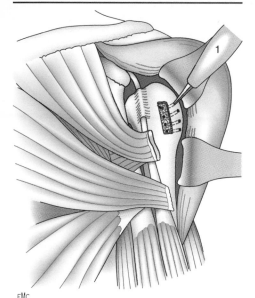

1 *Either the entire pectoralis major tendon (our preferred technique) or only the superior half, as described by Wirth and Rockwood [23], can be transferred to replace an irreparable subscapularis lesion. The pectoralis tendon is identified through a deltopectoral approach. The tendon is released at its insertion and freed from the surrounding tissue. If only the superior half of the pectoralis major tendon is transferred, the superior and inferior halves are divided medially for 8 to 10 cm. 1. Curved awl.*

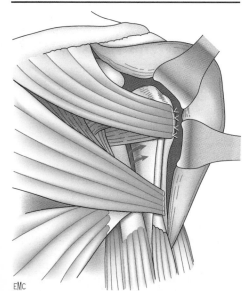

2 *The superior half of the pectoralis major tendon, as shown, (or the entire tendon) is transferred across the bicipital groove and transosseously fixed to a trough in the greater tuberosity.*

enough from the surrounding tissue so that it can be transferred across the bicipital groove to the greater tuberosity where it is fixed transosseously. If only the superior half of the pectoralis major tendon is transferred, the superior and inferior halves are divided medially for 8 to 10 cm (fig 2). Wirth and Rockwood [23] have reported satisfactory results in 5 out of 7 patients treated with transfer of the superior half of the pectoralis major for recurrent anterior glenohumeral instability, associated with an irreparable subscapularis lesion. Resch [20] has suggested that, especially in cases with associated anterior shoulder instability, the tendon can

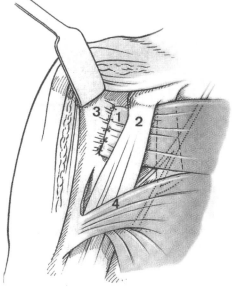

3 *Modification of transfer of pectoralis major by re-routing the tendon underneath the conjoined tendon according to the technique of Resch et al [20]. (Reproduced with permission from Resch H, Povacz P, Ritter E, Matschi W. Transfer of the pectoralis major muscle for the treatment of irreparable rupture of the subscapularis tendon. J Bone Joint Surg Am 2000 ; 82 : 372-382). 1. The upper one-half to two-thirds of the pectoralis major is released; 2. the tendon is passed underneath the conjoined tendon; 3. it is repaired to the lesser tuberosity; 4. inferior part of the pectoralis major.*

be brought laterally underneath the conjoined tendon to be reinserted at the lesser tuberosity (fig 3). With this re-routing, the tendon comes from more posteriorly, and the transfer should be better mechanically. The subjective outcome of 12 patients operated on with a pectoralis major transfer re-routed posteriorly to the conjoined tendon was reported satisfactory in 9 cases, and fair in 3 cases. The Constant and Murley score increased from 27% to 67% of normal [7]. All 4 pre-operatively unstable shoulders were stable at the time of the latest follow-up. There were no complications in this series.

Our personal experience with the conventional pectoralis transfer is good to fair. Repair of the subscapularis should always be attempted, as no muscle can really replace it. In our hands, the transfer has only been used for isolated subscapularis tears and has relieved pain and improved function substantially. However, in cases with static anterior subluxation of the humeral head, the transfer did not recentre this.

Supraspinatus

The supraspinatus alone is rarely torn and retracted to such a degree that it cannot be repaired. The supraspinatus is an optimal vector for abduction and is relatively strong and short. Two major proposals are known for its substitution: transfer of the trapezius and of the lateral deltoid. Both muscles are well suited in terms of amplitude and strength.

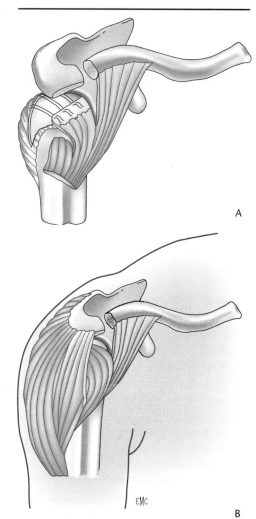

4 *A. Deltoid flap. An anterolateral strip of the deltoid is released from the acromion and sutured to the supraspinatus stump. Anterolateral view with lateral and posterior deltoid removed for demonstration. B. Anterolateral view after deltoid flap. In our experience, the deltoid flap yielded reliable pain relief without restoring satisfactory function. For failed painful deltoid flaps, revisions have shown to be difficult. We therefore do not use the deltoid flap anymore.*

TRAPEZIUS TRANSFER

The trapezius can be transferred with a technique which is similar to that in subscapularis deficiencies [19]. Instead of the lesser tuberosity, the tendon is implanted through the acromion split approach into the greater tuberosity [24]. The orientation of the transfer is not optimal as it pulls the head superiorly. There are only a few clinical results reported of this procedure, and they are somewhat controversial [24]. We have elected not to use this procedure for this indication until further results are available.

DELTOID FLAP

With the deltoid flap, an approximately 2.5 cm wide strip of the anterolateral deltoid is released from the acromion and then sutured to the supraspinatus stump or the superior aspect of the glenoid, thus providing a coverage of the humeral head and a dynamic abductor (fig 4) [1, 22]. Apoil

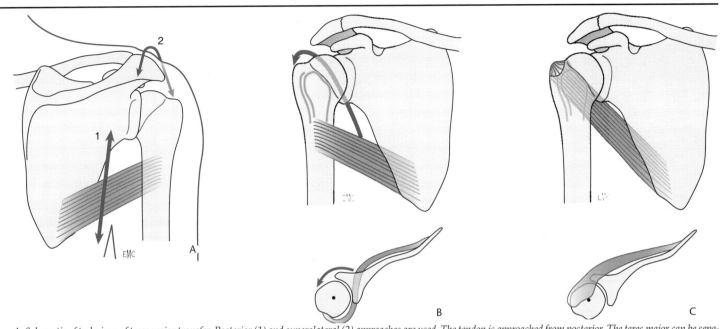

5 *A. Schematic of technique of teres major transfer. Posterior (1) and superolateral (2) approaches are used. The tendon is approached from posterior. The teres major can be separated from the latissimus dorsi by blunt dissection close to the inferior angle of the scapula at the origin of the teres major. The dissection is continued laterally with the arm in full internal rotation, and the tendon is then detached at its insertion at the humerus.*
B, C. Before (B) and after (C) transfer of teres major. The tendon is passed underneath the deltoid muscle towards the humeral head into the superolateral approach. Transosseous refixation is performed at the superolateral side of the humeral head.

and Augereau [1] have obtained excellent results in the treatment of massive tears with this technique. Gazielly [9] has recently summarised his own results in 20 cases. The overall results were definitely less good than those reported by Bigliani [3] for primary repair. Another study by Dierickx et al [8] also reported 20 cases with satisfactory results which, however, were no better than those of cuff debridement.

In our experience, we have only used the transfer for truly irreparable tears involving more than two complete tendons, and the results for this indication were good in terms of pain relief, but not better in terms of regaining function than cuff debridement or attempts at direct repair. We, personally, have had to revise three cases of failed deltoid flaps, which were sent to us for further treatment. All three cases were very painful and had an additional irreparable cuff tear. Whereas treatment of pain was possible, we could not regain satisfactory function in any of the three cases. We therefore do not continue to use the deltoid flap for irreparable tears.

Infraspinatus

The infraspinatus is almost never torn without a concomitant large tear of the supraspinatus. The infraspinatus is an external rotator and an elevator of the arm. Two muscles, the teres major and the latissimus dorsi, are used to substitute for the infraspinatus.

TERES MAJOR TRANSFER

The transfer of the teres major has been described by Combes and Mansat [5] and by Celli et al [4]. The teres major is like the

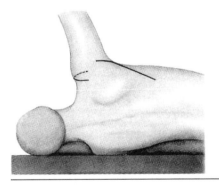
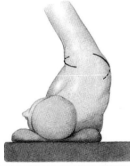

6 *Lateral decubitus position for transfer of latissimus dorsi. The arm is draped and remains free. Two incisions: one superolateral to approach the rotator cuff, the second posterior at the posterior axillary line for access to the insertion of the latissimus dorsi [10, 12].*

infraspinatus a scapulohumeral muscle with similar size and length. It can be transferred into the infraspinatus fossa with almost the same orientation as the infraspinatus (fig 5). Celli et al [4] reported the results of 6 patients treated with this transfer. All their patients had a massive rotator cuff tear with an irreparable infraspinatus rupture. They also had a concomitant supraspinatus tear which either could be directly repaired (4 cases) or treated by an additional trapezius transfer (2 cases). The Constant score [7] improved in all patients from an average of 40 points (27 to 54) before surgery to an average of 62 points (47 to 68) after surgery. Active external rotation improved by 35° in abduction and by 24° in adduction. One patient was very satisfied, 5 were satisfied at follow-up.

LATISSIMUS DORSI TRANSFER

The transfer of the latissimus dorsi was introduced as a salvage procedure to compensate for irreparable postero-lateral rotator cuff defects [10, 12]. The latissimus dorsi

is a relatively strong muscle with an extremely large amplitude which makes it better suited for transfer than the teres major [17]. The technique of the tendon transfer has been described in detail [10, 12]. The patient is in a lateral decubitus position with the trunk elevated (fig 6). A superolateral approach is used for an attempt at a conventional repair. If direct repair is impossible, a posterior approach along the posterior axillary line is performed, to identify the latissimus dorsi. The tendon is released from the humeral shaft, and the muscle is mobilised until the neurovascular pedicle can be identified (fig 7, 8). The tendon is then brought into the superolateral approach by pulling it upward between the deltoid and the teres minor (fig 9). It is then inserted at the very top of the humeral head. The end of the tendon is sutured to the subscapularis tendon and it comes to lie exactly at the insertion of the supraspinatus (fig 10). Herzberg [17] has studied the mechanical effects of transfer of the tendon to different sites at the humeral head, and has shown

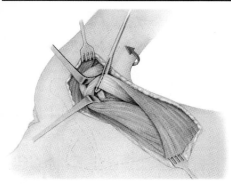

7   *The insertion of the latissimus dorsi is identified and released from the humeral shaft. The axillary nerve lies immediately adjacent to the proximal end of the tendon. The radial nerve curves around the humeral shaft immediately distal to the tendon. Both nerves are protected [10, 12].*

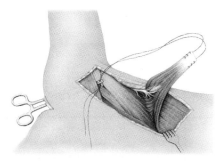

8   *The neurovascular pedicle is identified, and the latissimus is mobilised proximally to provide sufficient amplitude. Two non-absorbable sutures of size number 3 grasp the tendon. A clamp is passed underneath the deltoid muscle from the proximal to the distal incision, and the sutures with the latissimus dorsi tendon are re-routed medial to the axillary nerve, dorsal to the long head of the triceps, between the deltoid and the teres minor [10, 12].*

that the tip of the greater tuberosity and/or the region of the supraspinatus insertion are optimal.

We have recently reviewed the first consecutive 16 cases after a follow-up of 5.4 years (4.9 to 6.2). All had had chronic irreparable, massive rotator cuff tears and were treated with a latissimus dorsi transfer. Pain relief was excellent or good in 94% of the shoulders at rest, and in 75% on exertion. Painfree active flexion increased from 83° pre-operatively to 123° at follow-up. The

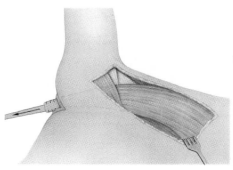

9   *The latissimus is pulled through the plane between the external rotators and the deltoid [10, 12].*

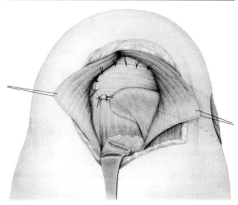

10   *For the superolateral approach, the acromial part of the deltoid has been detached with small bony fragments from the lateral acromion. In cases of osteoarthrosis of the AC joint, the 1.5 cm of the lateral clavicle are resected. The latissimus dorsi has been fixed medially to the tip of the greater tuberosity, posteriorly to the subscapularis tendon and laterally to the stump of the supraspinatus tendon [10, 12].*

mean active external rotation improved from 10° (-20° to 35°) pre-operatively to 23° (10° to 35°) postoperatively. The transfer successfully served as an external rotation tenodesis for the elevated arm. The function of the shoulders was assessed at follow-up by the Constant score. It averaged 60 points (29 to 87) and was calculated to be 73% of an age and gender matched normal shoulder [6]. The 12 shoulders with a functionally intact subscapularis scored an average of 83%, but those without an intact subscapularis scored only 54%. Latissimus dorsi transfers therefore yielded durably

good to excellent subjective and objective results in chronically painful, dysfunctional shoulders, with irreparable tears of the rotator cuff, if the subscapularis was intact. However, it was of no benefit in the presence of massive cuff tears with subscapularis insufficiency.

After 10 years of experience we know that the best indications for latissimus dorsi transfer are patients who can still elevate their arm, but only by internally rotating it. They are very weak in elevation and abduction and have complete loss of functional external rotation. It is this functional loss of external rotation (inability to reach forward with the hand, inability to stabilise the arm in space, e.g. in front of the mouth) which is consistently improved by this technique, provided the contraindications are respected. Contraindications for the latissimus dorsi transfer are subscapularis insufficiency, deltoid deficiency, and complete pseudoparalysis. If the patients can not actively elevate their arm pre-operatively, the results of the latissimus dorsi transfer are not predictable in terms of recovering function.

Conclusions

Although transfer surgery is currently only considered in irreparable tears, the authors feel that transfer surgery should always be considered if functional restoration is mandatory and significant muscular atrophy and/or degeneration are present. In our current practice, latissimus dorsi transfers for certain posterolateral cuff lesions, and pectoralis major transfers for certain subscapularis lesions, are best established and are also considered as an augmentation procedure if a primary repair is critical.

Acknowledgements – Figures 6 through 10 are reproduced by permission and were previously published in Gerber C, Vinh Tshertel R, Hess CW. Latissimus dorsi transfer for the treatment of massive tears of the rotator cuff. A preliminary report. *Clin Orthop* 1988 ; 232 : 51-61, and Gerber C, Hersche O. Tendon transfers for the treatment of irreparable rotator cuff defects. *Orthop Clin North Am* 1997 ; 28 : 195-203.

References

[1] Apoil A, Augereau B. Réparation par lambeau de déltoide des grandes pertes de substance de la coiffe des rotateurs de l'épaule. *Chirurgie* 1985 ; 111 : 287-290

[2] Apoil A, Dautry P, Moinet P, Koechlin PH. Le syndrome dit "de rupture de la coiffe des rotateurs de l'épaule". À propos de 70 observations. *Rev Chir Orthop* 1977 ; 63 (suppl II) : 145-149

[3] Bigliani LU, Cordasco FA, McIlveen SJ, Musso ES. Operative repair of massive rotator cuff tears: long-term results. *J Shoulder Elbow Surg* 1992 ; 1 : 120-130

[4] Celli L, Rovesta C, Marongiu C, Manzieri S. Transplantation of teres major for infraspinatus muscle in irreparable rotator cuff tears. *J Shoulder Elbow Surg* 1998 ; 7 : 485-490

[5] Combes JM, Mansat M. Lambeau du muscle grand rond dans les ruptures massives de la coiffe des rotateurs. In : Bonnel F, Blotman F, Mansat M éd. L'épaule. Berlin : Springer-Verlag, 1993 : 318-330

[6] Constant CR. Age related recovery of shoulder function after injury. [thesis], University College, Cork, Ireland, 1986

[7] Constant CR, Murley AH. A clinical method of functional assessment of the shoulder. *Clin Orthop* 1987 ; 214 : 160-164

[8] Dierickx C, Vanhoof H. Massive rotator cuff tears treated by a deltoid muscular flap. *Acta Orthop Belg* 1994 ; 60 : 94-100

[9] Gazielly DF. Deltoid muscular flap transfer for massive defects of the rotator cuff. In : Burkhead WZ ed. Rotator cuff disorders. Baltimore : Williams and Wilkins, 1996 : 356-367

[10] Gerber C. Latissimus dorsi transfer for the treatment of irreparable tears of the rotator cuff. *Clin Orthop* 1992 ; 275 : 152-160

[11] Gerber C, Hersche O. Tendon transfers for the treatment of irreparable rotator cuff defects. *Orthop Clin North Am* 1997 ; 28 : 195-203

[12] Gerber C, Vinh Tshertel R, Hess CW. Latissimus dorsi transfer for the treatment of massive tears of the rotator cuff. A preliminary report. *Clin Orthop* 1988 ; 232 : 51-61

[13] Gilbert A, Tassin JL, Benjeddou MS. Paralysie obstétricale du membre supérieur. *Encycl Méd Chir* (Éditions Scientifiques et Médicales Elsevier SAS, Paris), Pédiatrie, 4-002-R-05, 1985

[14] Goutallier D. Communication personnelle, Paris, 1995

[15] Goutallier D, Bernageau J, Patte D. L'évaluation par le scanner de la trophicité des muscles de la coiffe des rotateurs ayant une rupture tendineuse. *Rev Chir Orthop* 1989 ; 75 (suppl 1) : 126-127

[16] Goutallier D, Postel JM, Bernageau J, Lavau J, Voisin MC. Fatty muscle degeneration in cuff ruptures. *Clin Orthop* 1994 ; 304 : 78-83

[17] Herzberg G. Anatomical bases of musculotendinous transfers about the shoulder. Unpublished Data, University of Lyon, 1995

[18] Hoffer MM, Wickenden R, Roper B. Brachial plexus birth injuries: results of tendon transfer of the rotator cuff. *J Bone Joint Surg Am* 1978 ; 60 : 691-695

[19] Mikasa M. Trapezius transfer for global tear of the rotator cuff. In : Bateman JE, Wels RP eds. Surgery of the shoulder. Philadelphia : BCDecker, 1984

[20] Resch H, Povacz P, Ritter E, Matschi W. Transfer of the pectoralis major muscle for the treatment of irreparable rupture of the subscapularis tendon. *J Bone Joint Surg Am* 2000 ; 82 : 372-382

[21] Schmidt-Wiethoff R, Habermeyer P. Die Deltoideus-Lappenplastik bei der Massenruptur der Rotatorenmanschette. *Oper Orthop Traumatol* 1999 ; 11 : 255-267

[22] Takagishi N. A new operation for the massive cuff rupture. *J Jpn Orthop Assoc* 1978 ; 52 : 775-780

[23] Wirth MA, Rockwood CA Jr. Operative treatment of irreparable rupture of the subscapularis. *J Bone Joint Surg Am* 1997 ; 79 : 722-731

[24] Yamanaka K, Mikasa M. Trapezius transfer. In : Burkhead WZ ed. Rotator cuff disorders. Baltimore : Williams and Wilkins, 1996 : 374-379

Shoulder arthrodesis

B Wittner
U Holz

Abstract. – Arthrodesis of the shoulder joint is a salvage procedure for cases with chronic pain where arthroplasty is no longer an alternative. The functional limitations must be thoroughly discussed with the patient. The mechanical principles of the fusion are compression by lag screw and neutralisation by a plate. On the thoracic side, the plate must be fixed to the scapular spine and the socket of the glenoid. Protection of the osteosynthesis by casts is not necessary. Full range of motion exercises of the arm are possible very soon after the operation. In selected cases of failed arthroplasty of the shoulder joint, arthrodesis can be useful in allowing the patient to regain a stable and painfree arm.

Keywords: shoulder, osteoarthritis, arthrodesis, osteosynthesis, shoulder prosthesis, failed arthroplasty.

Introduction

Due to progress in arthroplasty of the shoulder joint, in the last two decades the indication for arthrodesis of this joint has become rare. Today's indications for this procedure are irreversible palsy of the upper arm plexus, failed stabilisation of a painful multidirectional unstable shoulder, failed arthroplasty of the shoulder joint and failed eradication of bacterial infection. Relative indications are osteoarthritis in shoulders with rotator cuff deficiency in young or middle-aged patients and genuine osteoarthritis of the shoulder joint in young patients. Contraindications for an arthrodesis of the glenohumeral joint are a stiff ipsilateral elbow or significant osteoarthritis of this elbow. The functional deficit in an arm with a stiff shoulder and a stiff elbow is not acceptable, and arthroplasty in the elbow with an ipsilateral arthrodesed shoulder will loosen early, due to the increased forces on the implants. A second relative contraindication for an arthrodesis of the shoulder is an arthrodesed contralateral shoulder. In these cases, the patient cannot manage the procedures of daily hygiene. However, in patients with severe painful multidirectional instability, there is sometimes no other possibility left, and the result may be acceptable [9].

Bernd Wittner, M.D.
Ulrich Holz, M.D., Professor.
Klinik für Unfall und Wiederherstellungschirurgie, Katharinenhospital,
70174 Stuttgart, Germany.

Prior to the procedure, it is of utmost importance to inform the patient about the expected result. Most functional deficits result from limitation of rotation: after shoulder arthrodesis, the mouth as well as the trouser pocket can normally be reached with the ipsilateral hand. Although this is the objective, not all patients will be able to comb their hair or reach the mid-line of the back. The abduction and flexion functions of the upper arm are limited below 90°. The patient should be aware of a possible shortening of the arm, which is without functional significance.

Surgical procedure

PREOPERATIVE WORK-UP, ANAESTHESIA AND POSITIONING

Diagnostic X-rays in standard true a.p. and axial views are usually sufficient to plan the operation. A CT scan may be useful in specific cases, for example after long-standing infection of the joint with considerable bone loss. Three to four units of blood should be available. The procedure is carried out under general anaesthesia with the patient in the "beach chair position". This makes it easier to adjust the position of the shoulder joint compared to a lateral decubitus position. The arm, shoulder and entire scapula are disinfected and draped so that the arm is freely mobile (*fig 1*). Special instruments are not necessary; the procedure can be performed with a standard operation

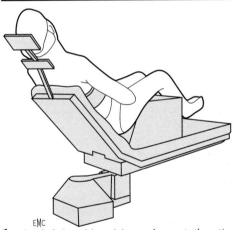

1 *Beach chair position, giving good access to the entire scapula, shoulder and arm.*

set for osteosynthesis with chisels of different sizes. A humeral head retractor facilitates access to the glenoid, but is not absolutely necessary. For stabilisation, we use a broad 4.5 mm AO-DC plate with 10 to 14 holes and cortical and cancellous bone screws. In cases where the humeral head and glenoid have good bone stock allowing good compression of the arthrodesis, a narrow 4.5 mm DC plate may be sufficient. When the procedure is carried out due to a failed arthroplasty, a broad plate is necessary to provide sufficient stability to the construct. The same is true in cases having considerable bone loss after infection or in cases with extremely soft bone, for example in patients with long-standing misuse due to upper brachial plexus palsy.

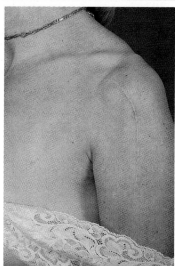

2 *Appearance after the transdeltoid approach. The bony structures of the shoulder girdle become obvious.*

SURGICAL APPROACH

Two approaches are possible: transdeltoid or deltoid-sparing. Placement of the implants is much easier with the transdeltoid approach than with the deltoid-sparing approach. However, after a transdeltoid approach, the part of the deltoid muscle which is ventral to the incision becomes atrophic, resulting in a cosmetic (but not a functional) disadvantage. This holds true especially in young patients: the contours of the bony structures become obvious (fig 2). Therefore, we use the transdeltoid approach in elderly patients, while we prefer the deltoid-sparing approach in younger patients with well-developed muscle contours of the shoulder.

Both approaches start with an incision from the medial aspect of the scapular spine to the acromion, and from there in a mid-line between the deltopectoral interval and the lateral shoulder line. In the lower third, the incision is directed slightly lateral (fig 3). The surfaces of the scapular spine and the acromion are exposed. In the lateral half of the incision in both directions, an epifascial flap is created to expose the ventral half of the deltoid muscle so as to gain access to the deltopectoral interval and the lateral shoulder line (fig 4). Through the deltopectoral interval, the shoulder joint is exposed by retracting the coracobrachial muscles and detaching the tendon of the subscapularis muscle from the lesser tuberosity. The shoulder is dislocated by maximal external rotation and the cartilage of the humeral head is exposed.

PROCEDURE

The cartilage is removed with a chisel. Hard subchondral bone must be maintained in as far as possible to allow good compression during osteosynthesis. With a humeral head retractor or two Hohmann retractors, the humeral head is displaced posteriorly and the cartilage of the glenoid removed (fig 5). The shoulder is now positioned for the

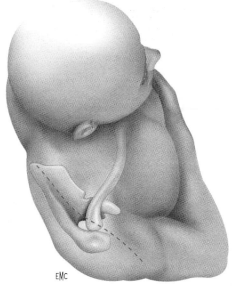

3 *Incision for shoulder arthrodesis.*

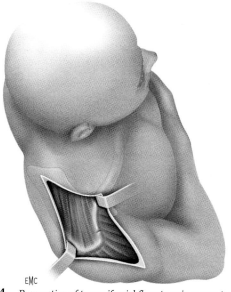

4 *Preparation of two epifascial flaps to gain access to the deltopectoral interval ventrally and the lateral shoulder line.*

arthrodesis. We prefer a position of 30° anteflexion, 20° abduction and 40° internal rotation [8]. It is necessary to keep the scapula in a neutral position at this stage of the procedure. While it is very important to achieve good contact and compression between the glenoid and humeral head surface, we do not force additional bony contact between the humeral head and the acromion in order to avoid cranialisation of the head. Because of the cosmetic result, we also do not osteotomise the acromion to force contact to the humeral head. In cases with arthritis due to cuff deficiency or where there is considerable bone loss (e.g. after failed arthroplasty), we allow this additional contact to facilitate bony fusion. While the desired shoulder position is held by the assistant, the humeral head is fixed to the glenoid by a 6.5 mm AO lag screw. The placement of this screw through the humeral

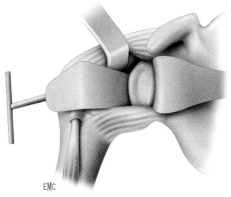

5 *The humeral head is displaced posteriorly for access to and removal of the cartilage of the glenoid.*

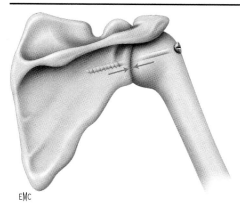

6 *The placement of the first lag screw is very important.*

head into the socket of the glenoid in the plane of the scapula is very important.

With a transdeltoid approach, the deltoid muscle is split from the acromion to its insertion in the plane of the scapula. The axillary nerve and artery are dissected. In the deltoid-sparing approach, the muscle is retracted laterally until the screw can be inserted through the middle of the humeral head into the glenoid. Partial release of the insertion of the muscle facilitates this manoeuvre. While drilling the hole for this screw, the plane of the scapula can be estimated with the index finger of the left hand. After insertion of the lag screw, X-ray control is helpful to make sure that the entire thread is in the glenoid only. A washer allows more compression of the arthrodesis, especially in osteoporotic bones (fig 6). The proper rotation of the humerus can now be checked by leading the hand of the patient to his draped face. During this manoeuvre, the surgeon must control carefully the fused bones with his palpating finger in order to prevent avulsion of the screw. The fixation with one lag screw is not very stable and the lever arm to the arthrodesis is quite long! Now a broad or (in good bone conditions) a narrow AO 4.5 DC plate is contoured along the spine of the scapula and the acromion to the humeral shaft. Good contouring is important to place the plate firmly on the bone along the entire distance. If the deltoid muscle is spared, its origin is released at the

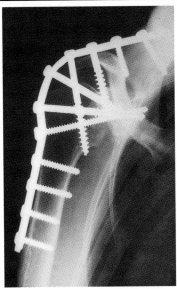

7 *X-ray of a plate arthrodesis of the shoulder: a minimum of two lag screws should penetrate the arthrodesis for solid compression. The placement of the screws in the scapular spine is important.*

anterolateral aspect of the acromion to allow penetration of the plate. In the humeral shaft, four to five firmly fixed screws should be used, and in the scapular part of the plate as many screws as possible. One or two additional screws through the plate should function as lag screws. Placement of the screws of the scapular part should be carried out carefully because this is the weakest part of the construct. The screws should have good bone grip. It is advisable to partially release the deltoid muscle so as to feel the plane of the spine of the scapula while drilling the holes. In this case, cortical bone screws allow a better grip than cancellous bone screws. In the lateral part, one screw should be placed in the base of the coracoid process and another in the glenoid socket (fig 7). Bone grafting is not compulsory, but advisable in cases with poor bone quality or bone defects. Then the supraspinatus tendon, if not absent, can be resected and bone grafts can be placed between the debrided humeral head and the debrided undersurface of the acromion.

The wound is closed over two suction drains. Refixation of the subscapularis tendon is not necessary. Most patients feel uncomfortable when the arm is placed in the neutral position several days after the operation; therefore, the arm is placed post-operatively on an abduction cushion.

POST-SURGICAL CARE

The arm remains placed on the abduction cushion (fig 8) for three to four days. After removal of the drainage at the second day, physiotherapy starts to mobilise the scapula. The scapulo-thoracic muscles are strengthened. Most patients experience pain at the medial border of the scapula until proper mobilisation of the scapula is achieved. Physiotherapy should include the elbow. Some patients feel comfortable

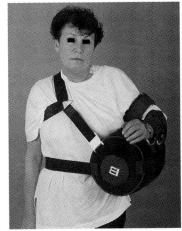

8 *After the procedure, the arm is placed on an abduction cushion for several days.*

wearing a sling between the exercises. At discharge from the hospital after 12 to 14 days, no support should be necessary.

As the plate is placed directly under the skin, especially at the medial border of the scapular spine, a painful bursitis sometimes develops. In severe cases, protection with a small cushion may be necessary to prevent pressure sores. Because of this problem, we prefer to remove the implant after two years when the arthrodesis is consolidated.

Failure and hazards

Early complications such as haematoma and infection are treated by revision according to the standards of revision surgery.

When using plate osteosynthesis, nonunion is very rare. If it occurs, re-osteosynthesis with compression and cancellous bone grafting is necessary. If the arthrodesis heals in an improper position, the patient cannot reach his mouth if there is pronounced internal rotation and cannot reach the body if the upper arm is rotated too externally. Patients with an arthrodesis in pronounced abduction complain of persistent pain at the medial border of the scapula. If these circumstances are recognised shortly after the operation, correction osteosynthesis to ensure the proper position is mandatory. If the malposition becomes evident after healing of the arthrodesis, correction osteotomy of the upper humerus may be necessary.

Some patients develop acromioclavicular joint pain due to increased scapular motion. In severe cases, lateral clavicle resection may be necessary. We do not suggest this as a routine procedure in arthrodesis of the shoulder [5].

The modified biomechanics after arthrodesis of the shoulder predispose to humeral shaft fractures. Therefore, the AO group has suggested routine bone grafting at the end of the plate to strengthen the humeral shaft at this location [4]. Conservative treatment of these fractures is possible only if a nearly anatomical position of the main fragments can be achieved. Special consideration

should be given to the proper rotation of the distal fragment. Due to the abduction position of the arthrodesis, conservative treatment is possible only with a shoulder spica. Given the problems in controlling proper rotation, open anatomical reduction and internal fixation with a plate should be considered in these cases.

Arthrodesis after failed arthroplasty

Arthrodesis after failed arthroplasty calls for some special comments. The incision should include the scar of the primary operation. The approach is the same as described above. After dislocation of the artificial joint, the stem and (if present) the glenoid of the endoprosthesis are removed. Bone cement with mal-vascularised bone is resected completely at the glenoid side. At the humeral side, only the upper easily accessible cement is removed. In non-infected cases[1], it is not necessary to remove the well-anchored cement in the shaft, due to the considerable risk of fracture of the humerus. As there is not enough bone stock left, compression arthrodesis is not possible. To allow screw fixation of the humerus to the glenoid, we interpose two or three tricortical bone blocks from the iliac crest. The bone graft is fixed together with a 3.5 cortical bone screw and is firmly pushed into the metaphyseal defect. At the free end, the bone block is shaped to fit with the surface of the remnants of the glenoid. Then the humerus is positioned for arthrodesis and fixed by a lag screw through the bone graft to the glenoid; osteosynthesis is finished as described above (fig 9).

In these cases, the post-operative treatment must be modified. The arm is placed on the abduction cushion for 6 weeks. After removal of the drainage, isometric physiotherapy is started to strengthen the scapulo-thoracic muscles. After three weeks, assisted active physiotherapy may begin. Between the exercises the arm is placed on the abduction cushion. After six weeks, the cushion is removed and exercises continue with full range of motion.

Results

Results after arthrodesis of the shoulder are rarely published and usually concern a small number of cases. Moreover, the results are not comparable due to different primary diseases. The functional result of this procedure in patients with brachial plexus

---

1. Infected cases are extremely rare. For such patients, we recommend a two-stage procedure. In the first operation, we remove the endoprosthesis with all the cement. Due to the extensive scarring, this procedure sometimes results in a painfree and stable shoulder [11]. For those patients who suffer from pain or instability [10], we recommend an arthrodesis after eradication of the infection.

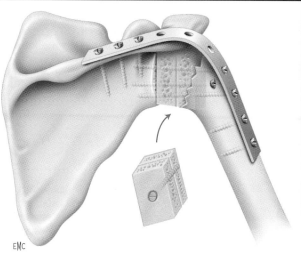
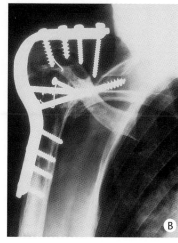

9 A. *Drawing of an arthrodesis after failed arthroplasty of the shoulder joint.*
B. *X-ray of an arthrodesis after failed arthroplasty.*

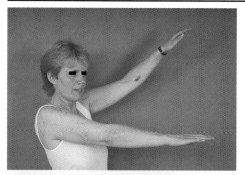
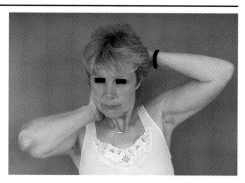
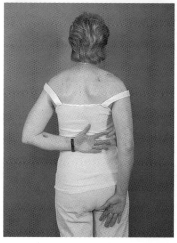

10 *Functional result after arthrodesis of night the shoulder.*

healed and all ten patients could manage their lives without external assistance (*fig 10*). Seven of the patients had no or only occasional mild pain. One complained of neuropathic pain resulting from brachial plexus injury, another complained of pain related to the implant but did not want plate removal, and one complained of pain at the medial border of the scapula. In the latter patient, the scapula lifted off the thorax with the arm in neutral position due to pronounced flexion position of the arthrodesis. In Richards' series [6], persistent pain after arthrodesis is not infrequent.

Conclusion

The functional deficits after arthrodesis of the shoulder are significant. Therefore this procedure is reserved as a salvage procedure for patients having pain that cannot be treated in another way or for patients with upper brachial plexus palsy having sufficient function of the hand to restore a stable arm. In most patients with severe pain in the shoulder joint, arthroplasty is the better choice. If arthrodesis is indicated, plate osteosynthesis leads to secure healing and allows functional post-operative treatment. After arthrodesis of the shoulder in the proper position, the patient is able to reach his face and ipsilateral ear, as well as his trouser pocket. Being able to comb his hair or attend to anal hygiene with the ipsilateral arm is desired, but this is not possible in all cases.

References

[1] Beltran JE, Trilla JC, Barjan R. A simplified compression arthrodesis of the shoulder. *J Bone Joint Surg Am* 1975 ; 57 : 538-541

[2] Cofield RH, Briggs BT. Glenohumeral arthrodesis. *J Bone Joint Surg Am* 1979 ; 61 : 668-677

[3] Kostuik JP, Schatzker J. Shoulder arthrodesis – AO technique. In : Bateman JE, Welsh RP eds. Surgery of the shoulder. Philadelphia : CV Mosby, 1984 : 207-210

[4] Müller ME, Allgöwer AM, Willenegger H. Manual der Osteosynthese, 2. Auflage. Berlin : Springer-Verlag, 1977 : 384-385

[5] Pipkin G. Claviculectomy as an adjunct to shoulder arthrodesis. *Clin Orthop* 1967 ; 54 : 145-159

[6] Richards RR. Glenohumeral arthrodesis. In : Iannotti JP, Williams GR eds. Disorders of the shoulder: diagnosis and management. Philadelphia : Lippincott, Williams and Wilkins, 1999 : 501-519

[7] Richards RR, Sherman RM, Hudson AR, Waddell JP. Shoulder arthrodesis in using a modified pelvic reconstruction plate: a review of eleven cases. *J Bone Joint Surg Am* 1988 ; 70 : 416-421

[8] Rowe CR. Arthrodesis of the shoulder used in treating painful conditions. *Clin Orthop* 1983 ; 173 : 92-96

[9] Rowe CR, Leffert RD. Advances in arthrodesis of the shoulder. In : Rowe CR ed. The shoulder. Edinburgh : Churchill Livingstone, 1988 : 507-519

[10] Sperling JW, Kozak TK, Hanssen AD, Cofield RH. Infection after shoulder arthroplasty. *Clin Orthop* 2001 ; 382 : 206-216

[11] Wallace WA. Revision shoulder replacement and rotator cuff problems. In : Wallace WA ed. Joint replacement in the shoulder and elbow. Oxford : Butterworth/Heinemann, 1998 : 81-95

palsy, with residual paresis of hand and elbow, or in patients with rheumatoid arthritis with functional deficits in the other joint of the arm, cannot be compared with patients after arthrodesis following infection of the glenohumeral joint or osteoarthritis due to a humeral head fracture.

The fusion rate after shoulder arthrodesis is high, regardless of the method of fixation. However, if screw fixation is used alone [1, 2] additional fixation in an spica cast is necessary. The same holds true if a reconstruction plate is used instead of the stronger narrow or broad DC plate [7]. The AO group has described plate fixation with one or two plates [3, 7] without additional external fixation. We have used the above-described technique in 16 cases. Of the ten patients we were able to re-examine at an average 5 years after the procedure, three have since died and three others live too far to come to follow-up. All of the arthrodeses

Late sequelae at the shoulder in obstetrical palsy in children

R Birch

Abstract. – Medial rotation contracture, posterior subluxation and posterior dislocation are a spectrum of the most common and most significant deformities present in obstetrical brachial plexus palsy. One third of children we saw required treatment by operation, most of these showing high levels of neurological recovery either spontaneously or after repair of the brachial plexus. Secondary bone changes involving the coracoid, the acromion, the glenoid, the head of the humerus and retroversion of the head on the shaft of the humerus are recognised and these progress with the evolution of the deformities. Severe deformation of the glenoid may involve defects of the postero-inferior wall and in these cases, a posterior bone block may be necessary to secure congruent reduction of the head of the humerus after relocation through an anterior approach. The recognition and treatment of this serious deformity require careful and prolonged observation and the recording of clinical findings by the treating clinician. Diagnosis depends on clinical examination, supplemented by plain radiographs. MR scan may contribute to the analysis of the severely deformed glenoid. Ultrasound is promising in confirming clinical evidence of the earliest changes in the first months of life.

Keywords: shoulder, obstetrical palsy, brachial plexus palsy, shoulder deformity, medial rotation contracture, posterior subluxation, posterior dislocation.

Shoulder: medial rotation contracture and posterior dislocation

This is the most common and most significant secondary deformity in obstetrical palsy (OBP). Fairbank wrote "the muscle which is most affected and offers the strongest bar to outward rotation is the subscapularis." [4] Sever [11] described radiological features, including "marked elongation of the coracoid process." Scaglietti [10], reporting Putti's work, thought that the deformity was caused by direct injury to the growing skeleton at birth: "the most constant and characteristic changes in the deformation of the angle of declination" (i.e. of retroversion of the head of the humerus upon the shaft). Controversy continues. Zancolli and Zancolli [13] thought that damage to the growth plate (epiphysiolysis) was the major factor. In the same volume Gilbert [5] wrote "posterior subluxation and deformity of the humeral head permanently worsens the prognosis. These anomalies, which have long been

Rolfe Birch, M.Chir., FRCS, The Royal National Orthopaedic Hospital Trust, Brockley Hill, Stanmore, Middlesex HA7 ALP, Great Britain.

considered the results of obstetrical palsy, are in fact the consequence of untreated contractures." These latter views are not incompatible; our experience suggests that both are correct and that they represent important contributions. It is with regret that we find it necessary to affirm that it is the responsibility of the treating clinician to recognise this serious complication in OBP and that it is his or her duty to follow these children carefully and for a sufficient length of time to be able to detect and treat it. Committee medicine leads to committee mistakes.

The methods used to record shoulder function are set out in Tables I, II (fig 1). Records are made at every attendance. Children aged more than 18 months usually perform various exercises eagerly and measurement of passive range is possible in younger children. Careful recording of clinical data is essential; without such records, comparison between different series is impossible and clinical activity valueless. The systems of functional analysis and measurement developed by Gilbert and Raimondi for the different segments of the upper limb are particularly valuable and are strongly recommended.

Over 400 children have required operation for medial rotation contracture, posterior

Table I. – Gilbert's chart for evaluation of shoulder examination [5].

Stage 0	Flail shoulder
Stage I	Abduction or flexion to 45 degrees. No active lateral rotation
Stage II	Abduction < 90 degrees. Lateral rotation to neutral
Stage III	Abduction = 90 degrees - Weak lateral rotation
Stage IV	Abduction < 120 degrees - incomplete lateral rotation
Stage V	Abduction > 120 degrees - Active lateral rotation
Stage VI	Normal

The suffix + is added to indicate sufficient medial rotation permitting the hand to come against the opposite shoulder.

Our convention restricts all children with no active or passive lateral rotation beyond neutral to Stage I - usually 1+ because adequate medial rotation is maintained.

subluxation or posterior dislocation since 1986. We are concerned with those children (the majority) who had good hand function and useful recovery in C5, C6 and C7 lesions, either spontaneously or after repair. The problem of the flail shoulder, seen in most severe neurological lesions, requires a quite different approach. Early experience with 86 cases treated by subscapularis recession and treatment of 59 cases of subluxation [1, 2] found a high incidence of

Table II. – A chart of shoulder range of movement in obstetrical palsy.

Range of Movement

Date	Forward Flexion		Lat Rotation		Inferior GH angle		Post GH Angle		Abduction		Medial rotation		Rotation forearm	
	Active	Passive	Active	Passive	Active	Passive	Active	Passive	Active	Passive	Active	Passive	Active	Passive

Value of active shoulder function = 1   2   3

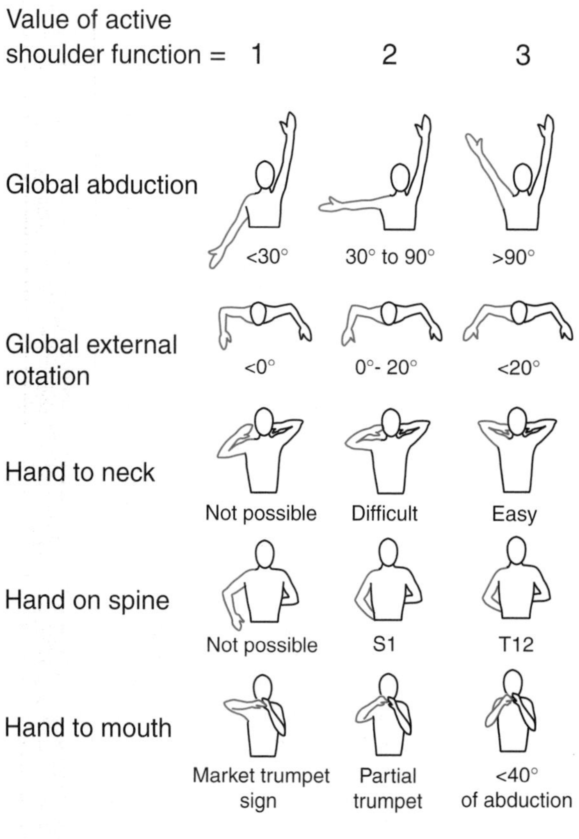

1 *The Mallet system of measuring function at the shoulder.*

Global abduction — <30°, 30° to 90°, >90°

Global external rotation — <0°, 0°- 20°, <20°

Hand to neck — Not possible, Difficult, Easy

Hand on spine — Not possible, S1, T12

Hand to mouth — Market trumpet sign, Partial trumpet, <40° of abduction

recurrence of the deformity in the former (29 cases) and frequent cases of loss of medial rotation in the latter. These findings have led to significant changes in our approach to a better understanding of the deformity of the glenoid in advanced cases and the high incidence of retroversion of the head of the humerus on the shaft (fig 2A, B).

The present data is based on an analysis of 166 children operated for the deformity between 1992 and 1996. All of these had at least useful neurological recovery, either spontaneously or after repair of the brachial plexus. Function of the hand and elbow was graded 4 or better. The range of elevation of the shoulder was over 130 degrees at final review. Forty-four children with more severe neurological injuries with paralysis have been excluded from this discussion. It is essential to distinguish between these two groups. The difficulties and methods of solution are quite different. In those children with severe neurological injury, the priority must be to improve innervation of the upper limb as much as is possible. In these cases muscle transfers are of limited palliative advantage although appropriate transfers to improve lateral rotation may prove necessary. Such muscle transfers were not needed in the 166 cases described here, all of whom regained functional lateral rotation. For many, the difficulty was in restoring medial rotation.

Amongst these children, there were 28 who had had previous subscapularis recession and 21 who had undergone a previous anterior operation. In 40 children, the deformity was detected at birth or shortly after and in 30 more it was recognised within the first year of life. However in 57 children, the deformity developed or progressed whilst under observation; in 20 the deformity occurred after repair of the upper trunk and it progressed in spite of continuing observation and assiduous exercises. In 11 of these children recovery had been so good that they were discharged from our clinic with normal or near normal function only to re-present later with the established deformity!

AETIOLOGY

The primary cause is, in many cases, the neurological lesion which invariably afflicts C5 and C6 irrespective of whether the rest of the plexus is damaged or not. There is paralysis of the lateral rotator muscles, infraspinatus and teres minor, innervated by the fifth cervical nerve. The medial rotators, the medial head of the pectoralis major and, above all, the subscapularis, innervated by the seventh and eighth cervical nerves, are never paralysed or only weakened for a short time so that their action is unopposed. Muscular imbalance is a potent cause for progressive deformity in the growing limb; the deformity at the shoulder is a reflection of this general principle. We have not encountered any cases of anterior dislocation of the shoulder.

The tempo of progression is not necessarily related to age. Marked secondary bone

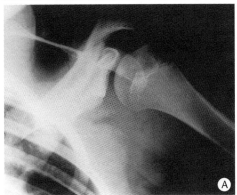 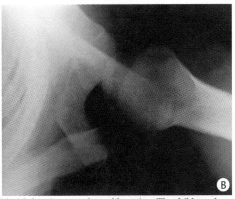

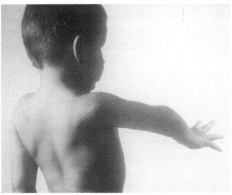

2 *A, B. AP and axial radiographs of shoulder in 12 year old girl showing complex subluxation. The child was born on the 9th May 1987 and ruptures of C5, C6 and C7 were repaired in August of that year. C8 and T1 were intact. Her function in June 1991 was: shoulder Gilbert 5+, Mallett 15; elbow 5; hand 5. Medial rotation contracture developed in 1993 and was treated by subscapularis recession in March 1994. By June 1995, function was good (Gilbert 5+, Mallett 15, abduction and forward flexion 160 degrees; lateral rotation 70 degrees, medial rotation 100 degrees, prono-supination 160 degrees) and she was discharged. She re-attended with recurrence of the deformity in March 1998. By this time, her shoulder function was graded at Gilbert 1+, Mallett 12; abduction and forward flexion were measured at 130 degrees; lateral rotation to –30 degrees. Medial rotation was 110 degrees and there was no active supination beyond neutral. The radiographs show overgrowth of the coracoid, double facet glenoid and the head of the humerus articulating with the false glenoid.*

This case exemplifies the slow evolution of the deformity, complicating otherwise successful repair, and it also exemplifies recurrence of deformity after initially successful subscapularis recession. The shoulder was relocated by the anterior approach described in the text. Function was improved but it did not reach the levels shown when she was first discharged from our care.

3 *Simple posterior dislocation in a 2 year old boy, with no significant secondary deformity of acromion, coracoid or glenoid. Retroversion of the head on the shaft of the humerus was estimated at 70 degrees.*

passive lateral rotation in the damaged upper limb is significant. We have encountered many serious errors in diagnosis because of incorrect examination and condemn the reprehensible practice of examining one limb alone or estimating the passive range of rotation with the arm in abduction. In older children the posture of the arm is characteristic; it lies in medial rotation with flexion and pronation at the elbow *(fig 3)*.

The contour of the shoulder is abnormal; the head is prominent behind the glenoid and palpation confirms any abnormalities of the coracoid and acromion. Measurements of the extent of the contracture indicate the amount of skeletal abnormality as well as of soft tissue contracture and differences between the active and the passive ranges give an indication of muscle weakness contribution to the observed defect. In nearly every case, a clear impression of the diagnosis and of the extent of secondary deformities can be achieved by physical examination and by plain antero-posterior and axial radiographs. The use of arthrograms and of MR and CT scans has been reported [9, 12].

The untreated deformity has very severe consequences for function in the upper limb as a whole. By late adolescence or early adult life, movements of the shoulder girdle are greatly restricted. The upper limb lies in fixed medial rotation; there is pain from the disorganised humeral joint; the flexion pronation posture of the elbow has become fixed. There may be subluxation of the head of the radius.

It is easy to miss the diagnosis before the first twelve months of life and our preliminary findings suggest that in those cases where the clinician has reason to be suspicious about the congruity of the shoulder, ultrasound examination is a suitable aid to diagnosis at this age.

Table III. – A clinical classification of shoulder deformity [1].

Type	Relation of head of humerus to glenoid	Clinical evidence	Radiological evidence	Supplementary investigations
Medial rotation contracture	Congruent.	Loss of passive lateral rotation of 30° or more.	Normal: coracoid may be elongated.	Ultrasound - congruent. MR scan may show retroversion of head upon shaft of humerus.
Simple subluxation	Head of humerus in false glenoid.	Lateral rotation to neutral. Head palpable posteriorly.	Incongruent. No other skeletal abnormality.	Ultrasound, CT and MR scans confirm incongruency: retroversion and "double facet" glenoid may be seen.
Simple dislocation	Head of humerus posterior to glenoid.	Fixed medial rotation contracture at about 30°. Head evidently lying behind glenoid.	Head of humerus behind glenoid. No other skeletal deformity.	Ultrasound, CT, MR scans confirm. Retroversion may be seen.
Complex subluxation	Head of humerus in false glenoid. Secondary bone deformity.	Lateral rotation to neutral or less. Overgrowth of coracoid and acromion palpable.	Extent of coracoid and acromion abnormality seen: "double facet" of glenoid.	Confirm incongruency and skeletal abnormality but may mislead about glenoid shape.
Complex dislocation	Head of humerus behind glenoid. Secondary bone deformity.	Fixed medial rotation contracture of 30° or more, obvious secondary bone changes.	Head of humerus behind glenoid: overgrowth of coracoid and acromion; abnormality of glenoid.	Confirm dislocation and extent of skeletal abnormality.

Note 1: In all cases, a flexion pronation posture of elbow and forearm is seen. In advanced cases, this deformity becomes fixed and may be associated with dislocation of the head of the radius.
Note 2: The extent of retroversion of the head on the shaft of the humerus cannot be measured accurately by any ancillary investigation, and it is best determined at operation of open reduction.

changes have been seen in children aged three years or less; on the other hand, dislocation in the presence of only minor deformities has been noted in children aged eleven or twelve. The deformity is progressive and ranges from medial rotation contracture to full posterior dislocation of the shoulder *(table III) (fig 2A, B)*.

DIAGNOSIS

The diagnosis is made by clinical examination. The infant is placed supine. The examiner holds both upper limbs with the elbows flexed to 90 degrees. **The arms are held adducted against the chest.** The upper limbs are gently rotated into lateral rotation. A diminution of the range of

THE OPERATION

■ *Subscapularis recession*

This was described by Carlioz and Brahimi [3]. Gilbert [5] emphasised that the operation should only be performed if the shoulder is congruent.

We performed 83 of these operations from 1987 to 1992. The initial results were promising but there has been a significant incidence of recurrence. Those surgeons inclined to this operation are advised to follow meticulously the indications and techniques of the originators. Above all, the operation should only be carried out when **the shoulder is congruent**. We add that the lateral rotator muscle must have recovered sufficiently to have restored balance but failing this, a supplementary latissimus dorsi transfer must be considered. As in all interventions in OBP, prolonged and careful follow up is essential.

■ *Correction of the deformity by the anterior approach*

The child is supine. Skin preparation and placing of towels are carried out so that the whole of the affected upper limb is accessible. An incision is made in the delto-pectoral groove. The cephalic vein is drawn medially, and the groove is opened to expose the coracoid process. Neither deltoid nor pectoralis major muscles are detached.

In most cases, the coracoid is long and inclined dorsally. An incision is made in the mid line of the longitudinal axis of the coracoid, preparing two flaps. The lateral flap consists of the periosteum and perichondrium, the coraco-humeral and the coraco-acromial ligaments. Lateral rotation is usually increased by 30-40 degrees upon elevation of this lateral flap, which suggests that the coraco-humeral ligament is an element in the contracture [8]. The medial flap, comprising the perichondrium and the periosteum, the pectoralis minor and coraco-clavicular ligaments, is detached from the coracoid which is now shortened to its base. Stay sutures are inserted into the two flaps. In a few cases of simple medial rotation contracture, no further steps need to be taken (fig 4, 5, 6).

The axillary fat pad is swept off the anterior face of the subscapularis muscle. It may be condensed, rather fibrous and adherent to the muscle in its superior part. Care must be taken to avoid damage to the neurovascular bundle. The thick glistening upper margin of the tendon of the suprascapularis is defined. The rotator interval is displayed. The subscapularis tendon can be drawn downwards with a skin hook, permitting limited inspection of the glenohumeral joint showing whether the head of the humerus is congruent within the glenoid or, as is usually the case, lying below and behind it. The upper part of the labrum is seen. The subscapularis is, on occasion, densely fibrous, a change which is perhaps consistent with post-ischaemic fibrosis [7].

In some early cases, before 1985, we performed a subscapularis tenotomy, sometimes combined with an anterior capsulotomy. This operation is needlessly destructive, and as Gilbert [6] emphasises, the subscapularis muscle is the most powerful

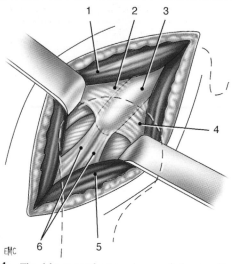

4   *The delto-pectoral groove is opened showing the elongated coracoid process. 1. Deltoid muscle; 2. coraco-humeral ligament; 3. elongated coracoid process; 4. pectoralis minor muscle; 5. pectoralis major muscle; 6. coracobrachialis, short head of the biceps.*

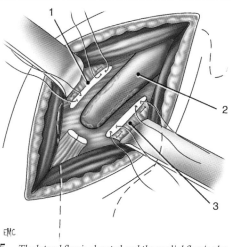

5   *The lateral flap is elevated and the medial flap is also detached to expose the coracoid itself. 1. Lateral flap including the periosteum, perichondrium, coracohumeral ligament, coraco-acromial ligament; 2. coracoid process exposed; 3. medial flap including the pectoralis minor, coracoclavicular ligament.*

medial rotator at the shoulder and it is essential for normal shoulder function. We now elongate the tendon in a Z-fashion. The upper flap is prepared by passing curved forceps underneath the superior part of the tendon and the upper one-third of the muscle, between it and the anterior face of the scapula. The flap is at least 2 cm long. This upper flap is then elevated, retaining its attachment to the lesser tuberosity (fig 7). The anterior capsule is preserved. A further gain in lateral rotation occurs after this manoeuvre and this may be all that is required in simple medial contracture. It is a mistake to stop here in cases of established subluxation or posterior dislocation. The lower flap of the muscle is prepared. Curved forceps are passed from below, being careful of the circumflex nerve and vessels, and the muscle is detached from its insertion onto the lesser tuberosity, preserving the capsule. Stay sutures are inserted into both flaps; the

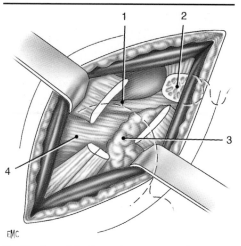

6   *The fat pad is dissected away to reveal the upper margin of the subscapularis tendon and the rotator interval. The coracoid has been shortened to its base. 1. Rotator interval. Superior lip of glenoid; 2. coracoid process shortened to its base; 3. axillary fat pad and neurovascular bundle; 4. subscapularis muscle.*

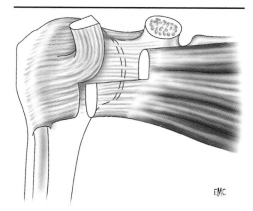

7   *The subscapularis muscle is divided in a Z-fashion, the upper flap is elevated, retaining its attachment to the lesser tuberosity and the lower flap is detached from the lesser tuberosity. The flaps should be at least 2 cm in length; the capsule should be preserved.*

arm is now put into full lateral rotation; the head of the humerus will be seen to glide back into the true glenoid where it is grasped by the labrum and secured by the anterior capsule (fig 8). In long-standing dislocations, the anterior translation of the head of the humerus means that the subscapularis flaps must be of sufficient length to permit repair. Capsulotomy is never necessary to secure relocation of the shoulder. The careful preparation of subscapularis flaps of sufficient length is of critical importance.

Anterior dislocation is an iatropathic disaster and it is caused by capsulotomy. Poor formation of the labrum, seen in a small number of cases, is a contributing factor.

At this stage, it may be apparent that overgrowth of the acromion is preventing congruent reduction of the head into the true glenoid. Resection by bone nibblers of the small anterior wedge of the acromion is permissible, but in more advanced cases showing downward prolongation of the acromion, our experience with osteotomy of the acromion has been negative.

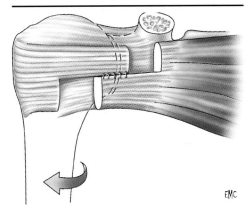

8 *Repair of subscapularis flaps after relocation of the head of the humerus into the glenoid.*

The surgeon must now make a formal record of the abnormalities displayed:

– the condition of the deltoid and pectoralis muscles;

– the length, breadth and inclination of the coracoid, and whether it abuts against the head of the humerus in attempted lateral rotation;

– the contribution of the coraco-humeral ligament to the contracture;

– variations in the course of the tendon of pectoralis minor which may be seen traversing the coracoid rather than inserting onto it;

– the state of the subscapularis muscle;

– the condition of the labrum;

– the depth and breadth of the true glenoid. The glenoid is usually well formed although at times it may be small and it is very rarely flat. There is usually a visible distinction between true and false sockets;

– the location of the false glenoid socket and the presence or absence of an intervening cartilaginous ridge between this and the true socket;

– overgrowth of the acromion;

– abnormality of the anterior part of the head of the humerus;

– the stability of reduction between full lateral rotation and medial rotation. Re-dislocation of the head of the humerus into the false glenoid socket or behind it at neutral rotation or even in the inner range of lateral rotation is one indication of retroversion;

– retroversion of the head upon the shaft of the humerus. We estimate this by grasping the head of the humerus between the index finger and thumb of one hand, to define the coronal plane of the head and grasping the epicondyles of the humerus with the finger and thumb of the other hand. The coronal planes of the head of humerus and the distal humerus are parallel in the normal infant shoulder. Retroversion of the head in excess of 30 degrees is significant; retroversion in excess of 50 degrees demands de-rotation osteotomy.

Table IV. – Secondary bone deformities in 166 shoulders.

Coracoid overgrowth	Moderate	90	Head of humerus	Conoid	25
	Severe	36		Flattened	9
				Trench defect	7
Acromion overgrowth	Anterior spur only	36			
	Of whole acromion	9			
Glenoid	Double facet	99	Retroversion	30 to 50 degrees	20
	Planar	22		50 to 70 degrees	36
	Severe postero-inferior defect	16		70 to 90 degrees	27

Planar and posterior defects co-exist in the severely deformed glenoid.

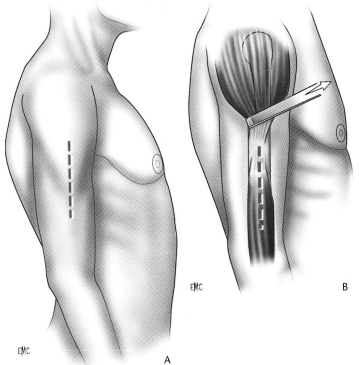

9 *Medial rotation osteotomy.*
A. Incision.
B. Exposure of humerus.

A summary of the significant secondary bone disorders is set out in table *IV*.

■ *De-rotation osteotomy*

De-rotation osteotomy of the humerus is an essential part of the operation in about one-third of operated cases. Since 1993, we have combined this procedure with the relocation of the head of the humerus. The shaft of the humerus is exposed between the pectoralis major and the deltoid tendons. This approach is chosen to avoid the risk of undue torsion on the radial nerve through the conventional mid lateral approach. The periosteum is elevated from the shaft of the bone; a small plate is applied to the shaft and secured in its upper part with one screw *(fig 9)*. A drill hole is then placed into the distal shaft, at the calculated angle for medial rotation of the distal fragment of the humerus *(fig 10)*. The plate is removed, the humerus is cut in the plane between the second and third holes of the 4-hole plate, the distal part of the limb is rotated medially so that the drill holes are in alignment and the plate is applied *(fig 11)*.

The stability of the shoulder is now re-examined. Usually lateral rotation to at least 50 degrees is still possible; the shoulder remains congruent in the glenoid to about 70 degrees of medial rotation.

The subscapularis flaps are now repaired with strong non-absorbable sutures. This usually enhances the shoulder stability. The flaps elevated from the coracoid are repaired. The wound is closed. The arm is immobilised in a plaster of Paris jacket, as a waistcoat around the body, with the upper limb in maximum lateral rotation and the forearm in supination. The arm is maintained at no more than 30 degrees of abduction.

At six weeks the plaster is removed and the patient starts exercises aiming to regain active elevation and lateral rotation. About two weeks after plaster removal, the patient concentrates more vigorously on regaining medial rotation.

In cases where de-rotation osteotomy has not been performed, it may become apparent that there was, after all, significant retroversion of the head of the humerus or there is a defect in active medial rotation. This is demonstrated by the inability of the child to bring the hand comfortably onto the body or behind his or her back. Attempting medial rotation provokes apparent winging of the scapula (reduced posterior postero-

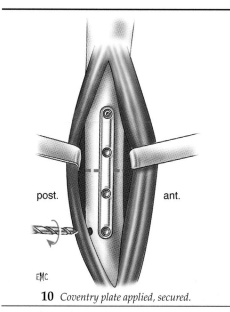

10 *Coventry plate applied, secured.*

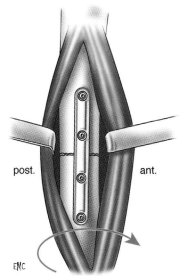

11 *Medial rotation osteotomy. Fixation after osteotomy and medial rotation of distal fragment.*

glenohumeral angle). De-rotation osteotomy is a simple enough matter; the child's arm is protected with a plaster of Paris back slab within a body sling for between four and six weeks.

The mid lateral approach was used for about the first 20 cases of de-rotation osteotomy. In three cases partial radial palsy occurred, and in one of these, full extension of digits was never recovered. In another child, the brachial artery was injured. The more proximal approach is safer *(fig 12)*.

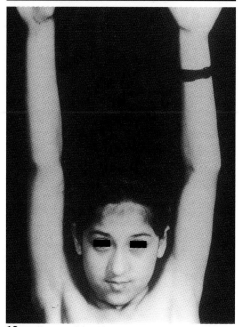

12 *Full range of shoulder movements in this 12 year old girl six years after relocation of a complex dislocation of the right shoulder.*

Results of this procedure in 166 cases operated between 1992 and 1996 are set out in table V. Results have been gratifying and so far seem to be lasting but we do not know the real long-term outcome of this intervention and will not be in a position to evaluate this for another five to ten years. We have not found it necessary to detach the pectoralis major, nor has the operation been combined with latissimus dorsi transfer for the enhancement of lateral rotation.

LATE OR PALLIATIVE OPERATIONS

Our attempts to correct severe overgrowth of the acromion (9 cases) have failed. Seven children with established posterior dislocation in whom earlier attempts of relocation had failed, and in whom it was clear there was a severe postero-inferior defect of the glenoid, were treated by a bone block fixed to the glenoid outside the capsule. The approach was in the plane between the infraspinatus and the teres minor and we now combine this step with anterior relocation in these advanced cases. It is likely that later reconstructive operations will prove inevitable in these children and we hope that by improving anatomical relations, later arthrodesis or arthroplasty will be practical propositions. Only time will tell. We see no place at all for primary interventions on the dislocated shoulder solely through the dorsal approach. We are uncertain about the place of lateral rotation osteotomy.

Conclusions

The treatment of this complex deformity is difficult. Insidious progression presents a pitfall for the unwary clinician. Prolonged and careful clinical review is essential; this should be done by the clinician responsible for the child's care. We urge adoption of the systems for functional assessment outlined in this article. Each case must be taken on its merits and each requires appropriate modification of the operating technique outlined above.

Acknowledgements – Preliminary drawings by Mr Tony Kochlar and Dr Bhupinderman. Photographs by Uta Boundy and Dirk De Camp of the Photographic Department of The Royal National Orthopaedic Hospital. Data and manuscript prepared by Mrs Margaret Taggart.

Table V. – *Results of surgery for 166 shoulders with a minimum follow-up of 3 years.*

			Gilbert and Mallett Score			
Gilbert score	Pre-op	mean	1.7	Post-op	mean	4.5
Mallett score	Pre-op	mean	9.3	Post-op	mean	13.3
			Active Movements			
Active elevation (forward flexion)	Pre-op	mean	110	Post-op	mean	131
Active medial rotation	Pre-op	mean	91	Post-op	mean	82
Active lateral rotation	Pre-op	mean	- 12	Post-op	mean	48
Active pronosupination	Pre-op	mean	99	Post-op	mean	151

Note: The low pre-operative Gilbert score reflects the modified system used in our Unit.

References

[1] Birch B, Bonney G, Wynn Parry CJ. Surgical disorders of the peripheral nerve. Edinburgh : Churchill Livingstone, 1998 : chap 10

[2] Birch R, Chen L. The medial rotation contracture of the shoulder in obstetric brachial plexus palsy. *J Bone Joint Surg Br* 1996 ; 78B (suppl 1) : 68

[3] Carlioz H, Brahimi L. La place de la désinsertion interne du sous-scapulaire dans le traitement de la paralysie obstétricale du membre supérieur chez l'enfant. *Ann Chir Infant* 1986 ; 12 : 159

[4] Fairbank HA. Subluxation of shoulder joint in infants and young children. *Lancet* 1913 ; 1 : 1217-1223

[5] Gilbert A. Obstetrical brachial plexus palsy. In : Tubiana R ed. The hand. vol. IV. Philadelphia : WB Saunders, 1993 ; chap 38 : 576-601

[6] Gilbert A. Paralysie obstétricale du plexus brachial. In : Alnot JY, Narakas A éd. Les paralysies du plexus brachial. Monographie de la société française de chirurgie de la main. Paris : Expansion Scientifique Française, 1995 : 270-281

[7] Landi A, Schoenhuber R, Funicello R, Rasio G, Esposito M. Compartment syndrome of the scapula. *Ann Hand Surg* 1992 ; 11 : 383-388

[8] Musa P. Observation made by Dr Musa in the course of a demonstration operation at the Symposium of study of OBPP, Heerlen. The Netherland, 1997

[9] Pearl ML, Edgerton BW. Glenoid deformity secondary to brachial plexus birth palsy. *J Bone Joint Surg Am* 1998 ; 80 : 659-667

[10] Scaglietti O. The obstetrical shoulder trauma. *Surg Gynecol Obstet* 1938 ; 66 : 868-877

[11] Sever JW. Obstetrical paralysis. Report of eleven hundred cases. *JAMA* 1925 ; 85 : 1862-1865

[12] Waters PM, Smith GR, Jaramillo D. Gleno-humeral deformity secondary to brachial; plexus birth palsy. *J Bone Joint Surg Am* 1998 ; 80 : 668-677

[13] Zancolli EA, Zancolli ER. Palliative surgical procedures in sequelae of obstetrical palsy. In : Tubiana R ed. The hand. vol. IV. Philadelphia : WB Saunders, 1993 ; chap 38 : 602-623

Early sequelae of the shoulder in obstetrical palsy

A Gilbert

Abstract. — After spontaneous recovery or surgical repair of the obstetrical brachial plexus, sequelae at the shoulder level may be disabling and can be treated surgically.
Lack of passive medial rotation should be rapidly treated by subscapularis release in order to avoid secondary joint incongruence. The paralytic shoulder can be improved by a latissimus dorsi transfer or trapezius transfer. These operations give constant improvement but the results are better in the young. Lack of appropriate rehabilitation and disuse will lead to decreased mobility, recurrence of the medial rotation contracture and joint anomalies with retroversion of the glenoid and posterior subluxation of the humeral head.

Keywords: shoulder, obstetrical palsy, internal rotation contracture, external rotation palsy, abduction palsy, muscle transfer, tendon transfer, soft tissue release.

Early sequelae

After an obstetrical lesion of the brachial plexus, spontaneous recovery [8] or repair of the plexus will generally allow good function of the shoulder. However, in both cases there are patients in whom muscle recovery will be late or incomplete [6]. Function of the lateral rotators usually comes back very late, but the medial rotators are not paralysed and recover quickly. There is an imbalance between the muscular groups. The internal rotators tend to be hyperactive and can become contracted; medial rotation contracture is a common feature and can be limited by physiotherapy, but sometimes the imbalance is so strong that the joint becomes fixed in internal rotation.

This internal rotation contracture may occur very early at 6-8 months, but more often at 16-20 months.

This position can become deleterious after some time and provokes anomalies of the joint, the first of which is flattening with posterior subluxation of the humeral head [1, 2, 3, 4]. After several years, the head is deformed, posteriorly dislocated, and the glenoid is small, flattened and retroverted. At this stage very little can be done. This will happen over 8-10 years. It seems that up to approximately 3 years, the deformity

of the joint is limited, allowing a useful release. It is mandatory to treat this contracture rapidly when it occurs. After no more than 3 months of unsatisfactory physiotherapy, surgery is the only solution [3, 9, 11].

In the young child the main cause of internal rotation is the contracture of the subscapularis. Joint contracture is not a primary cause and the bone anomalies (coracoid) occur later.

In the past several techniques have been described:

– Sever proposed sectioning the subscapularis tendon, associated with capsular resection.

– Saloff-Coste [10] prefers lengthening the tendon.

These techniques are very effective but their main drawback is the loss of internal rotation. Carlioz [2] proposed the release of the subscapularis muscle from the scapula as this preserves the function of the muscle.

TECHNIQUE OF SUBSCAPULARIS RELEASE

This operation is only possible if the joint remains congruent and the humeral head is round. It is necessary to verify this anatomy preoperatively; arthroscan and magnetic resonance imaging are the most precise methods.

The child is positioned on his back with the shoulder elevated by a large cushion; the shoulder should be free. The incision is made along the axillary border of the

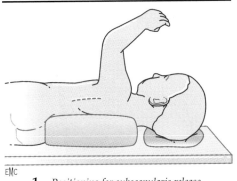

1   *Positioning for subscapularis release.*

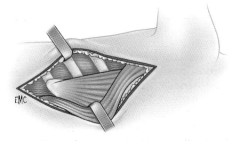

2   *The latissimus dorsi is retracted.*

scapula with the arm in abduction (*fig 1*). The anterior border of the latissimus dorsi is identified and retracted posteriorly (*fig 2*). The angle of the scapula then sticks out and is transfixed by a strong suture which is used for traction (*fig 3*). The deep surface of the blade of the scapula and the subscapularis are seen. The angular part of the muscle attachment is divided (*fig 4*). The teres major, which is quite close, should be respected.

Alain Gilbert, M.D., Institut de la Main, 6, square Jouvenet, 75016 Paris, France.

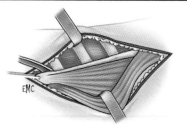

3   *Placement of a traction suture in the scapula.*

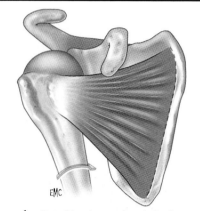

4   *Detaching the muscle at its border.*

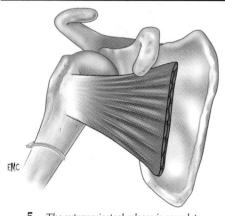

5   *The extraperiosteal release is complete.*

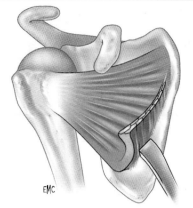

6   *At the end of the detachment, external rotation is free.*

7   *Cast immobilisation for 3 weeks.*

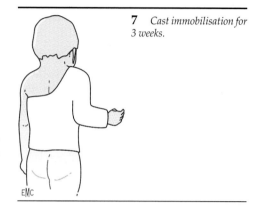

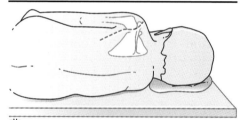

8   *Positioning and incision for latissimus dorsi transfer.*

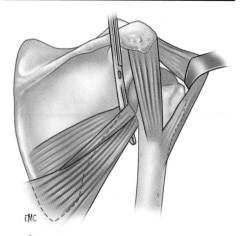

9   *Isolation of the latissimus dorsi tendon.*

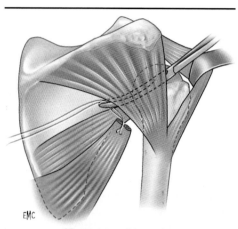

10   *Division of the tendon.*

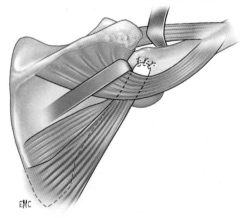

11   *Fixation to the humeral head.*

The subscapularis is then released progressively, remaining extraperiosteal. The fibrous bands are sectioned one by one (fig 5). The detachment should be complete, particularly at the superomedial angle of the scapula. (Detachment that goes too far medially may injure the serratus anterior or the superior border of the pedicle of the subscapularis and should be avoided.) The result is an immediate gain of motion at the end of the detachment, often surpassing 60 to 70 degrees. It is never necessary to open the joint capsule (fig 6).

A drain is left for 48 hours. A cast is applied, with the elbow at the child's side in a position of maximal external rotation for 3 weeks (fig 7), after which physiotherapy is started.

After removal of the plaster, intensive physiotherapy is initiated. It is crucial to maintain the good external rotation obtained by surgery, but passive rotation will only be maintained if the external rotator muscles become active. If, after 5 or 6 months, there is still no active lateral rotation and progressive loss of passive rotation, a tendon transfer should be performed. If this is not done in time, the contracture will recur.

In our series, about 50% of patients recovered active rotation after simple release [5]. Some of the others ought to have undergone a muscle transfer, but only 20% accepted it or were followed closely enough. When the patient is a foreigner or if the family does not seem to be compliant, it is better to associate a latissimus dorsii transfer at the same time as the release.

For others, the transfer will be performed on a supple joint after a minimum of 6 month's physiotherapy.

TECHNIQUE OF LATISSIMUS DORSI TRANSFER [7]

The patient is positioned on the opposite side with the affected arm and shoulder prepped and draped free. An incision is made vertical and posterior to the shoulder and following the lateral border of the scapula (fig 8).

The latissimus dorsi muscle is freed from the teres major and the scapula and its tendon of insertion on the humerus is isolated (fig 9). The tendon is divided at its insertion to the humerus, and the muscle is freed, taking care to preserve its neurovascular pedicle. A transdeltoid incision between the middle and posterior parts of the deltoid provides access to the humeral head and to the insertion of the external rotators (fig 10). The latissimus dorsi tendon is then passed under the posterior deltoid and fixed either to the rotator cuff or directly to the humeral head in the young child (fig 11). A stout non-resorbable suture is used to fix the transfer

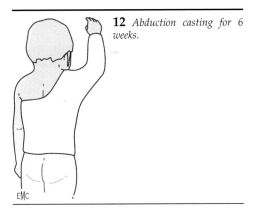

12 *Abduction casting for 6 weeks.*

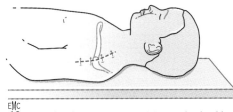

13 *Transfer of the trapezius: incision on the shoulder.*

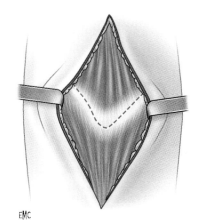

14 *Release of the trapezius.*

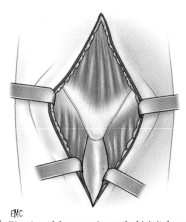

15 *Fixation of the trapezius to the bicipital groove.*

while holding the shoulder in 120 degrees of abduction and external rotation. The infant is immobilised in a cast in this position for 6 weeks (fig 12).

RESULTS

The results of the latissimus dorsi transfer are encouraging. We reviewed a series of 150 cases and 122 were followed-up over an average of 5-8 years and a minimum of 3 years.

The average age at operation was 3.6 years. The results showed an average improvement of abduction of 29 degrees at one year, 31 degrees at 3 years but only 15 degrees at 5 years, demonstrating that with time and disuse, many of these children lose abduction. The external rotation was improved in almost all cases (83% at 5 years).

In severe cases where the latissimus dorsi is very weak, the trapezius may be used. Its action will be more of abduction and it will provide less external rotation, but in most cases, by choosing its insertion carefully, it will be possible to correct some of the internal rotation deformity.

Technique of trapezius transfer

The patient is installed in a lateral position with the arm free. A V-Y incision is drawn on the shoulder; the anterior incision is made on the clavicle, the posterior incision on the spine of the scapula. The skin is incised but not lifted from the muscle. The trapezius is detached from its bony insertions on the clavicle and the scapula. The muscle should be extensively dissected, freeing it completely from the clavicle and from the spine of the scapula. The musculocutaneous flap is lifted as a whole. The flap is limited by the deep vascular pedicle where dissection should stop (fig 13, 14).

Distally, the tendon is lifted with the periosteum of the acromion. A T-shaped incision is made on the deltoid; the muscle is usually denervated. The two flaps are detached from the acromion. The humeral head is held in rotation and the bicipital groove becomes lateral. The trapezius tendon will be fixed on the anterior lip of the bicipital groove. The arm is held in abduction and external rotation. Fixation is made through the bone; this is best done with a bone anchor. The two deltoid flaps are closed over the trapezius tendon. The skin can be closed in a V fashion. The arm is immobilised in a cast in abduction and external rotation for 6 weeks (fig 15, 16).

This transfer has been described numerous times with different techniques of insertion. In the young infant it is possible to fix the transfer directly to the humerus without elongating it.

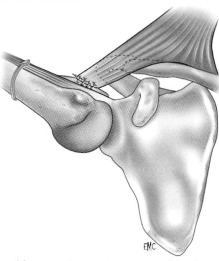

16 *Positioning in abduction-external rotation.*

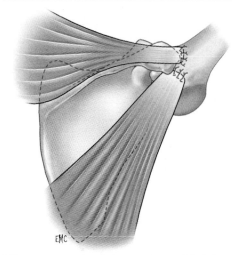

17 *Double transfer of the trapezius and latissimus dorsi.*

POST-OPERATIVE CARE

The following important points should be respected.

The splint is left for 6 weeks and is then opened, allowing physiotherapy in the splint for another 2 weeks.

Re-education of the muscle progresses slowly and starts in the supine position, eliminating gravity. Muscle strengthening may take 6 to 10 months.

The muscle has to be worked intensively as it is usually too weak to give good abduction. After several months, the average abduction is around 40 degrees.

In weak shoulders with limited abduction, it may be necessary to associate two transfers at the same time. The muscles the most often used are the latissimus dorsi and the trapezius (fig 17). Other authors [3] have used the levator scapulae muscle with the latissimus dorsi.

References ➤

References

[1] Babbitt DP, Cassidy RH. Obstetrical paralysis and dislocation of the shoulder in infancy. *J Bone Joint Surg Am* 1968 ;
50 : 1447-1452

[2] Carlioz H, Brahimi L. La place de la désinsertion interne du
sous-scapulaire dans le traitement de la paralysie obstétricale du membre supérieur chez l'enfant. *Ann Chir Infant*
1986 ; 12 : 159-170

[3] Egloff DV, Raffoul W, Bonnard C, Stalder J. Palliative surgical
procedures to restore shoulder function in obstetric brachial palsy: critical analysis of Narakas's series. *Hand Clin*
1995 ; 11 : 597-606

[4] Fairbank HA. Birth palsy : subluxation of the shoulder joint
in infants and young children. *Lancet* 1913 ; 1 : 1217

[5] Gilbert A, Romana C, Ayatti R. Tendon transfers for shoulder paralysis in children. *Hand Clin* 1988 ; 4 : 633-642

[6] Gilbert A, Tassin JL. Réparation chirurgicale du plexus brachial dans la paralysie obstétricale. *Chirurgie* 1984 ; 110 :
70-75

[7] Hoffer MM, Wichenden R, Roper B. Brachial plexus birth
palsies : Results of tendon transfer to the rotator cuff. *J Bone
Joint Surg Am* 1978 ; 60 : 691-695

[8] Mallet J. Paralysie obstétricale. *Rev Chir Orthop* 1972 ; 58
(suppl 1) : 115

[9] Price AE, Grossman JA. A management approach for secondary shoulder and forearm deformities following obstetrical brachial plexus injuries. *Hand Clin* 1995 ; 11 : 607-617

[10] Saloff-Coste J. À propos du traitement des paralysies
obstétricales du plexus brachial : désinsertion du sous-
scapulaire sans capsulotomie. *Rev Chir Orthop* 1966 ; 52 :
395-400

[11] Zancolli EA, Zancolli ER. Palliative surgical procedures in
sequelae of obstetrical palsy. *Hand Clin* 1988 ; 4 : 643-669

Paralytic shoulder in the adult

L Celli
C Rovesta
MC Marongiu
A Celli

Abstract. – The paralytic shoulder in adults is the loss of mobility and stability of the scapulothoracic and scapulohumeral joints with a secondary peripheral nerve lesion.
On the basis of our experience over the last 25 years of treating damaged peripheral nerves, we describe the surgical treatment for the reparable and irreparable nerve lesions around the shoulder in post-traumatic and postneuritic pathology.
For reparable nerve lesions, we present the surgical treatment for the reconstruction procedure of the XI cranial nerve, the suprascapular and axillary nerves. In irreparable nerve lesions, we describe the main palliative procedures for recovering the principle muscle functions in:
– the scapular thoracic joint: muscular transfer in trapezius, rhomboid and serratus anterior muscle palsy,
– the scapular humeral joint: muscle transfer in supraspinatus and infraspinatus muscle palsy.

© 2001, Editions Scientifiques et Médicales Elsevier SAS. All rights reserved.

Keywords: shoulder, paralysis, muscle transfer, long thoracic nerve palsy, XI cranial nerve palsy, axillary nerve palsy, suprascapular nerve palsy.

Introduction

A paralytic shoulder means loss of mobility and stability of the scapulothoracic and scapulohumeral joints caused by post-traumatic or post-neuritic lesions involving the peripheral nerves around the shoulder girdle. Isolated nerve injuries to the shoulder can be caused by a variety of types and degrees of lesions: traumatic (fractures, acute instability, iatrogenic); microtraumatic entrapment with or without a cyst (suprascapular and axillary nerve); neuropathic (Parsonage-Turner syndrome).

In this chapter we analyse the paralytic shoulder in adults involving isolated nerve lesions of the scapulothoracic and scapulohumeral joints and requiring surgical treatment [1]. In particular, we deal with lesions of the XI cranial nerve and the long thoracic nerve for the scapulothoracic joint, and lesions of the suprascapular and axillary nerves concerning the scapulohumeral joint.

Luigi Celli, *Professor, Chief of Orthopaedic and Traumatological Department.*
Claudio Rovesta, *M.D.*
Maria Carmen Marongiu, *M.D.*
Andrea Celli, *M.D.*
University of Modena and Reggio Emilia, Department of Surgery and Emergency Services, Polyclinic, Largo del Pozzo, 71, 41100 Modena, Italy.

We do not analyse the problems of surgical treatment of complete shoulder palsy after cervical and brachial plexus lesions.

Controversy exists regarding the management and progress of isolated nerve injuries to the shoulder in adults. Some authors have recommended observation and a rehabilitation programme after lesions, whereas others advocate early surgery (within 6 months) for the treatment of nerve lesions, and late surgery (after 12 months) with muscle transfer when palsy is irreversible. We recommend a period of six months of non-operative treatment following nerve injuries. Operative exploration and early nerve repair may be indicated when the aetiology, entity and location of the lesion can be determined. However, if symptoms persist, with pain and loss of function despite adequate time after conservative treatment or failed nerve reconstruction, muscular transfer must be used.

Palliative surgery is suggested if:

– the joints are not stiff;

– the palsy involves only one or two muscles and the other muscles of the shoulder have normal strength and function;

– the transfer is similar in contraction, length and synergic activity to the paralysed muscle;

– the patients understand and co-operate in the rehabilitation programme after surgery.

Reparable and irreparable nerve lesions of the scapulothoracic and scapulohumeral joints

SCAPULOTHORACIC NERVE LESIONS

Palsy of the trapezius, rhomboid and serratus anterior muscles is the most common cause of scapular winging. Muscle atrophy and the clinical aspect of the scapulothoracic joint, with the arm at the side and elevated, confirm the diagnosis. The scapula is depressed and translated laterally with the lower corner rotated laterally when the XI cranial nerve is injured (*fig 1A*). The scapula assumes a different position when the long thoracic nerve is injured, with a superior elevation, the lower corner rotated medially and the medial border rotated outward (*fig 1B*). Patients with scapulothoracic palsy suffer pain and weakness and have difficulty in raising their upper limb.

LONG THORACIC NERVE LESIONS

Long thoracic nerve lesions are relatively common [6, 18] and only play a role in early

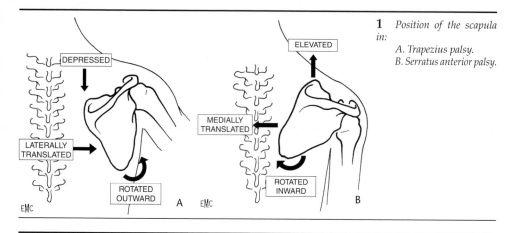

1 Position of the scapula in:

A. Trapezius palsy.
B. Serratus anterior palsy.

Surgical techniques for transfer to the sternal part of the pectoralis major and teres major muscles for dynamic scapular stabilisation

PECTORALIS MAJOR TRANSFER IN SERRATUS ANTERIOR PALSY

This technique was written by Marmor and Becthol [13]. The patient is in a beach-chair (fig 2A) or lateral decubitus position. The skin incision is about 10-15 cm long crossing the axilla from the pectoralis major muscle at the front to the lower tip of the scapula (fig 2B). The sternal part of the pectoralis major is identified and its tendon is removed from its humeral insertion. The lower part of the pectoralis major must be extended with a fascia lata graft (6 x 15 cm). Subsequently, the lower border of the scapula is exposed and the transfer is passed through a hole made in the lower corner of the scapula and inserted with non-absorbable sutures in the tendon of the pectoralis major near the bone of the scapula (fig 2C). Postoperative treatment requires immobilisation of the patient with the upper limb in adduction and in a neutral position for 6 weeks. Following this, it is useful to apply a custom scapulothoracic orthosis that presses the scapula against the chest wall during the rehabilitation programmes.

TERES MAJOR TRANSFER IN SERRATUS ANTERIOR PALSY

This technique was described by Hass [7]. The patient is in a beach-chair or contralateral decubitus position; two skin incisions are required.

The first skin incision, 10-15 cm long, is made above the posterior pillar of the axilla (fig 3A). The tendon of the teres major must be separated from the latissimus dorsi tendon and detached from the humerus (fig 3B).

The teres major is passed to the lateral wall of the chest.

The second small skin incision, at the level of the 4th and 5th ribs over the anterior margin of the lateral aspect of the thorax, permits the insertion into the rib bone (fig 3C).

Excessive tension over the neurovascular pedicle of the teres major must be avoided when the tendon is transferred to the front.

Postoperative treatment requires immobilisation of the shoulder in a soft bandage with the upper limb adducted in neutral rotation for 5-6 weeks, followed by a rehabilitation programme of 2-3 months, keeping the scapula pressed against the thorax using a custom orthosis.

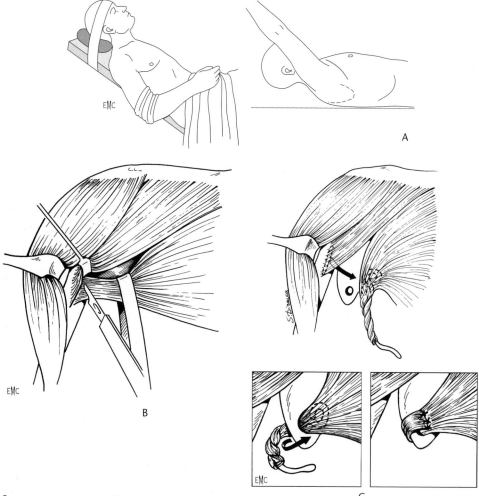

2 Transfer of the pectoralis major in serratus anterior palsy.
A. Patient position and skin incision.
B. The sternal part of the pectoralis major is identified and removed from its humeral insertion.
C. The transfer is extended with a fascia lata graft and inserted in a hole made in the lower corner of the scapula.

surgery in cases of brachial plexus lesions. Since it is often difficult to recognise the cause of the trauma and site of the lesion, we have never performed a nerve reconstruction when the lesion is isolated. Such a reconstruction is only possible in iatrogenic lesions or in direct lateral thoracic wall traumas. Neuritic pathologies (Parsonage-Turner syndrome) which frequently lead to paralysis of the serratus anterior muscle play a role in rehabilitation, but not in surgery.

An operation to correct winging of the scapula is required when serratus anterior paralysis is stabilised and the patients suffer disabling pain and dysfunction of the shoulder. Different operations have been classified in the literature: scapulothoracic fascial sling suspension, scapulothoracic fusion or muscle transfer. Different muscle transfers are used including the pectoralis major, the pectoralis minor, the teres major, the rhomboid muscle and combinations of all these.

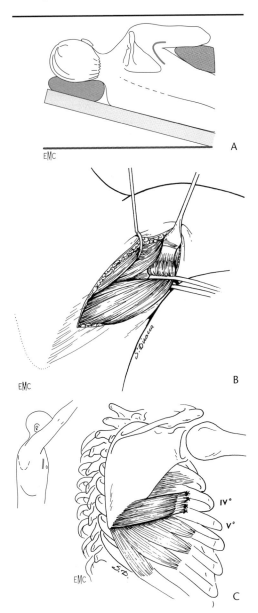

3 *Transfer of the teres major in serratus anterior palsy.*
A. Patient is in the lateral decubitus position; the first incision is made above the posterior pillar of the axilla.
B. The tendon of the teres major is detached from the humerus.
C. The second small skin incision is made in the lateral wall of the chest. The teres major tendon is transferred to the front and inserted in the 4th-5th rib bone.

XI cranial nerve lesions

A direct laterocervical trauma can damage the XI cranial nerve (nervus accessorius spinalis), although the most common cause of such lesions is iatrogenic as a result of a laterocervical biopsy [9]. The clinical aspect depends on the location of the lesion. In fact, when the injury involves only the cranial portion of the nerve, the trapezius muscle becomes paretic and its function is partially preserved. Such lesions do not often require surgery. Nevertheless, when the lesion is low in the laterocervical space and involves both the cranial and cervical components, trapezius muscle paralysis is total and requires surgery. In this case the patient's

ability to raise his arm is reduced and secondary pathologies can arise as a result of acromiohumeral impingement and outlet syndromes.

SURGICAL MANAGEMENT FOR REPARABLE NERVE LESIONS

The patient is placed in a contralateral decubitus position (fig 4A). The surgical incision runs along the posterior edge of the sternocleidomastoid muscle and the upper edge of the trapezius muscle, partially following the scar left by the previous surgery (fig 4B). The proximal stump of the nerve is isolated at the posterior edge of the muscle, while the distal stump is identified at the point where it enters the trapezium, approximately 4-5 cm from the posterior edge of the clavicula and the anterior margin of the trapezius (fig 4C). Nerve continuity is reconstructed by a sural nerve graft (usually 5-8 cm long).

SURGICAL MANAGEMENT FOR IRREPARABLE NERVE LESIONS

If, in early surgery, it is impossible to find the distal stump of the nerve, if nerve reconstruction proves unsuccessful or the lesion cannot be reconstructed, we recommend a transfer operation. The transfer of the levator scapulae muscle from the scapula to the acromion is performed to obtain recovery of the upper trapezius muscle function and to transpose the rhomboid muscles lateral to the scapular body so as to recover function of the middle and lower parts of the trapezius [2, 5].

Levator scapulae and rhomboid minor and major transfers in trapezius palsy

SURGICAL MANAGEMENT (EDEN–LANGE TECHNIQUE) [10]

The patient is placed in contralateral decubitus position with the thorax and the head raised 15°-20° (fig 5A).

Two skin incisions are necessary; the first incision is made along the medial scapula border from the upper to the lower corner. The levator scapulae is identified at the superior angle of the scapula and the insertions of the rhomboid minor muscle at the medial border of the spina and the rhomboid major muscle at the medial border of the infraspinatus fossa are differentiated (fig 5B).

The lateral transfer of these muscles allows function of the upper, middle and inferior portions of the trapezius to be recovered.

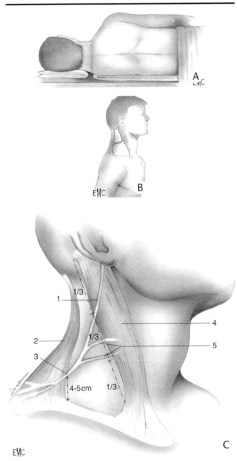

4 *Surgical management for reparable lesions of the XI cranial nerve.*
A. The patient is placed in a contralateral decubitus position.
B. The surgical incision runs along the posterior edge of the sternocleidomastoid muscle and the upper edge of the trapezius muscle, partially following the scar left by the previous surgery.
C. The proximal stump of the nerve is isolated at the posterior edge of the muscle, while the distal stump is identified at the point where it enters the trapezium, approximately 4-5 cm from the posterior edge of the clavicula and the anterior margin of the trapezius. 1. Accessory nerve, cranial level; 2. trapezius muscle; 3. accessory nerve; 4. sternocleidomastoid muscle; 5. accessory nerve, cervical level.

With the second skin incision of about 5-6 cm along the posterior and lateral margins of the acromion, the levator scapulae is transferred to the posterior tip of the acromion and inserted with non-absorbable sutures through two or three holes in the bone (fig 5C).

When the levator scapula is dissected proximally before being transferred, care needs to be taken at the dorsal scapular nerve.

When the levator scapulae is transferred to the acromion it becomes a substitute for the upper portion of the trapezius.

Subsequently, the tendinous attachments of the rhomboid minor and major, with or without a small piece of the medial border of the scapula bone, are transferred laterally and fixed to the bone of the supraspinatus and infraspinatus fossa (fig 5C).

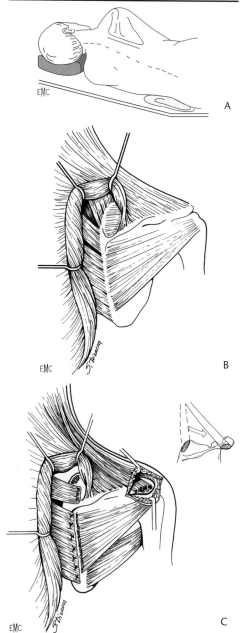

5 *Transfer of the levator scapulae and the rhomboid minor and major in trapezius palsy.*

A. The patient is placed in a contralateral decubitus position and two skin incisions are required.

B. The first incision along the medial scapula border allows identification of the insertions of the levator scapulae, rhomboid minor and major muscles.

C. The second skin incision along the posterior and lateral margins of the acromion enables the levator scapulae tendon to be transferred. The tendinous attachment of the rhomboid minor and major are transferred laterally and fixed into the bone of the suprapinatus and infraspinatus fossa.

Under these conditions, the rhomboid muscles are suitable to substitute for the middle and lower portions of the trapezius.

In the postoperative programme, the upper limb must be immobilised in a thoraco-brachial cast in approximately 60°-70° abduction and 30°-40° anteposition for 4-5 weeks.

The rehabilitation programme starts with passive motion exercises and then active exercises are gradually added.

Scapula humeral nerve lesions

The importance of the deltoid, supraspinatus and infraspinatus muscles in providing active elevation of the arm is readily appreciated when the loss of function of these muscles in the paralytic shoulder is considered. In normal function, the scapulohumeral joint requires coordinated action among many muscles of the scapular girdle muscles. The three heads of the deltoid and rotator cuff muscles work in synergy during shoulder movements. In patients with isolated and complete paralysis of the deltoid, active elevation can be preserved by compensatory action of the rotator cuff, but these patients will still have considerable deficits in abduction strength and humeral extension with early fatigability.

The suprascapular nerve provides scapulohumeral stability in the upward and anteroposterior directions and active movements in abduction and external rotation. The supraspinatus muscle is the stabilising muscle and can be considered the pivot of scapulohumeral movement, modifying the forces of the deltoid that tends to decentralise the head of the humerus. The infraspinatus muscle is the main external rotator of the shoulder.

A patient with supraspinatus and infraspinatus muscle palsy loses (or suffers reduction of) the capacity of abduction and external rotation of his arm. Shoulder abduction can be preserved only when the deltoid muscle functions well (M_5) and the upper portion of the subscapularis muscle and the long head of the biceps tendon have the capacity to avoid upper subluxation of the humeral head.

In these conditions, the active movement of abduction is without strength and the patient might lose this movement if there is a tear in the subscapularis tendon which, over time, becomes overloaded by repetitive motion.

In infraspinatus muscle palsy, the patient preserves the capacity of external rotation of the arm when the teres minor muscle and the posterior part of the deltoid muscle function well (M_5). This active movement is possible only when the shoulder is in more than 40°-60° arm abduction.

On the basis of these considerations, we believe that in an irreversible nerve lesion where the supraspinatus and infraspinatus muscle do not have sufficient re-innervation, it is useful to improve or recover abduction and external rotation of the shoulder by a muscle transfer. However, when the deltoid muscle has irreversible palsy, the use of a transfer is questionable. Axillary and suprascapular nerve lesions are commonly caused by trauma to the shoulder. These are more often seen in association with fractures, dislocations, or surgical procedures to the shoulder. Injuries of these nerves may be isolated or occur in association with one another, or with brachial plexus lesions. In repetitive activities of athletes or workers, with or without a ganglion cyst, the axillary nerve may be entrapped in the quadrilateral space and the suprascapular nerve in the suprascapular and spinoglenoid notches. In these cases, irreversible muscle paralysis may occur due to lesions caused by compressed or stretched nerves.

Axillary nerve lesions

Axillary nerve lesions can be isolated or associated with the suprascapular nerve [4, 11]. Compressive canalicular lesions in Velpeau's quadrilateral space are quite unusual. Nevertheless, this is the level that presents the greatest number of traumatic lesions. When the trauma involves a forced abduction and retroposition of the arm in external rotation, the axillary nerve can be damaged by a scissor-like pinching between the tricipital tendon and the humeral bone [1, 4]. This mechanism becomes even more damaging if the humeral head is dislocated downward and forward, stretching the vasculonervous structures. Dislocation of the shoulder can cause an isolated axillary nerve lesion in patients under 30 years of age in about 30% of cases. In those over 40 years old, scapulohumeral dislocation can cause not only a nerve lesion but also a rotator cuff tear. In these cases, we can sometimes see the "terrible triad": simultaneous scapulohumeral dislocation, rotator cuff tear and axillary nerve lesion. A post-traumatic shoulder paralysis, subsequent to dislocation or fracture of the scapular-clavicular skeleton, can arise through an associated suprascapular and axillary nerve lesion. Such a lesion must always be suspected when a patient with evident deltoid paralysis also shows a total inability to abduct and externally rotate his arm. It is important to remember that if the suprascapular and infraspinatus muscles function, the patient can abduct and externally rotate the arm even if the deltoid muscle is paralysed. In most lesions diagnosed as isolated axillary nerve injuries, the suprascapular nerve lesion is wrongly identified because the damaged nerve often remains in continuity and spontaneously recovers in just a few months: axillary nerve lesions are likely to recover spontaneously within a period of 4-6 months. The absence of any significant EMG re-innervation signs after that period of time indicates that surgery is required.

SURGICAL MANAGEMENT FOR REPARABLE AXILLARY NERVE LESIONS

The patient is placed in a supine decubitus position. There are two possible routes of access to the axillary nerve: the axillary approach and the deltopectoral approach

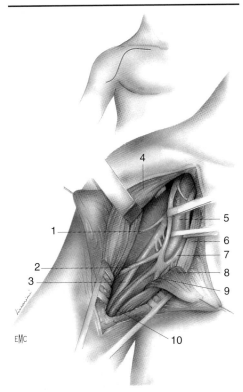

6 *Axillary nerve. Anterior approach: the incision runs parallel to the deltopectoral sulcus. After pulling the deltoid and the pectoralis major muscles aside, the pectoralis minor muscle is detached from the coracoid so that it can be reinserted later. The vasculonervous structures of the brachial plexus are identified; the lateral cord is isolated and pulled aside with soft rubber laces. Once the subclavian artery has been isolated, the posterior cord is visible with small nerve branches running to the subscapular and latissimus dorsi muscles. The axillary nerve originates from the posterior cord high up in the vicinity of the clavicle. 1. Axillary nerve; 2. musculocutaneous nerve; 3. radial nerve; 4. deltoid muscle; 5. subclavian artery;*
6. pectoralis major muscle; 7. medial cord; 8. pectoralis minor muscle; 9. ulnar nerve; 10. median nerve.

with a secondary retrodeltoid access. The axillary approach can be used in young women. However, in muscular patients, the axillary approach makes it difficult to view the point where the nerve originates from the posterior cord and its terminal branches divide in the retrodeltoid region. We consider the double approach, with anterior and posterior access, to be the technique of choice.

■ *Anterior approach to isolate the axillary nerve*

The incision runs parallel to the deltopectoral sulcus (fig 6). After pulling the deltoid muscle and the pectoralis major aside, respecting the cephalic vein, the pectoralis minor muscle is detached from the coracoid so that it can be reinserted later. Once the subclavian artery has been isolated, the posterior cord is visible with small nerve branches running to the subscapular and latissimus dorsi muscle. The space in front of Velpeau's quadrilateral can be prepared once the musculocutaneous nerve has been isolated and pulled aside. It is usually at this level that a neuroma characterising the lesion can be palpated and isolated.

■ *Posterior approach to isolate the axillary nerve*

The incision, approximately 10 cm long, is arched and runs parallel to the lower margin of the posterior deltoid muscle (fig 7). Detaching the subcutaneous layer and cutting the fasciae, the space between the deltoid muscle, tricipital muscle fasciae and humerus is exposed. This exposes the point where the axillary nerve emerges, divided only into its terminal branches. The first, more superficial, is a sensitive branch supplying the deltoid region. The motor branches (2 or 3) are deeper and surrounded by numerous veins and small arterial branches (branches of the posterior circumflex artery). After recognising where the nerve is interrupted and after dissecting the nerve stumps, the continuity is reconstructed with 2-3 sural nerve grafts, approximately 10-15 cm long. Before suturing the nerve grafts, they are run from the posterior region through Velpeau's quadrilateral to the anterior region. Postoperatively, the limb is immobilised with a Velpeau bandage for approximately 3 weeks. A rehabilitation programme is then started.

SURGICAL MANAGEMENT FOR IRREPARABLE NERVE LESIONS

The latissimus dorsi bipolar transplant can be used for muscle transfer in irreversible deltoid muscle paralysis. The humeral tendon – approximately 20 cm of latissimus dorsi muscle mass with its neurovascular pedicle – is transferred and reinserted into the deltoid insertion area. Itoh et al [8] reported 8 cases where this technique gave good functional results. We have performed this type of transplant in 2 cases with modest results (more aesthetic than functional). Nevertheless, this initial experience taught us the technical difficulties involved in giving the transplant the right tension so that adequate contraction and force can be achieved.

Suprascapular nerve lesions

Isolated traumatic lesions of the suprascapular nerve are unusual and are generally associated with lesions of the brachial plexus and axillary nerve. Such lesions are more frequently found in canalicular nerve compression of the coracoid notch and spinoglenoid space [19, 22]. When the nerve is compressed at the coracoid notch, diagnosis is based on the presence of hypotrophy of the supraspinatus and infraspinatus muscles, rendering shoulder abduction and external rotation exhausting. EMG and NMR evaluations of the supraspinatus fossa are essential for diagnosis as they show the presence of cystic

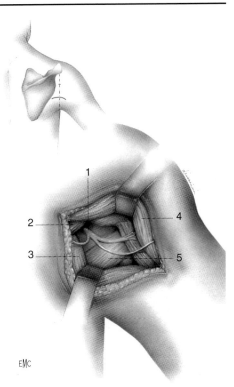

7 *Axillary nerve lesions. Posterior approach: the second incision, approximately 10 cm long, is arched and runs parallel to the lower margin of the posterior deltoid muscle. Detaching the subcutaneous layer, the space between the deltoid muscle, tricipital muscle fasciae and humerus is exposed. This exposes the point where the axillary nerve emerges, divided into its terminal branches. 1. Axillary nerve, 2. teres minor muscle; 3. long head of the triceps muscle; 4. deltoid muscle; 5. teres major muscle.*

ganglia. Isolated hypotrophy of the infraspinatus muscle with limited active external rotation of the arm, while abduction ability and strength is preserved, should lead the surgeon to suspect compression within the spinoglenoid notch of the nerve branch for the infraspinatus muscle. Surgical treatment must isolate the nerve inside the coracoid and spinoglenoid notches.

SURGICAL MANAGEMENT FOR REPARABLE NERVE LESIONS

Different surgical approaches have been described – the anterior approach [15], the posterosuperior approach [20, 21], the posterior approach [17] – but we will consider the superior approach [12], viewing the suprascapular nerve at the suprascapular notch, and the modified posterior approach, isolating the nerve in the suprascapular and spinoglenoid notches.

The superior surgical approach was described by Mansat in 1983 [12].

The patient is positioned in a lateral decubitus or dorsal decubitus position. The retroclavicular skin incision is parallel to the trapezius fibres and split for approximately 4-5 cm until the nerve can be seen at the suprascapular notch.

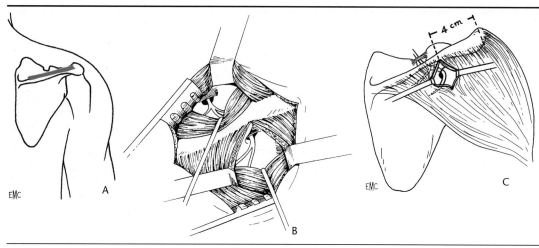

8 *Suprascapular nerve lesion: the modified posterior approach. The patient can be placed in a lateral decubitus or beach-chair position. The skin incision is made parallel to the spina of the scapula for a length of 10-12 cm (A). The suprascapular nerve at the suprascapular notch can be seen after the trapezius muscle is elevated at the upper part and the supraspinatus is retracted at the lower part (B). The deltoid fibres are split for a length of 2-3 cm at 4 cm from the posterior lateral corner and this makes the suprascapular nerve at the spinoglenoid notch visible (C).*

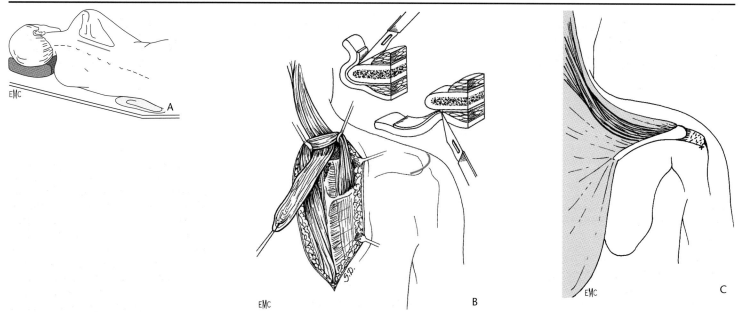

9 *Levator scapulae transfer for supraspinatus muscle.*
A. The patient is placed in a contralateral decubitus position. Two skin incisions are required.
B. The first incision along the vertebral margin of the scapulae enables the transplant to be taken. The tendon insertion of the levator scapulae is extended along the supra- and infraspinatus fasciae, preserving the connections between the

periosteum and the tendon of the levator scapulae with the muscular fascia, even on the internal border of the scapula.
C. The second skin incision along the lateral border of the acromion is required to expose the tendon of the rotator cuff muscle. The tendon transfer with the periosteal fascial flap is transferred to the humeral insertion of the supraspinatus muscle under the trapezius muscle and the acromion.

In the modified posterior approach *(fig 8)*, the patient can be positioned in a lateral decubitus or beach-chair position. The skin incision is made parallel and slightly above the spina of the scapula for a length of 10 to 12 cm. The trapezius is elevated from the scapular spina and the supraspinatus is retracted distally; this allows release of the nerve in the suprascapular notch.

When the suprascapular nerve is entrapped in the spinoglenoid notch, the same posterior skin incision is used, and at 4 cm from the posterior lateral corner of the acromion, the deltoid is split in line with its fibres over a length of 2-3 cm.

When the deltoid fibres are retracted, the spinoglenoid notch should be seen. The inferior transverse scapular ligament is removed under direct view. If the ganglion cyst is visible, the nerve should be dissected, freed from the cyst and the cyst from its origin at the glenohumeral joint.

SURGICAL MANAGEMENT FOR IRREPARABLE NERVE LESIONS

The levator scapulae or anterior and middle parts of the trapezius tendon can be used as a substitute for the supraspinatus muscle, and the teres major transfer can replace the infraspinatus muscle.

Finally, in young adult patients with a well-functioning deltoid muscle, a double transfer can be performed: trapezius for the supraspinatus and teres major for the infraspinatus muscle.

Levator scapulae transfer for supraspinatus muscle

Saha [18] used the transfer of the levator scapulae for treatment of the paralytic

shoulder. The levator scapulae has a short tendon inserted on the periosteum of the superior and medial angle of the scapula. This anatomical condition allows transfer of the muscle to the posterior and lateral part of the acromion (Eden-Lange technique), but often the tendon is too short to be transferred to the side of the supraspinatus tendon on the greater tuberosity.

Since 1987 [3] we have been using the original surgical technique for lengthening the short tendon of the levator scapulae with the supraspinatus and infraspinatus fascia, preserving the connections between the periosteum and the muscular fascia.

The patient is placed in a contralateral decubitus position *(fig 9A)*. Two skin incisions are required. The first incision, 10-12 cm in length along the vertebral margin of the scapulae, enables the transplant to be taken after isolating the lower margin of the

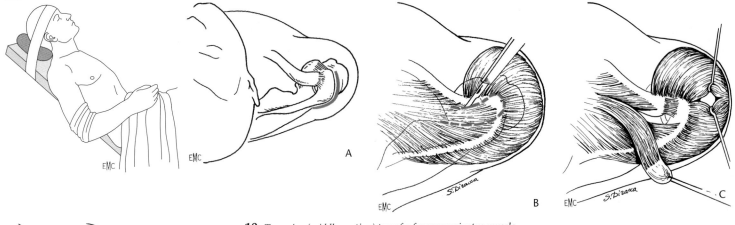

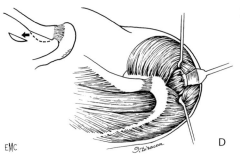

10 *Trapezius (middle portion) transfer for supraspinatus muscle.*
A. The patient is placed in the beach-chair position. The skin incision is made from the lateral and posterior margins of the acromion to the middle level of the scapula spina (about 10-12 cm long).
B. The middle part of the tendon insertions are detached from the acromion and the acromioclavicular joint.
C. The deltoid fibres are split for 2-3 cm along the anterior corner of the acromion.
D. Before transferring the transplant to underneath the acromioclavicular arch on the supraspinatus tendon, it is useful to bevel the posterior prominent portion of the clavicle. The transfer is sutured on the supraspinatus tendon and the greater tuberosity.

trapezius. Detaching it for approximately 5 cm from the spina of the scapula, it is possible to see the insertion of the levator scapulae and the rhomboid muscle as well as the fascia of the supra- and infraspinatus muscles.

To extend the insertion of the levator scapulae distally, the fascia of the supra- and infraspinatus muscles is detached 3-4 cm from the internal border of the scapula, preserving the adipose tissue covering the fascia. The connections between the periosteum and the fascia and the elevator scapulae tendon are preserved.

The periosteum is accurately detached from the bone of the scapula for 1 cm at the upper part and 1 cm at the posterior part *(fig 9B)*, so that the levator tendon may be removed with a long periosteal-fascial flap which preserves the tendon vascularisation with the suprafascial tissue.

The second skin incision along the external border of the acromion (about 5 cm) is required to expose the rotator cuff tendons. The transplant with the periosteal fascial flap is transferred to the supraspinatus tendon under the trapezius and the acromion *(fig 9C)*.

The suture of the transplant on the supraspinatus area (tendon and bone) is made with the shoulder at 40°-60° abduction and 30° degrees flexion.

Postoperatively, the shoulder is immobilised in a thoracobrachial cast for 5 weeks, allowing free movement of the elbow, followed by a rehabilitation programme for 2-3 months.

Trapezius (middle portion) for supraspinatus muscle

For the paralytic shoulder, different methods have been described in the past to transfer the trapezius muscle from the acromioclavicular insertion to the humerus bone. In these older techniques, all of the trapezius muscle was transferred to the humerus bone near the deltoid insertion above the acromioclavicular arch.

Mayer (1916) described the trapezius transfer by extension with fascia lata. Bateman (1954) transferred the trapezius with the bone of the acromion and the spina of the scapula and Saha (1967) with the bone of the clavicula and acromion.

These techniques are rarely used today since the trapezius muscle transfer for the deltoid muscle, when there is no supraspinatus muscle, only results in a tenodesis effect blocking the humeral head in the upper part of the glenoid. In the surgical technique we describe, the middle part of the trapezius insertion is transferred to the supraspinatus muscle, passing through the subacromial space only when the deltoid muscle functions well [14].

In these conditions, the biomechanical action of the trapezius transfer is to depress and fix the humeral head in the glenoid surface so that the deltoid muscle is able to abduct the arm.

The patient is placed in the beach-chair position. A skin incision of about 10-12 cm is made from the anterior border, along the external posterior margin of the acromion to the middle level of the scapular spina *(fig 10A)*. After isolating the upper muscular

fibres of the trapezius, only the middle part of the tendon insertion is detached from the acromion and the acromioclavicular joint *(fig 10B)*. Thus the balance of the scapula is preserved with the function of the posterior part of the trapezius. The deltoid is then split in line with its fibres for 2-3 cm along the anterior corner of the acromion. When the deltoid fibres are retracted, the insertion of the supraspinatus muscle should be seen *(fig 10C)*. Before transferring the transplant to underneath the acromioclavicular arch on the supraspinatus tendon, it is useful to bevel the posterior prominent portion of the clavicle *(fig 10D)*, allowing the transfer a new wide passage. With the arm on the side, the transfer is sutured on the supraspinatus tendon and the greater tuberosity. The upper limb is immobilised in a cast in about 60° abduction and 30° flexion for five weeks. Passive and active exercises are then started.

Teres major transfer to the infraspinatus muscle

We describe the standard surgical procedure for teres major transfer to the infraspinatus to recover active external rotation of the shoulder.

The patient is in a prone position with the thorax relieved with a small cushion in such a way that the upper limb can move freely in abduction and external rotation and in adduction and internal rotation.

The skin incision of about 10-15 cm is made along the lower border of the deltoid muscle *(fig 11A)*. With the arm in adduction and internal rotation, the long head of the triceps

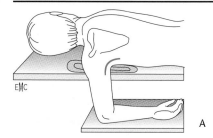

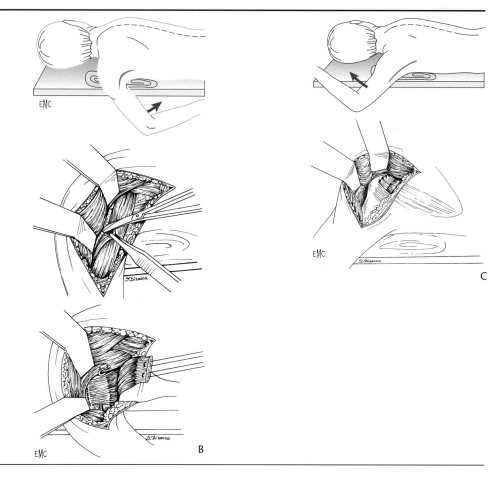

11 *Teres major transfer for the infraspinatus muscle.*
A. The patient is in a prone position with the upper limb free. The skin incision is made along the lower border of the deltoid muscle (10-15 cm long).
B. The long head of the triceps muscle is released and reflected laterally with the arm in adduction and internal rotation. The teres major is separated from the latissimus dorsi tendon and detached from the humerus.
C. The arm is placed in abduction and external rotation and the deltoid muscle is retracted. The teres major tendon is passed under the deltoid muscle and inserted in the infraspinatus tendon.

muscle is released and reflected laterally; this enables the teres major tendon to be separated from the latissimus dorsi tendon and detached from the humerus (fig 11B). At this point, care must be taken to isolate and protect the neurovascular pedicle at the medial third of the muscle, the radial nerve below, and the axillary nerve above the tendon. The arm is then placed in abduction and external rotation and the deltoid muscle is retracted; in this way the infraspinatus muscle can be seen. The teres major tendon is passed under the deltoid muscle and inserted in the infraspinatus tendon (fig 11C). Postoperatively, the upper limb is immobilised for 4 weeks in a spica cast with the arm in neutral rotation and 40°-60° abduction.

Conclusion

For a paralytic shoulder in the adult, it is important to remember that treatment of nerve lesions with a direct surgical approach is always necessary after a nerve lesion where the patient has not recovered muscle innervation and function within 6 months.

In irreparable nerve lesions or in nerve reconstruction failures, muscle transfer may be advisable when:

– patients have lost an important shoulder function (for example: abduction or external rotation) and are young adults and workers;

– the shoulder has only isolated nerve lesions and the muscle transfer must recover precise movements (e.g. external rotation) and defined sectors of shoulder stability (e.g. antero-posterior stability).

In the flaccid shoulder, for total muscle paralysis the use of transfers is often unsuccessful in recovering movements, since the single muscle transfer is only capable of producing the scapulohumeral tenodesis effect. In the choice of the muscle to transfer, it must be remembered that the transfer can recover the function of one muscle, but that every movement of the shoulder depends on the synergy of at least a couple of muscles.

The transfer can produce shoulder movements only when joint stability has been recovered. This is possible if its contraction strength is adequate to recover a good balance with the other muscles of the shoulder.

Bunnell said that muscular transfer is equal to a balancing operation. To summarise the transfer techniques described in this chapter:
– in trapezius palsy: levator scapulae and rhomboid muscle transfer, only when the serratus anterior has good innervation and function;
– in serratus anterior palsy: pectoralis major or teres major transfer, only when the trapezius and rhomboid muscles have good innervation and function;
– in supraspinatus and infraspinatus palsy: levator scapulae or trapezius (anterior and middle portion) transfer, only when the deltoid and subscapularis muscles have good innervation and function;
– in deltoid muscle palsy: latissimus dorsi transfer (bipolar transfer), only when the supraspinatus and infraspinatus muscles have good innervation and function.
Finally, in patients with brachial plexus lesions without any recovery of the scapulohumeral muscle, combinations of two or more muscle transfers may be used to obtain joint stability and limited active control of the shoulder, essential for daily activities. The use of transfer combinations in shoulder palsy is not reported in the literature and we have performed only a few. However, we think that in the future this choice could be an alternative to arthrodesis of the scapulohumeral joint.

References

[1] Alnot JY, Narakas A. Traumatic brachial plexus injuries. Paris : Expansion Scientifique Française, 1996

[2] Bigliani LU, Perez-Sanz JR, Wolpe IN. Treatment of trapezius paralysis. *J Bone Joint Surg Am* 1985 ; 67 : 871-877

[3] Celli L, De Luise G, Marinelli M. Irreparable lesions of the rotator cuff method of reconstruction by transposition of the levator muscle of the scapula. In : The shoulder: periarticular degenerative pathology. Berlin : Springer-Verlag - Auro Gaggi, 1990 : 123-128

[4] Celli L, Rovesta C, Marongiu MC, Mingione A. Peripheral nerve lesion in anterior scapulo-humeral dislocation. In : Alnot JY, Narakas A eds. Traumatic brachial plexus injuries. Paris : Expansion Scientifique Française, 1996 : 212-217

[5] Dewar FP, Harris RI. Restoration of function of the shoulder following paralysis of the trapezius by fascial sling fixation and transplantation of the levator scapulae. *Ann Surg* 1950 ; 132 : 1111-1115

[6] Foo CL, Swann M. Isolated paralysis of the serratus anterior. A report of 20 cases. *J Bone Joint Surg Br* 1983 ; 65 : 552-556

[7] Hass J. Muskelplastik bei Serratuslahmung (Ersatz des gelahmten Musculus Serratus Anterior durch den Musculus Teres Major). *Z Orthop Chir* 1931 ; 55-617

[8] Itoh Y, Sasaki T, Ishiguro T et al. Transfer of latissimus dorsi to replace a paralysed anterior deltoid. *J Bone Joint Surg Br* 1987 ; 69 : 647-650

[9] King R, Motta G. Iatrogenic spinal accessory nerve palsy. *Ann R Coll Surg Engl* 1983 ; 65 : 35-37

[10] Lange M. Die Behandlung der irreparablen Trapeziuslahmung. *Langenbecks Arch Klin Chir* 1951 ; 270 : 437-439

[11] Leffert RD. Neurological problems. In : Rockwood-Matsen WB ed. The shoulder. Philadelphia : WB Saunders, 1990 : vol 2 : 750-773

[12] Mansat M, Mansat CH, Guirand B. Pathologie de l'epaule et syndromes canalaires. In : Sougnet R éd. Syndromes canalaires du membre supérieur. Paris : Expansion Scientifique Française, 1983 : 31-33

[13] Marmhor L, Becthol CO. Paralysis of the serratus anterior due to electric shock relieved by transplantation of the pectoralis major muscle: a case report. *J Bone Joint Surg Am* 1963 ; 45 : 156-160

[14] Mikasa M. Trapezius transfer for global tear of the rotator cuff surgery of the surgery of the shoulder. Burlington : BC Decker, 1984 : 196-199

[15] Murray JW. A surgical approach for the entrapment neuropathy of the suprascapular nerve. *Orthop Rev* 1974 ; 3 : 33-35

[16] Narakas AO. Les atteintes paralytiques de la ceinture scapulo-humerale et de la racine du membre. In : Tubiana R éd. Traité de chirurgie de la main. Paris : Masson, 1981 : 113-155

[17] Post M. Orthopaedic management of neuromuscular disorders. In : The shoulder: operative technique. Baltimore : Williams and Wilkins, 1988 : 201-233

[18] Saha AK. Surgery of the paralysed and flail shoulder. *Acta Orthop Scand [suppl]* 1967 ; 97 : 5-90

[19] Sunderland S. Nerve and nerves injury. Edinburgh : Churchill Livingstone, 1978

[20] Swafford AR.. Suprascapular nerve entrapment: a case report. *J Hand Surg Am* 1982 ; 7 : 57-60

[21] Thompson RC Jr, Schneider W, Kennedy T. Entrapment neuropathy of the inferior branch of the suprascapular nerve by ganglia. *Clin Orthop* 1982 ; 166 : 185-187

[22] Vastamaki M. Suprascapular nerve entrapment. In : Norris TR ed. Shoulder and elbow. American Academy of Orthopaedic Surgeons, 1997 : 265-268

Nerve entrapments around the shoulder

M Vastamäki

Abstract. — *Suprascapular nerve entrapment in the suprascapular notch is the most common nerve disorder around the shoulder and often requires operative treatment. Spinoglenoid notch entrapment of the suprascapular nerve is often caused by a ganglion cyst arising from the glenohumeral joint. Isolated palsy of the long thoracic nerve, giving rise to a winging scapula (serratus palsy), requires tendon transfer in severe chronic cases. In accessory nerve palsy, appropriate surgical treatment of the nerve is mandatory, but if it fails, tendon transfers may be helpful. Quadrilateral space syndrome (entrapment of the axillary nerve) is less common and is easy to treat surgically.*

Keywords: shoulder, nerve entrapment, nerve palsy, suprascapular nerve, serratus palsy, winging scapula, accessory nerve, trapezius palsy, quadrilateral space syndrome, axillary nerve, musculocutaneus nerve.

Introduction

Nerve entrapments around the shoulder are a more common cause of shoulder disorders than is usually recognised. The nerves most often affected are the suprascapular, long thoracic, accessory and axillary nerves. The most common disorder is suprascapular nerve entrapment, which accounts for some 1 to 2% of all shoulder disorders [12]; the second most common disorder concerns the long thoracic nerve (i.e. serratus palsy). Axillary nerve entrapment (i.e. the quadrilateral space syndrome) is the least frequently seen.

Suprascapular nerve entrapment (SNE)

The suprascapular nerve is derived from the upper trunk of the brachial plexus (C5-C6), enters the supraspinatus fossa through the suprascapular notch, passes below the superior transverse scapular ligament, supplies one or two branches to the supraspinatus muscle, and after passing into the infraspinatus fossa around the lateral margin of the scapular spine (spinoglenoid notch), supplies the infraspinatus muscle. The suprascapular notch may be low and narrow and the nerve can be adherent to the notch (suprascapular notch entrapment, SNES), or the nerve may be tethered by the spinoglenoid ligament or a ganglion cyst arising from the glenohumeral joint to the spinoglenoid notch (spinoglenoid notch entrapment, SNEI). In this case, only the infraspinatus muscle is affected [5].

CLINICAL FEATURES AND DIAGNOSIS

In clinical examination of SNES, tenderness over the suprascapular notch, in the triangle between the clavicle and the scapular spine, is an almost invariable sign *(fig 1)*. The power of active abduction and external rotation is usually reduced. The spinati muscles, particularly the infraspinatus, may be atrophied *(fig 2)*. Pain in SNEI is usually milder than in SNES. It is located in the infraspinatus area. Local findings in SNEI are not very prominent, except atrophy of the infraspinatus muscle, which may be quite remarkable. The diagnosis of SNE is based on a careful and thorough history, physical examination and electroneuromyography. Positive ENMG findings such as delayed conduction velocity and fibrillation potentials are decisive.

After clinical examination and ENMG, if the infraspinatus muscle alone is affected, the possible presence of a ganglion should be

Martti Vastamäki, M.D, Orton Orthopaedics Hospital, Invalid Foundation, Tenholantie 10, FIN-00280 Helsinki, Finland.

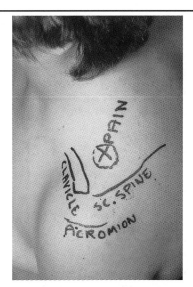

1 *Painful area in suprascapular nerve entrapment.*

checked by magnetic resonance imaging (MRI). If no ganglion exists, the cause of the disorder may be spinoglenoid ligament compression or scar formation and tethering of the nerve after strenuous activities such as volley ball [6, 12].

OPERATIVE TREATMENT

If conservative treatment such as rest, analgesics, physical therapy, and local injections have failed, operative treatment, i.e. decompression of the nerve, should be

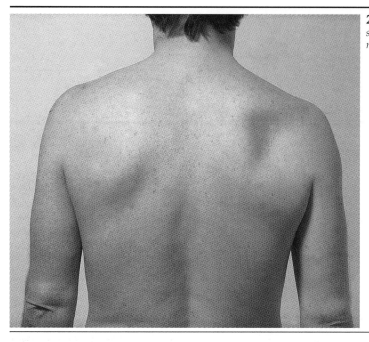

2 *Infraspinatus atrophy in suprascapular nerve entrapment.*

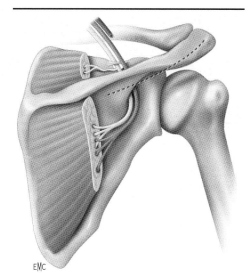

4 *Skin incision for spinoglenoid notch exploration.*

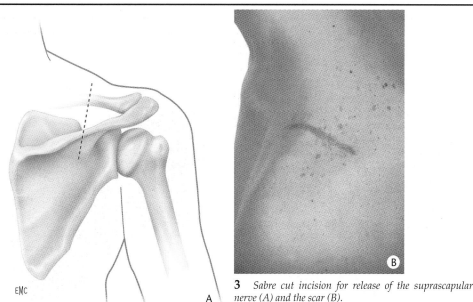

3 *Sabre cut incision for release of the suprascapular nerve (A) and the scar (B).*

offered. Cases caused by acute trauma or exceptional single exertion without any marked anatomical compression may recover with conservative treatment.

■ *Surgical technique in SNES*

There are two main approaches to treat suprascapular notch compression: the posterior approach advocated by Clein [3] and the cranial approach used by the author [12]. The posterior approach is safer and provides a better view, especially in heavily-built patients, but requires more tissue resection.

The cranial approach is simpler and in most cases offers a sufficient view of the suprascapular notch. The patient lies in the lateral decubitus position on a vacuum mattress. The arm is draped free. The skin incision of 8-10 cm is a sabre cut just over the suprascapular notch, 3 cm medial to the acromioclavicular joint *(fig 3)*. A

subcutaneous pouch is developed. The trapezius muscle is divided along its fibres to within 5 cm of its lateral end. The supraspinatus fat is moved aside and the supraspinatus muscle is retracted backward. The index finger is used to locate the superior transverse scapular ligament. The suprascapular nerve is most suitably identified by means of electrical stimulation, if the nerve is still functioning. The ligament can be cleaned with a moist cottonoid to show its glistering white structure. The ligament is sectioned, taking care not to damage the nerve, the suprascapular artery and veins. The artery and veins are located immediately superficial to the ligament. Normally, a bloodless field is easy to maintain. Additional exploration of the nerve or neurolysis is not necessary. The author does not recommend a primary notch resection. After making sure of decompression of the nerve, the trapezius

muscle is approximated by one or two loose stitches and the wound is closed without drainage. After operation, no sling or other bandage is used, and unlimited motion of the arm is allowed.

In the procedure for the posterior approach, the patient is placed in a semi-prone position with the arm draped free. The skin incision is made parallel and slightly cephalad to the spine of the scapula and is approximately 10 to 12 cm long. The trapezius is elevated sharply from the scapular spine. As the fibres of the trapezius and periosteum are elevated, a thin, fatty layer is observed between the undersurface of the trapezius and the supraspinatus muscle. The trapezius muscle is retracted cephalad with a wide blunt retractor. Blunt dissection is carried out with a wet finger; the suprascapular ligament overlying its notch is palpated. The ligament is released sharply while protecting the suprascapular nerve beneath. The trapezius muscle is then reattached to the spine of the scapula using no. 2 non-absorbable sutures placed through drill holes in the scapular spine. The wound is closed in a routine manner and a sling is used for immobilisation for 1 to 2 weeks postoperatively, until pain from the operation has subsided. Active motions are allowed within 10 to 14 days postoperatively and are increased as pain allows [8].

During surgery for SNEI, the patient lies in the lateral decubitus position. The skin incision goes along the lateral scapular spine *(fig 4)*; the deltoid muscle is released subperiosteally from its insertion to the lateral scapular spine and posterior acromion for 6-7 cm and is split at the posterior corner of the acromion for 5 cm. The infraspinatus muscle is gently retracted to expose the spinoglenoid notch and the infraspinatus branch of the suprascapular nerve. The nerve may be difficult to find and is identified most suitably by means of electrical stimulation, if the nerve is still functioning. The nerve is freed from scar tissue, if present, and the spinoglenoid

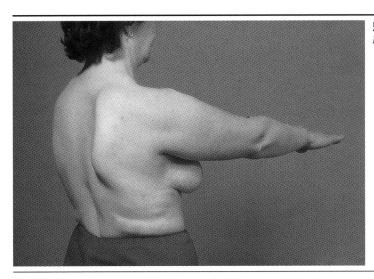

5 *Serratus palsy (Grade III).*

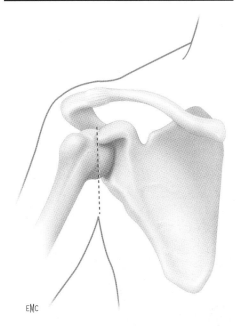

6 *Deltopectoral skin incision for pectoralis major transfer.*

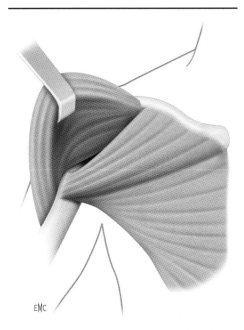

7 *Sternal and clavicular heads of the pectoralis major. The sternal head passes underneath the clavicular head.*

ligament is sectioned, if it exists. If there is a ganglion cyst, it should be resected and the root of the ganglion, if detected, should be ligated. The cause of the cyst, usually a labral lesion in the glenohumeral joint, should also be treated. It is also possible to carry out arthroscopic debridement of the labral tear responsible for the cyst, leaving the cyst to resolve spontaneously [2].

Serratus palsy

A lesion of the long thoracic nerve causes isolated paralysis of the serratus anterior muscle, giving rise to a winging scapula, which results from the posterior displacement of the vertebral border and the inferior angle of the scapula *(fig 5)*. The aetiologies of paralysis of the serratus anterior are multiple. Most authors have found acute or recurrent trauma to be the most frequent causative factor. In addition, neuralgic amyotrophy, toxic, infectious or hereditary brachial plexus neuropathy, anaesthesia, associated and unrelated surgical operations, use of crutches, a pressing cast, and sleeping position have been mentioned as aetiological factors [13]. However, there are many cases without an attributed cause. Because of its vertical course to the axilla, the long thoracic nerve is prone to being stretched if the shoulder is depressed or if the neck is flexed to the opposite side. The nerve is also susceptible to compression if lateral pressure is exerted against the scapula.

In order to better classify serratus paralysis, the author devised a new grading system in 1985 [10]. Four grades are used. Grade I is the least severe stage with a slight scapular winging of 1-2 cm in forward flexion. In Grade II, scapular winging is 2-3 cm and active forward flexion is limited. In Grade III, the winging is 4-5 cm, flexion is to the horizontal level and abduction is limited. In the most severe, Grade IV, winging is maximal as in Grade III and abduction is also severely limited. In the author's personal series of 197 patients, the most

common aetiology for serratus palsy was some kind of exertion (forward lifting, volleyball, etc.) or trauma (a fall or a blow) [13]. The most applied treatment was derotation of the scapula by means of a protective brace. Of course, the patients were ordered to avoid all movements causing scapular winging, especially lifting objects in forward flexion of the arm. The author has not explored or decompressed the long thoracic nerve in serratus palsy, but in some cases, this might be beneficial. This may be especially so if the aetiology is a dynamic fascial sling, as reported by Hester et al [7], or some other verified or supposed entrapment site of the long thoracic nerve. When the palsy has not recovered or improved enough within two years, the author has performed a muscle transfer in appropriate cases, first using the pectoralis minor tendon, and later the sternal part of the pectoralis major.

OPERATIVE TECHNIQUE

The patient is positioned on the operating table on the unaffected side. Two skin incisions are necessary: one deltopectoral to expose the humeral insertion of the pectoralis major muscle, and one posterior in the axilla to expose the lateral border of the scapula. It is important to drape to the posterior midline so that the scapula can be manipulated during the procedure. A 10 cm deltopectoral incision is made in the axillary skin crease *(fig 6)*. The deltopectoral interval is developed, taking the cephalic vein laterally. The pectoralis major tendon is identified at its humeral insertion. The sternal head passes deep to the clavicular head *(fig 7)*. The interval between the two heads is identified by abduction and external rotation of the arm and developed bluntly using the index finger. The sternal head tendon is cut directly off the bone and a traction suture is placed in the tendon. The sternal head muscle belly is freed as far medially as possible. The inferior lateral border of the scapula is exposed through the same approach or through a 8 cm dorsal incision, used by the author. The author

started these procedures by using the pectoralis minor tendon; at that time two approaches were needed, which still seems comfortable. The overlying muscles are divided along the course of their fibres. The lateral border of the inferior scapula is exposed subperiosteally some 3-4 cm cranially from the inferior corner, and a 6 mm drill hole is placed 1-1½ cm medial to the lateral border.

A tunnel is created between the lateral border of the scapula and the deltopectoral approach using the fingers. The plantaris longus tendon is harvested next. A 3 cm incision is made behind the medial malleolus. The plantaris longus tendon is identified just anterior to the Achilles tendon; it is cut and harvested using a long

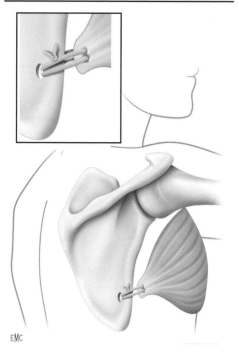

8 *Fixation of the pectoralis major using a free plantaris longus tendon graft. Insert: A gap of some 4 cm is extended by a 4 folded graft.*

tendon stripper. Normally, a 25-30 cm tendon just suitable for this kind of transfer is obtained. If the plantaris longus tendon is lacking, the long extensors of the second and third toes or a fascia lata autograft may be used.

The plantaris longus tendon graft is passed through the mobilised pectoralis major tendon and the hole in the scapula twice or three times, if possible (fig 8). The scapula is reduced manually to the pectoralis tendon. Before suturing the graft, it is important to check the tightness of the transfer. Passive forward flexion of the arm should be at least 120°. Otherwise, the transfer may be too tight. Normally, a gap of 2-3 cm exists between the pectoralis tendon and the scapula, and the graft extends the transfer. Postoperatively, a shoulder sling is used for 6 weeks, and after that, progressive range of motion and strengthening exercises are started. Return to manual labour is allowed after 3 to 4 months [4, 9, 11, 16].

Accessory nerve palsy

The superficial course of the accessory nerve in the posterior cervical triangle makes it particularly susceptible to injury during a lymph node biopsy, removal of tumour masses and other operative procedures in this region (fig 9). The nerve may be damaged by section or constriction due to ligature or scar tissue. It is a rather thin nerve, 1-3 mm in diameter. A small branch from the transverse cervical artery may accompany the nerve or closely approximate its course. During lymph node biopsy, control of this vessel has often implicated the accessory nerve by forceps or ligation

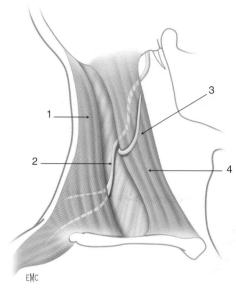

9 *Anatomical distribution of the accessory nerve. 1. Trapezius muscle; 2. accessory nerve; 3. great auricular nerve ; 4. sternocleidomastoid muscle.*

injury. The trapezius and sternocleidomastoid muscles are innervated by the accessory nerve. In addition, the trapezius muscle also receives direct innervation from the cervical nerves.

Paresis of the trapezius muscle is a dominant diagnostic sign. Paresis involves lowering of the shoulder and causes the scapula to slip away from the median line. The loss of the bulk of the trapezius muscle leaves a hollow in the supraclavicular region. Sometimes, it is impossible to find the atrophy without abduction of the arms. A positive abduction test is a typical finding. When performing the test, the examiner holds the patient's wrist firmly at the side. The patient then attempts abduction against this resistance. The test is positive with a flaring of the entire vertebral border of the scapula and a virtual dislocation of the scapula upon the thoracic cage. Of course, active motion of the arm is affected.

When the diagnosis of the lesion has been made, surgical intervention should be considered. Spontaneous regeneration of the accessory nerve is very unlikely. Conservative treatment may strengthen the auxiliary muscles of the shoulder but it never compensates for the loss of the trapezius.

Most often, the cause of injury is compression of the nerve by scar tissue or a suture. In such cases, careful external neurolysis is enough. Neurorrhaphy or reconstruction of the nerve with free nerve grafts may be necessary in appropriate cases [11, 14].

SURGICAL TECHNIQUE

Accessory nerve palsy is almost invariably iatrogenic, and results mainly from lymph node biopsy. The patient usually has a 2-3 cm transverse scar in the posterior

cervical triangle. The lesion, mostly compression by scar tissue, is located just at the site of the scar. It may, however, be very difficult to find the correct nerve, because many sensory nerves also cross the area. The author usually utilises the old scar: the incision is extended 1-2 cm over the old scar and then a subcutaneal pouch is developed upwards and downwards to a healthy area in order to find the accessory nerve. The other possibility is to make a vertical incision of 5 cm in the middle of the old scar. This gives a safer approach to the nerve, but also a less cosmetic scar. Loupe or microscope magnification is necessary. Finding the accessory nerve in the small area (5 x 5 cm) may require up to 1 or 2 hours, as it is important to proceed very carefully. After detecting the correct nerve, external neurolysis is performed, and the nerve is followed until it enters the trapezius muscle.

Chronic trapezius palsy

In chronic trapezius palsy without any possibility of nerve recovery, surgical options may be divided into static and dynamic procedures. Static procedures include scapulothoracic fusion and other static methods to stabilise the scapula. They are not indicated for patients with isolated accessorius palsy, but can be appropriate in neuromuscular disorders such as facioscapulohumeral dystrophy. Dynamic procedures include transfer of the levator scapulae with or without transfer of the rhomboid muscles (Eden-Lange method).

The procedure is indicated for healthy and active patients with isolated total trapezius palsy and severe dysfunction of the shoulder. The operation may also give good results in older patients (up to 60-65 years), but is most favourable in younger patients. Before surgery, patients should be treated with rehabilitation exercises for at least 6 months to determine the true extent of the disability.

SURGICAL TECHNIQUE

The entire shoulder girdle and upper extremity are draped free to allow free manipulation of the shoulder during the procedure. The head of the table is raised some 15°. A 15 cm incision is made along the medial scapular border starting from just above the superior medial angle of the scapula (fig 10). After releasing the atrophied trapezius muscle from its scapular insertion, the levator scapulae, rhomboideus minor and rhomboideus major are identified, separated from each other, and released from the scapula using an osteotome. Then the muscles are dissected medially for a few centimetres to achieve an appropriate amplitude for transfer. The supraspinatus and infraspinatus muscle bellies are bluntly elevated from their respective fossae for half the width of the scapula, the rhomboideus

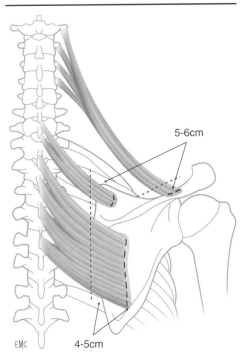

10 *Skin incision and completed transfer of the levator scapulae and rhomboids in accessory nerve palsy.*

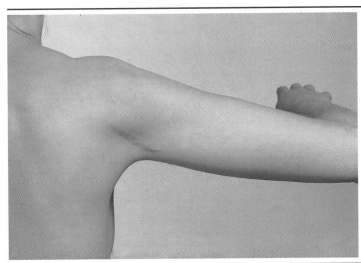

11 *Scar over the quadrilateral space after release of the axillary nerve.*

minor is transferred to the supraspinatus fossa and the rhomboideus major to the infraspinatus fossa. Two drill holes are made in the supraspinatus fossa and 3-4 drill holes in the infraspinatus, some 4 cm lateral to the medial border of the scapula. The transferred muscles with the bony insertions are sutured using no. 1 or 2 non-absorbable sutures with a large curved needle that passes through the drill holes. The spinati muscles are imbricated over the repair [15]. A separate 5 cm incision is made above the spine of the scapula, starting from the lateral spine and continuing medially. The trapezius, deltoid, and supraspinatus are elevated off the spine of the scapula and 2 drill holes are made in the scapular spine some 5 cm lateral to the superior medial corner of the scapula. A tunnel for the passage of the levator scapulae is developed through the paralysed trapezius. The levator scapulae is transferred through the tunnel and sutured to the scapular spine through the drill holes. Normally, the levator scapulae can be transferred 4 to 5 cm lateral from its genuine origin. An abduction pillow of 60° is used for 4 weeks. In some cases, the author has also used only a sling with acceptable results. Passive ROM exercises are started after the first postoperative week and strengthening exercises after 4 weeks.

Axillary nerve entrapment (quadrilateral space syndrome)

The axillary nerve innervates the deltoid and teres minor muscles and may be compromised during humeral dislocation or its too aggressive reduction. In such cases, the problem is always stretching, or even disruption, of the nerve. Axillary nerve entrapment in the quadrilateral space is caused by compression of surrounding tissues (humeral bone, teres major and minor, and the long head of the triceps muscle). Compression may be enforced by scar tissue, perhaps produced after strenuous exercises such as javelin throwing [1].

The most prominent symptom is a dull ache in the posterior aspect of the shoulder. The patient is able to indicate very precisely the site of pain and this point of maximum pain is also easy to find upon palpation. When the symptoms begin, the deltoid muscle is not seriously affected, but the velocity of conduction of the axillary nerve is affected. There are no sensory findings.

Chronic pain and ache on the posterior aspect of the shoulder may be very disturbing and may resist all conservative treatment modalities such as physical therapy, massage, injections, etc. In such cases, surgery is indicated even though the deltoid muscle is not affected.

SURGICAL TECHNIQUE

The incision is vertical on the proximal posterior aspect of the arm just over the quadrilateral space and the posterior border of the deltoid (*fig 11*). The deltoid is gently retracted upwards and the quadrilareral space, the axillary nerve and the posterior circumflexa artery are identified. In a typical entrapment case, the axillary nerve is tethered by scar tissue to the surrounding tissues for a length of 3 to 4 cm and therefore it cannot glide during movements of the arm. The nerve is simply freed off the surrounding scar and tissues. The circumflexa artery may be occluded but does not require any treatment.

Musculocutaneal nerve entrapment

Musculocutaneal nerve problems are usually iatrogenic and mostly diagnosed after certain shoulder stabilising procedures using the conjoined tendons. The musculocutaneal nerve passes in some instances rather close to the coracoid process and may be kinked, compressed or stretched during the conjoined tendon transfer. The symptoms are typical: loss of strength of the biceps until total paralysis and loss of sensation on the radial aspect of the forearm. The entrapment site may be painful. ENMG examination proves the diagnosis. Surgical intervention is almost invariably necessary.

SURGICAL TECHNIQUE

The approach is deltopectoral. The musculotaneal nerve is explored medial to the conjoined tendons and between the pectoralis major and minor muscles where it emerges from the lateral cord of the brachial plexus and before it pierces the coracobrachialis muscle some 3 to 5 cm distal to the coracoid process. The nerve is freed.

References ➤

References

[1] Cahill BR, Palmer RE. Quadrilateral space syndrome. *J Hand Surg Am* 1983 ; 8 : 65-69

[2] Chochole MH, Senker W, Meznik C, Breitenseher MJ. Glenoid-labral cyst entrapping the suprascapular nerve: dissolution after arthroscopic debridement of an extended SLAP lesion. *Arthroscopy* 1997 ; 13 : 753-755

[3] Clein LJ. Suprascapular entrapment neuropathy. *J Neurosurg* 1975 ; 43 : 337-342

[4] Connor PM, Yamaguchi K, Manifold SG, Pollock RG, Flatow EL, Bigliani LU. Split pectoralis major transfer for serratus anterior palsy. *Clin Orthop* 1997 ; 341 : 134-142

[5] Cummins CA, Messer TM, Nuber GW. Suprascapular nerve entrapment. *J Bone Joint Surg Am* 2000 ; 82 : 415-424

[6] Ferretti A, Cerullo G, Russo G. Suprascapular neuropathy in volleyball players. *J Bone Joint Surg Am* 1987 ; 69 : 260-263

[7] Hester P, Caborn D, Nyland J. Cause of long thoracic nerve palsy: A possible dynamic fascial sling cause. *J Shoulder Elbow Surg* 2000 ; 9 : 31-35

[8] Post M. Diagnosis and treatment of suprascapular nerve entrapment. *Clin Orthop* 1999 ; 368 : 92-100

[9] Vastamäki M. Pectoralis minor transfer in serratus anterior paralysis. *Acta Orthop Scand* 1984 ; 55 : 293-295

[10] Vastamäki M. Serratus anterior paralysis. [abstract]. Presented at the Fifty-sixth Annual Meeting of the American Academy of Orthopaedic Surgeons, Las Vegas, Nevada, February 24-28, 1989

[11] Vastamäki M. Accessory nerve palsy and serratus palsy. *Ann Chir Gynecol* 1996 ; 85 : 167-171

[12] Vastamäki M, Goransson H. Suprascapular nerve entrapment. *Clin Orthop* 1993 ; 297 : 135-143

[13] Vastamäki M, Kauppila L. Etiologic factors in isolated paralysis of the serratus anterior muscle: a report of 197 cases. *J Shoulder Elbow Surg* 1993 ; 2 : 240-243

[14] Vastamäki M, Solonen KA. Accessory nerve injury. *Acta Orthop Scand* 1984 ; 55 : 296-299

[15] Wiater JM, Bigliani LU. Spinal accessory nerve injury. *Clin Orthop* 1999 ; 368 : 5-16

[16] Wiater JM, Flatow EL. Long thoracic nerve injury. *Clin Orthop* 1999 ; 368 : 17-27

Congenital elevation of the scapula (Sprengel's deformity)

J Le Saout

Abstract. – Congenital elevation of the scapula is an anomaly of the scapula and its muscle attachments. The scapula is hypoplastic, elevated and adducted, with an abnormal prominence in the supraclavicular fossa.

Muscle imbalance involves the levator scapulae, upper and middle fibres of the trapezius, and rhomboïd muscles. An omovertebral bone is sometimes present.

The Woodward procedure is presented. It consists of release of the origin of the trapezius and rhomboid muscles, sectioning of the levator scapulae, removal of the omovertebral bone, freeing of fibrous adhesions in the anterior portion of the scapula to allow the scapula to move downward, and finally, reattachment of the trapezius and rhomboid muscles in a more caudal position, that is, two interspinous spaces inferior to their point of origin.

Brachial palsy is the major risk of this procedure, because it induces a retropulsion of the clavicle.

It is possible to associate an extraperiostal resection of the supraspinatous portion of the scapula.

© 2000, Editions Scientifiques et Médicales Elsevier SAS. All rights reserved.

Keywords: shoulder, congenital elevation of the scapula, Sprengel's deformity, Woodward procedure.

Introduction

Congenital elevation of the scapula, usually known as the Sprengel shoulder, is not a common deformity. In this condition, elevation of the scapula is associated with local anomalies of the spine and particularly of the rib cage. The Woodward procedure, which was described by its author in 1961, is presented below [19]. In this procedure, lowering of the scapula is associated with myoplasty of the trapezius, so that the two main causes of discomfort are treated conjointly (cosmetic considerations and limitation of abduction).

It is also possible to associate other procedures from other techniques: partial resection of the scapula [14, 18], osteotomy of the clavicle (Huc-Ombredanne), wrist traction [5].

Anatomical considerations

NORMAL ANATOMY

The scapula is attached to the trunk by a superficial muscle, the trapezius (*fig 1*), and by deeper muscles, namely the two rhomboid muscles and the levator scapulae (*fig 2*).

ANATOMICAL CHANGES RESULTING FROM CONGENITAL ELEVATION OF THE SCAPULA (*fig 3*)

In this condition, a regional deformity is associated with anomalies of the scapula and its muscle attachments.

The scapula may be hypoplastic; it is elevated and somewhat adducted, which forms an abnormal prominence in the supraclavicular fossa.

Muscle imbalance involves the levator scapulae, upper and middle fibres of the trapezius, and rhomboid muscles. Fibrous adhesions are also found between the anterior portion of the scapula and the chest, and an omovertebral bone is sometimes present, extending from the medial angle of the scapula to the cervical spine.

Some authors have also described a fibrocartilagenous bar connecting the scapula with the clavicle [10].

Before describing the surgical procedure, two specific points merit emphasis:

■ *Track of the spinal accessory nerve* (*fig 4*)

The spinal accessory nerve supplies the sternocleidomastoid and the trapezius. It

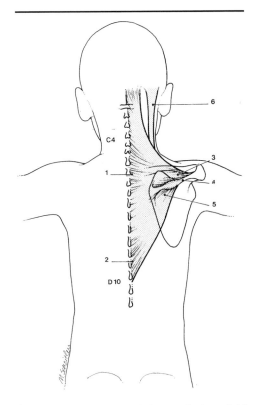

1 *The normal anatomy of the scapula (superficial muscle: trapezius). 1 and 2. Triangular fibrous bands at their vertebral origin; 3. clavicular attachment; 4 and 5. attachments to the scapular spine; 6. sternocleidomastoid muscle.*

Jacques Le Saout, M.D, Service d'orthopédie, Clinique Pasteur-Saint-Esprit, 34, rue du Moulin à Poudre, 29200 Brest, France.

All references to this article must include: Le Saout J. Congenital elevation of the scapula (Sprengel's deformity). Editions Scientifiques et Médicales Elsevier SAS (Paris). All rights reserved. Surgical Techniques in Orthopaedics and Traumatology, 55-210-C-10, 2000, 4 p.

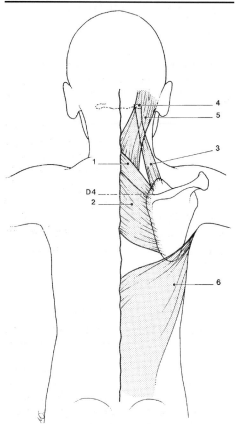

2 *Normal anatomy: deep muscles (after resection of trapezius and sternocleidomastoid). 1. Rhomboideus minor; 2. rhomboideus major; 3. levator scapulae; 4. transverse process of atlas; 5. splenius capitis; 6. latissimus dorsi. The medial angle of the scapula is at the level of the spinous process of T4.*

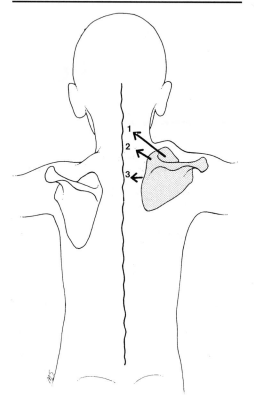

3 *Anatomical changes resulting from congenital elevation of the scapula: the scapula is hypoplastic and somewhat adducted, and forms a prominence in the supraclavicular fossa. 1. Upper fibres of trapezius; 2. levator scapulae and omovertebral bone (when present); 3. middle fibres of trapezius and rhomboid muscles. Fibrous adhesions are also found between the anterior portion of the scapula and the chest.*

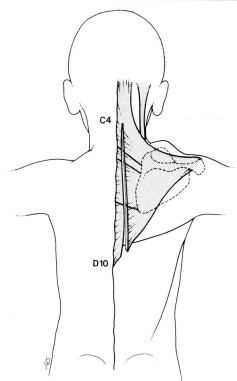

5 *Dissection of the trapezius-rhomboid muscle layer within 10 mm of the midline.*

vertebra. The skin is detached from the trapezius as far as the spinal border of the scapula.

■ Dissection of the trapezius-rhomboid layer

The trapezius and rhomboid muscles are released within about 10 mm of the spinous processes (*fig 5*). Sharp dissection is carried out over the entire length of the skin incision, and the whole muscle sheet is raised. Inferiorly, it is separated from the latissimus dorsi by blunt dissection. The two muscles are retracted laterally, which allows for resection of the fibrous adhesions between the anterior portion of the scapula and the chest (*fig 6*). This gives access, in the upper part of the incision, to the omovertebral bone, when present, and to the levator scapulae.

■ Excision of the omovertebral bone

Once the trapezius has been retracted, the omovertebral bone is fully exposed and can be sectioned inferiorly at the omovertebral bone/scapula junction. It is then resected step by step until completely excised.

■ Sectioning of the levator scapulae (*fig 6*)

The levator scapulae should be sectioned within one or two finger breadths of the scapula. Care should be taken to avoid damage to the spinal accessory nerve.

runs along the undersurface of the sternocleidomastoid, obliquely crosses the supraclavicular fossa inferiorly and posteriorly, and then passes under the trapezius, about 2 to 3 cm above the clavicle.

■ Risk of brachial plexus palsy

Brachial palsy is the major risk of this procedure. The lowering of the scapula induces retropulsion of the clavicle which may result in compression of the brachial plexus.

An omoclavicular bar, when it is missed, may play an important role in causing brachial plexus palsy [10].

Woodward procedure

MAIN SURGICAL STEPS

This procedure consists of releasing the origin of the trapezius and rhomboid muscles, sectioning the levator scapulae, removing the omovertebral bone, when present, freeing fibrous adhesions in the anterior portion of the scapula to allow the scapula to move downward, and, finally, reattaching the trapezius and rhomboid muscles in a more caudal position, that is, two interspinous spaces inferior to their point of origin.

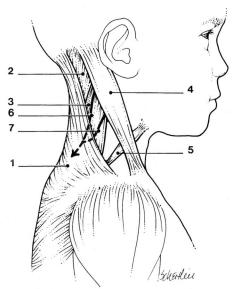

4 *Spinal accessory nerve. 1. Trapezius; 2. splenius; 3. levator scapulae; 4. sternocleidomastoid; 5. omohyoid; 6. spinal accessory nerve; 7. anastomotic branch of the accessory nerve arising from the superficial cervical plexus.*

■ Patient positioning

The patient is placed prone on the operating table.

■ Skin incision

A skin incision extends from the fourth cervical vertebra to the tenth thoracic

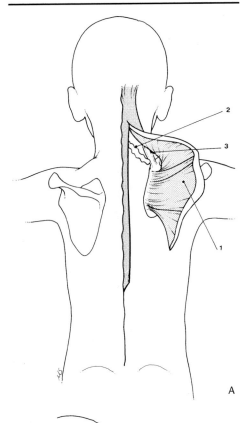

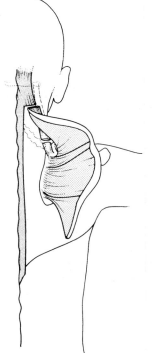

6 *A. The trapezius-rhomboid muscles (1) are retracted as a single sheet, which provides full exposure of the omovertebral bone, when present (2), and the levator scapulae (3), and allows resection of the fibrous adhesions between the anterior portion of the scapula and the chest.*
B. Excision of the omovertebral bone, sectioning of the levator scapulae, transection of the upper fibres of the trapezius.

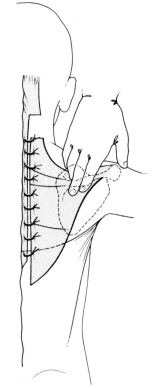

7 *Reattachment of the trapezius-rhomboid muscle sheet in a more caudal position. Reattachment can be adjusted to allow for counter-rotation of the scapula and correction of the varus tilt of the glenoid.*

■ Sectioning the upper part of the trapezius

The upper fibres of the trapezius are split transversely, beyond the spinal accessory nerve so as to preserve innervation of the muscle.

■ Scapular lowering and reattachment of the trapezius-rhomboid muscle sheet *(fig 7)*

The scapula can be moved downwards and rotated in a counter direction in order to correct the varus tilt of the glenoid. Palpation of the radial pulse is recommended during this manoeuvre. The trapezius-rhomboid muscle sheet can now be reattached in a more caudal position, that is, two interspinous spaces inferior to its point of origin. This avoids excessive downward displacement which may cause brachial plexus complications. Reattachment is performed using absorbable interrupted sutures. Tension on reattached structures can be adjusted as needed from above downward, so as to facilitate counter-rotation of the scapula and correction of the varus shift of the glenoid. During reattachment, the scapula should be maintained in the correct position. Suction drains are placed where detachments have been performed.

Modified Woodward procedure [1]

In addition to the Woodward procedure, excision of the medial border of the scapula and resection of the supraspinous portion are performed.

The muscles attached to the superior and medial borders of the scapula are reflected extra-periosteally so as to facilitate bony excision. Superiorly, the scapula is excised, medial to the suprascapular notch. Approximately one centimetre of the medial border is excised.

Osteostomy of the clavicle is sometimes performed to prevent complications, such as damaging the plexus [7].

Procedure with only a cosmetic repair [1, 7]

Cases with minor deformities (Cavendish types 1 and 2) [3] can be treated by resection only of the prominent part of the superior angle of the scapula. This is only a cosmetic repair: the incorrect rotation of the scapula and the functional deficit of the shoulder movements are not corrected.

Postoperative management and results

POSTOPERATIVE IMMOBILISATION

A Velpeau® bandage (with the elbow at the side in flexion) is applied and worn for three weeks.

REHABILITATION

Three weeks after the operation, physical therapy is initiated to recover normal abduction motion.

OUTCOME *(fig 8)*

In general, there is greater functional than cosmetic improvement, as the latter may be incomplete. Outcome is influenced by the degree of elevation and, above all, by the presence of severe vertebral abnormalities, which are an unfavourable element. It seems that outcome is not influenced by the age of the patient at the time of surgery, nor by the presence of an omovertebral bone. However, the recommended age for the operation is 5 to 6 years.

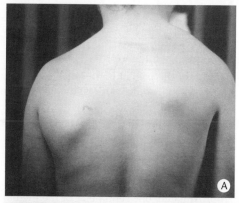

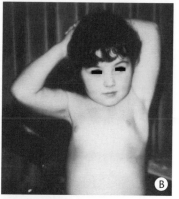

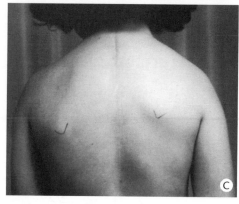

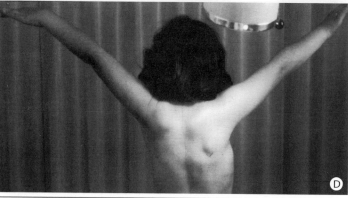

8 *Grade 2 elevation* [12] *in a five and a half year old child:*
A. Posterior view showing the elevation of the right scapula and the supraclavicular bulging.
B. Limitation of abduction in the right shoulder.
C, D. Postoperative result: visible cosmetic improvement and restoration of normal function of the shoulder.

References

[1] Borges JL, Shah A, Torres BC, Bowen JR. Modified Woodward procedure for Sprengel deformity of the shoulder: long-term results. *J Pediatr Orthop* 1996 ; 16 : 508-513

[2] Carson WG, Lovell WW, Whitesides TE. Congenital elevation of the scapula. Surgical correction by the Woodward's procedure. *J Bone Joint Surg Am* 1981 ; 63 : 1199-1207

[3] Cavendish ME. Congenital elevation of the scapula. *J Bone Joint Surg Br* 1972 ; 54 : 395-408

[4] Ciaudo O, Bensahel H, Desgrippes Y, Csukonyi Z. Réflexions thérapeutiques sur la surélévation congénitale de l'omoplate ; à propos de 16 cas. *Chir Pédiatr* 1984 ; 25 : 58-63

[5] Erceg M, Biocic M. Congenital elevation of the scapula (Sprengel's deformity). *Acta Med Croatica* 1998 ; 52 : 73-75

[6] Gandin J. Traitement chirurgical de la surélévation congénitale de l'omoplate : 4 observations. *Chirurgie* 1972 ; 98 : 674-677

[7] Greitemann B, Rondhuis JJ, Karbowski A. Treatment of congenital elevation of the scapula. 10 (2-18) year follow-up of 37 cases of Sprengel's deformity. *Acta Ortho Scand* 1993 ; 64 : 365-368

[8] Hammer DL, Hall JE. Sprengel's deformity associated with multidirectional shoulder instability. *J Pediatr Orthop* 1995 ; 15 : 641-643

[9] Klisic P, Filipovic M, Uzelac O, Milinkovic Z. Relocation of congenitally elevated scapula. *J Pediatr Orthop* 1981 ; 1 : 43-45

[10] Mikawa Y, Watanabe R, Yamano Y. Omoclavicular bar in congenital elevation of the scapula. A new finding. *Spine* 1991 ; 16 : 376-377

[11] Picault C, Daudet MS. Cas de surélévation congénitale de l'omoplate, Traités par la technique de JW Woodward. *Rev Chir Orthop* 1966 ; 52 : 96-97

[12] Rigault P, Pouliquen JC, Guyonvarch G, Zujovic J. Surélévation congénitale de l'omoplate chez l'enfant. Étude anatomo-pathologique et thérapeutique à propos de 27 observations. *Rev Chir Orthop* 1976 ; 62 : 5-26

[13] Ross DM, Cruess RL. The surgical correction of congenital elevation of the scapula. A review of 77 cases. *Clin Orthop* 1977 ; 125 : 17-23

[14] Schrock RD. Congenital elevation of the scapula. *J Bone Joint Surg* 1926 ; 8 : 207-215

[15] Serafin J, Sotirow B. Élévation congénitale de l'omoplate. *Rev Chir Orthop* 1966 ; 52 : 477-484

[16] Thuilleux G, Brevet JP. Surélévation congénitale de l'omoplate. *Encycl Méd Chir* (Éditions Scientifiques et Médicales Elsevier SAS, Paris), Appareil locomoteur, 5-202-B-10, 1975 : 1-6

[17] Von Bazan UB. The association between congenital elevation of the scapula and diastematomyelia : a preliminary report. *J Bone Joint Surg Br* 1979 ; 61 : 59-63

[18] Wilkinson JA, Campbell D. Scapular osteotomy for Sprengel's shoulder. *J Bone Joint Surg Br* 1980 ; 62 : 486-490

[19] Woodward JW. Congenital elevation of the scapula. Correction by release and transplantation of muscle origins; a preliminary report. *J Bone Joint Surg Am* 1961 ; 43 : 219-228

Conservative surgery for oncological pathology of the shoulder

A Taminiau

Abstract. – Limb salvage procedures in primary bone tumours of the scapula and proximal humerus, if oncologically adequate, offer attractive prospects regarding function and aesthetics of the shoulder girdle. Good insight into the anatomy is required to obtain safe resections and good functional results. Reconstruction after tumour resection in the shoulder girdle is, in many cases, restricted to soft tissue. For resections involving the glenohumeral joint, several options are available to achieve shoulder function such as custom-made prostheses, allografts and composites of these. Procedures and risk areas are described for different sites.

The choice of when and which procedure must be performed depends mainly on the site, extension and diagnosis of the tumour. The more extensive the resection of bone and soft tissue (muscle, nerve, ligaments) and reconstruction, the more shoulder function is affected after surgery. Regardless of the type of reconstruction, the main goal is to create a stable shoulder with good elbow and hand function.

© 2001, Editions Scientifiques et Médicales Elsevier SAS. All rights reserved.

Keywords: shoulder, oncological pathology, limb salvage, clavicle resection, glenoid resection, upper humerus resection.

Introduction

Malignant bone and soft tissue tumours of the shoulder girdle are a unique clinical and surgical challenge. The mutilating consequences of amputation of the upper extremities have given rise to several accepted surgical procedures in which extremity as well as function can be salvaged to a certain extent. Shoulder resections of individual bones or part of the scapula, clavicle and humerus have been performed for many years. Although prognosis is related to the grade of malignancy, local tumour control is also important for the outcome.

With the use of modern imaging techniques (MRI, CT) preoperatively, the tumour extension can be visualised in greater detail. The surgical staging system by Enneking [1] is used to define the stage of the disease in primary bone tumours. This staging system refers to the grade of the tumour, the tumour extension into the surrounding compartments and the presence or absence of metastases.

The classification of the defined margin is indicative of the adequacy of the procedure. The oncological surgical status is based on the margin achieved by surgery: intralesional, marginal, wide and radical, and can be limited by the extent and localisation of bone tumours in the shoulder region. For adequate local tumour control the resection margins have to be wide, which means the specimen must be taken out en-bloc, with a cuff of normal tissue all around it, including the biopsy tract. Surgical planning is based on the tumour extension visualised by different methods. The prerequisites for considering limb salvage surgery are diagnosis, extension into bone and soft tissue, the involvement of neurovascular structures and muscles (rotator cuff, deltoid). After tumour resections of the shoulder region, bony reconstruction is not always necessary. In most cases reattachment of the soft tissues, sometimes with augmentation of artificial material or allograft tendon material, is advocated to achieve stability of the shoulder. For example, resections of the clavicle, the blade of the scapula or the acromion are usually only replaced by muscle and soft tissue. Even after total scapulectomy, stabilisation of the humerus can be created by its fixation to the chest or remaining clavicle [2, 4, 5].

However, in cases of resection of the glenoid or proximal humerus, stabilisation of the shoulder is required. Several options are available such as custom-made prostheses, allografts and combinations, all with the goal of achieving stability of the shoulder and good elbow and hand function. Shoulder function is in general restricted [1, 2, 3, 4, 5].

Insight into the anatomical situation of the shoulder region determines the surgical options for the possible resection of each site. For the shoulder, the major structures of interest are divided into different categories:

– bones: clavicle, scapula and humerus;

– muscle: the abductor muscle compartment includes the deltoid and rotator cuff muscles;

– vascular structures: brachial artery and vein, cephalic vein and axillary artery;

– nerves: brachial plexus including axillary and suprascapular nerves.

Staging system

Staging of tumours is important for comparing tumour and patient data and results. However, it does not enable the classification of the procedure to be evaluated.

The Enneking [1] staging system is based on the localisation of the tumour and the extent of the tumour process in the surrounding structures. To characterise the magnitude of the tumour process, the relationship to

Antonie H M Taminiau, M.D., Ph.D, Department of Orthopaedics, Leiden University Medical Centre, Leiden, The Netherlands.

anatomical compartments (intracompart-mental vs. extracompartmental) and the ultimate stage type are based on the extension of tumour-bearing tissue in five distinct regions in the humerus and scapula:

– S-I: blade and spine of the scapula;

– S-II: acromion and glenoid complex;

– S-III: epiphysis of the humerus;

– S-IV: metaphysis of the humerus;

– S-V: diaphysis of the humerus.

The different types are modified according to the extension into soft tissues:

– A: abductor mechanism intact (function after surgery);

– B: abductor mechanism disrupted (no function after surgery).

Classification of shoulder resections

For a classification of the very diverse limb salvaging procedures for patients with primary bone tumours in the shoulder region, the system proposed by Malawer [3] is based on possible surgical procedures in these cases.

In more detail, the Malawer staging system is a surgical classification system for shoulder girdle resections by limb salvaging procedures [3]. There are six types of different surgical procedures, according to the magnitude of the resection and the status of the abductor mechanism:

– Type I: intra-articular proximal humeral resection;

– Type II: partial scapular resection;

– Type III: intra-articular total scapulectomy;

– Type IV: extra-articular total scapulectomy and humeral head resection;

– Type V: extra-articular humeral and glenoid resection;

– Type VI: extra-articular humeral and total scapular resection.

Each type is modified by the status of the abductor mechanism (deltoid muscle): A: intact, B: partial or complete resection. The presence or absence of the abductor mechanism is the key factor for functional outcome and is therefore the major variable. Conservative surgical procedures are best determined by the site and grade of the lesion, the anatomy involved, key risk areas for the resection and possible options for reconstruction.

However, Malawer's classification of the surgical resections does not totally cover shoulder resections. Depending on the anatomical site, tumour extension and the stage of different, often low-grade tumours, the clavicle as well as the acromion and glenoid should be entered as separate parts. Resections of the shoulder region for bone tumours are discussed, focussing on the involved bony parts (clavicle, scapula, humerus).

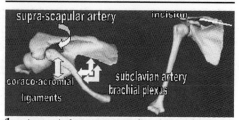

1 *Anatomical structures and excision related to a clavicle resection.*

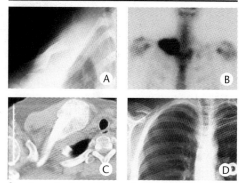

2 *A proximal clavicle resection.*
A. X-ray of a proximal clavicle, osteolytic process.
B. Clavicle hot spot on the scintigraphy.
C. CT scan - osteosarcoma.
D. Post operative view after resection.

Procedures

PROXIMAL CLAVICLE

■ *Anatomical structures of interest*

– Muscle: sternocleidomastoideus, trapezius, pectoralis;

– Bone: first rib, sternum;

– Ligament: costoclavicular;

– Vascular: subclavian artery and vein;

– Nerve: brachial plexus;

– Joint: sternoclavicular.

Resection: sternoclavicular resection.

Key risk areas: vascular structures.

Reconstruction: reinsertion of the sternocleidomastoideus.

Functional results: normal shoulder function (*fig 1*).

■ *Exposure*

This incision is in line with the clavicle, with dissection of the muscles, identification of the subclavian artery and vein and osteotomy or disarticulation of bone and/or joint of the affected bone (clavicle/sternum). The resected specimen is removed and the muscles are reinserted to the remaining clavicle. Bone reconstruction is no more advantageous than leaving the remaining distal clavicle loose. If the scapuloclavicular ligaments are detached, reinsertion of these ligaments to the distal clavicle is advocated, if possible. The function of the shoulder is generally unrestricted, as is known from cases of congenital clavicle deficiency (*fig 2*).

DISTAL CLAVICLE

■ *Anatomical structures of interest*

– Muscle: sternocleidomastoideus, trapezius, pectoralis, subclavius deltoideus;

– Bone: clavicle, acromion;

– Ligament: coracoclavicular, coraco-acromial;

– Vessel: subclavian artery and vein, suprascapular artery;

– Nerve: brachial plexus, suprascapular;

– Joint: acromioclavicular.

Resection: distal clavicular resection.

Key risk areas: subclavian artery and vein, suprascapular artery, coracoclavicular and coraco-acromial ligaments, brachial plexus, suprascapularis nerves, acromioclavicular joint.

Reconstruction: reinsertion trapezius and deltoid muscle, ligament stabilisation from proximal clavicle to scapula.

Functional results: normal shoulder function.

■ *Exposure*

The incision is in line with the clavicle as for the proximal site, with dissection of the muscles, identification of the subclavian artery and vein, subscapular artery and brachial plexus. Due to the rigid fixation of ligaments to the scapula, its dissection should be carried out carefully, eventually achieving a wide margin by taking the insertion from the scapula. Osteotomy or disarticulation of bone and/or the joint of the clavicle and acromion is performed with removal of the resected specimen. The muscle is reinserted to the remaining clavicle and the deltoid fixed to the trapezius muscle. If possible, the proximal part of the clavicle should be fixed to the scapula by the remaining ligaments, by graft or by other ligament reconstruction. Bone reconstruction is no more advantageous than leaving the remaining proximal clavicle loose. The function of the shoulder is generally unrestricted, as is known from cases of congenital clavicle deficiency (*fig 3*).

Scapula blade (type II)

■ *Anatomical structures of interest*

– Muscle: trapezius, deltoid, levator scapulae, rhomboideus major/minor serratus anterior, latissimus dorsi, subscapularis, supraspinatus, infraspinatus, teres major/minor, triceps;

– Vascular: subscapular, suprascapular artery and vein, axillary artery;

– Ligament: coracoclavicular, coraco-acromial;

– Nerve: brachial plexus, suprascapularis, subscapularis, axillary;

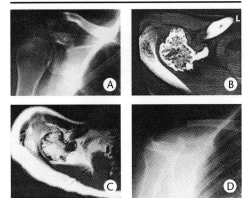

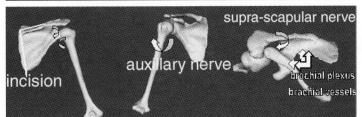

4 *Anatomical structures and excision related to scapula resection.*

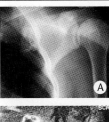

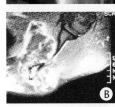

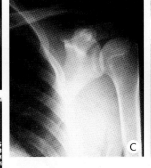

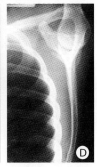

5 *A scapular blade resection.*
A. X-ray of the scapula showing calcifications on the margo vertebralis.
B. MRI scapula with chondrosarcoma extending into the soft tissue on both sides.
C. Status after partial scapular blade resection.
D. X-ray showing full abduction.

3 *A distal clavicle resection.*
A. X-ray of the distal clavicle, soft tissue calcification.
B. CT-scan for suspected cartilaginous tumour.
C. MRI distal clavicle chondrosarcoma.
D. Status after resection of the distal clavicle and reinsertion of the coracoclavicular ligaments.

– Joint: acromioclavicular, glenohumeral.

Resection: partial blade resection (exclusion of the glenoid).

Key risk areas: subscapular, suprascapular artery and vein, axillary artery; brachial plexus, suprascapular, subscapular, axillary nerves; glenohumeral joint.

Reconstruction: the muscles are reinserted into the remaining part of the scapula.

Functional results: if the glenoid humeral joint can be saved, excellent and/or good function is possible, depending on the remaining part of the scapula (fig 4).

■ *Exposure*

The skin incision extends from the inferior angle of the scapula over the margo vertebralis, curving over the spine of the scapula towards the acromion. The trapezius is detached, exposing the margo vertebralis, and the deltoid, rhomboid, infra- and supraspinatus muscles are cut, treating the extension of the dissection as well as the serratus, teres and levator scapulae muscles with care. The blade of the scapula is now exposed and the scapula is osteomised, leaving the glenoid and as much as is oncologically acceptable in situ. After removal of the specimen, the remaining muscles are reinserted to the glenoid area, using all the muscles to balance the glenohumoral joint (fig 5).

Scapula (acromion) (type II)

■ *Anatomical structures of interest*

– Muscle: trapezius, deltoid, rotator cuff;

– Ligament: coraco-acromial;

– Nerve: suprascapularis;

– Joint: acromioclavicular, glenohumeral.

Resection: acromion (exclusion of the glenoid).

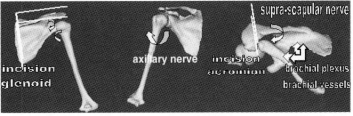

6 *Anatomical structures and excision related to acromion resection.*

Key risk areas: suprascapular artery and vein, suprascapular nerve, glenohumeral joint.

Reconstruction: reinsertion of the deltoid and trapezius muscles to the remaining part of the scapula and to one another.

Functional results: if the glenohumeral joint can be saved, excellent and/or good function is possible, depending on rotator cuff and muscle reattachment (fig 6).

■ *Exposure*

The incision is curved over the acromion, or over the spina scapula towards the acromion if an extended dissection is necessary. The deltoid and trapezius muscles are detached. The collum scapulae is explored between the tendons of the supra and infraspinatus muscles. It is important to be aware of the suprascapular nerve curving just underneath the collum scapulae. The acromioclavicular joint is visualised and the affected bony parts are osteomised. After removal of the specimen the deltoid muscle is reconstructed to the trapezius and to the remaining part of the acromion. No other bone reconstruction is necessary (fig 7).

Scapula (glenoid)

■ *Anatomical structures of interest*

– Muscle: trapezius, deltoid, latissimus dorsi, subscapularis, supraspinatus, infraspinatus, teres major/minor, triceps;

– Vascular: subscapular, suprascapular artery and vein, axillary artery;

– Ligament: glenohumeral, coracoclavicular, coraco-acromial;

– Nerve: brachial plexus, suprascapularis, subscapularis, axillary nerve;

– Joint: acromioclavicular, glenohumeral joint.

Resection: glenoid resection.

Key risk areas: subscapular, suprascapular artery and vein, axillary artery; brachial plexus, suprascapular, subscapular, axillary nerves, glenohumeral joint.

Reconstruction: reconstruction of the glenoid to the remaining part of the scapula by custom-made prosthesis or bone graft as well as stabilisation of the glenohumeral joint.

Functional results: limited, stable functions, depending on stability, joint reconstruction and the remaining muscles (rotator cuff/deltoid).

■ *Exposure*

The skin incision extends from the inferior angle of the scapula over the margo vertebralis, curving over the spine of the scapula towards the acromion. The trapezius is detached, exposing the margo vertebralis, and the deltoid and infra-supraspinatus muscles are cut. The infraspinatus muscle is reflected upward, taking care to protect the suprascapular nerve. The teres muscles and

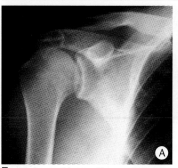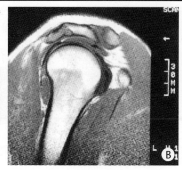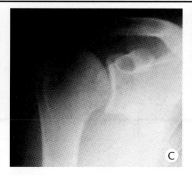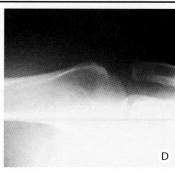

7   *An acromion resection.*
   A. X-ray of the shoulder.   *B. MRI acromial chondrosarcoma.*   *C. Status after acromion resection.*   *D. Active abduction.*

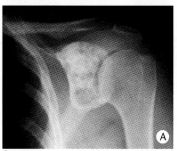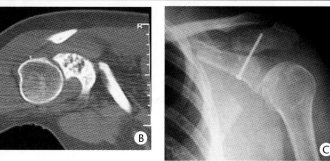

8   *A glenoid resection.*
   A. X-ray of a glenoid myxoid chondrosarcoma.
   B. CT-scan intracompartimental extension.   *C, D. X-rays after resection and reconstruction with allografts of the glenoid radius.*

triceps are detached, exposing the collum scapulae and glenoid. If the coracoid process is involved, this should be visualised by a separate, anterior incision detaching the biceps and coracobrachial muscles. If the glenohumoral joint is not involved, a posterior arthrotomy is performed. The glenoid is usually osteomised at the collum scapulae, with removal of the specimen.

There are three options for reconstruction: flail shoulder joint, allograft and a custom-made prosthesis. The choice depends on experience and is still classified as experimental.

Muscle reconstruction is carried out as anatomically as possible (fig 8, 9).

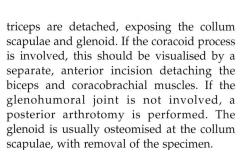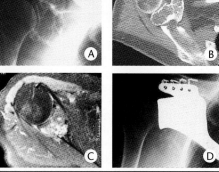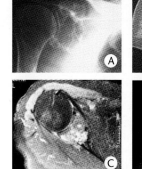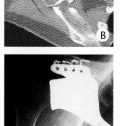

9   *A glenoid resection.*
   A. Chondrosarcoma of the glenoid.
   B. C-scan showing no invasion of the glenohumeral joint.
   C. MRI.
   D. Custom-made glenoid prosthesis.

Humerus (transarticular)

■ Anatomical structures of interest

– Muscle: deltoid, pectoralis major, pectoralis minor, latissimus dorsi, subscapularis, supraspinatus, infraspinatus, teres major, teres minor, triceps, biceps, coracobrachialis;

– Vascular: brachial artery and vein, axillary artery, cephalic vein;

– Ligament: coracoclavicular, coraco-acromial;

– Nerve: brachial plexus, axillary, musculocutaneous, medianus, radialis, ulnaris;

– Joint: glenohumeral joint.

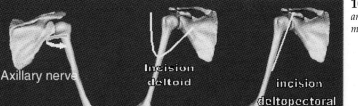

10 *Anatomical structures and excision related to a humerus resection.*

Resection: partial humerus resection (excluding the glenoid).

Key risk areas: deltoid, subscapularis, supraspinatus, infraspinatus, teres major, teres minor, triceps, biceps, coracobrachialis; brachial artery and vein, axillary artery, cephalic vein, and the brachial plexus; axillary, musculocutaneous, medianus, radialis, ulnaris nerves.

Reconstruction: allograft/composite allograft prosthesis, tumour prosthesis, reattachment capsule, cuff, muscles.

Functional results: good function possible depending on stability, joint reconstruction and remaining muscles (rotator cuff/deltoid) (fig 10).

■ Exposure

The incision runs over the deltopectoral groove, curving at the point of insertion of the deltoid posteriorly and upwards in the interval between the deltoid and triceps.

Detachment of the deltoid (if oncologically possible) and elevation of the cranial deltoid. Attention must be paid to the neurovascular

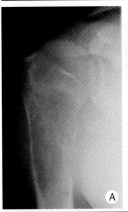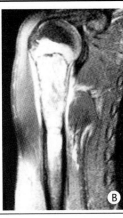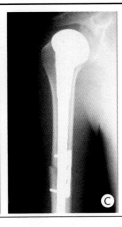

11 *A proximal humerus resection.*
A. X-ray of a proximal humerus osteosarcoma.
B. MRI showing no joint involvement.
C. Postoperative view, after resection and allograft composite prosthesis reconstruction.

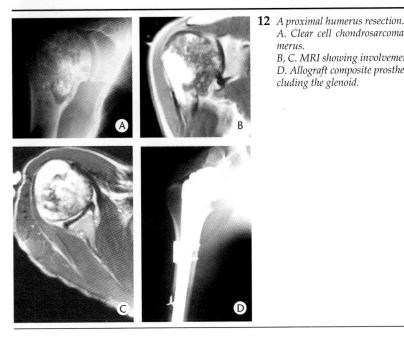

12 *A proximal humerus resection.*
A. Clear cell chondrosarcoma of the proximal humerus.
B, C. MRI showing involvement of the joint.
D. Allograft composite prosthesis reconstruction including the glenoid.

– Ligament: coracoclavicular, coraco-acromial;

– Nerve: brachial plexus, axillary, musculocutaneous, medianus, radialis, ulnaris;

– Joint: glenohumeral joint.

Resection: partial proximal humerus resection including the glenohumeral joint.

Key risk areas: deltoid, subscapularis, supraspinatus, infraspinatus, teres major, teres minor, triceps, biceps, coracobrachialis; brachial artery and vein, axillary artery, cephalic vein, and the brachial plexus; axillary, supraspinal, infraspinal, musculocutaneus, medianus, radialis, ulnaris nerves.

Reconstruction: allograft/composite allograft, prosthesis, tumour prosthesis, capsule, cuff, muscle reattachment.

Functional results: function is usually stable, with a stiff shoulder joint, depending on stability, muscle attachment and joint reconstruction.

■ *Exposure*

As for the proximal humerus, exposure with extension to the glenoid and collum scapulae.

For the reconstruction there are three options: flail shoulder joint, allograft and custom-made prosthesis. The choice depends on experience and is still classified as experimental.

Muscle reconstruction must be as anatomical as possible *(fig 12)*.

structures (musculocutaneous, radialis, ulnaris) and to visualising the insertion of the pectoralis, latissimus dorsi, teres major and minor muscles. The insertions are detached and the axillary nerve and vessels are explored. The joint capsule can be incised and, after osteotomy, the proximal humerus is removed. Reconstructive options are allografts, vascularised fibula grafts, allograft composites and prostheses and custom-made or modular prostheses. Allografts give the advantage of muscle, ligament, and capsule attachment,. Vascularised grafts are considered if the deltoid muscle must be removed with the specimen, and in young children. An extended incision into the deltopectoral groove can also be made *(fig 11)*.

Humerus including the glenohumeral joint

■ *Anatomical structures of interest*

– Muscle: deltoid, pectoralis major, pectoralis minor, latissimus dorsi, subscapularis, supraspinatus, infraspinatus, teres major, teres minor, triceps, biceps, coracobrachialis;

– Vascular: brachial artery and vein, axillary artery, cephalic vein;

References

[1] Enneking WF, Dunham W, Gebhardt MC, Malawer M, Pritchard DJ. A system for the functional evaluation of reconstructive procedures after surgical treatment of tumors of the musculoskeletal system. *Clin Orthop* 1993 ; 286 : 241-246

[2] Linberg BE. Interscapulo-thoracic resection for malignant tumors of the shoulder joint region. *Clin Orthop* 1999 ; 358 : 3-7

[3] Malawer MM, Meller I, Dunham WK. A new surgical classification system for shoulder girdle resections. Analysis of 38 patients. *Clin Orthop* 1991 ; 267 : 33-44

[4] Mnaymneh W, Malinin T, Mnaymneh LG, Benedetto P. Scapular allografts. A report of two cases. *Clinl Orthop* 1991 ; 262 : 124-128

[5] O'Connor MI, Sim FH, Chao EYS. Limb salvage for neoplasms of the shoulder girdle. Intermediate reconstructive and functional results. *J Bone Joint Surg Am* 1996 ; 78 (12) : 1872-1888

Forequarter amputation

W Winkelmann

Abstract. — If a malignant bone or soft tissue tumour of the proximal arm or the shoulder region has invaded major parts of the shoulder muscles, and especially if the tumour has infiltrated the great vessels and the brachial plexus, an amputation is the only option for obtaining adequate surgical margins. The forequarter or interscapulothoracic amputation consists of removal of the entire upper limb and the shoulder girdle on the involved side. The line of the amputation is the interval between the scapula and the thoracic wall. Sometimes, parts of the thoracic wall must be included in the amputated specimen. The large tumours have often penetrated the skin, which requires individual skin incisions and skin flaps for wound closure.
This amputation is very mutilating and fitting a prosthesis is difficult. Most patients do not wear a prosthesis.

Keywords: shoulder, tumours, forequarter amputation, interscapulothoracic amputation.

Indications

Forequarter amputation is indicated for malignant tumours of the proximal upper arm and shoulder region with involvement of the shoulder joint and the regional vessels as well as the brachial plexus. This is the only option if adequate surgical margins are to be obtained.

Positioning and skin incisions

The patient is placed in a mobile lateral position on the unaffected side. The cervicothoracic part of the incision begins in the middle of the clavicle, extending laterally to the acromion, where it curves posteriorly to the lateral border of the scapula; it then curves to the middle of the scapula. The axillary incision begins again in the middle of the clavicle, extends along the deltopectoral groove, crosses the anterior axillary fold and extends to the dorsal aspect of the arm and joins the posterior incision *(fig 1)*.

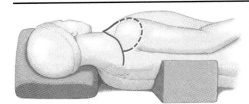

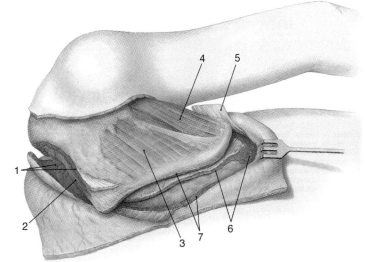

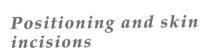

1 *Positioning of the patient and skin incisions. (Reproduced with permission from Winkelmann W. Interscapulothorakale Amputation. In Bauer R, Kerschbaumer F, Poisel S eds. Orthopädische Operationslehre 3; Schulter und obere Extremität. © Georg Thieme-Verlag, 1997.)*

2 *Posterior approach. 1. Trapezius m.; 2. supraspinatus m.; 3. infraspinatus m.; 4. teres major m.; 5. latissimus dorsi m.; 6. serratus anterior m.; 7. rhomboideus m. (Reproduced with permission from Winkelmann W. Interscapulothorakale Amputation. In Bauer R, Kerschbaumer F, Poisel S eds. Orthopädische Operationslehre 3; Schulter und obere Extremität. © Georg Thieme-Verlag, 1997.)*

Surgical technique

After mobilising the flaps and dividing the fascia in line with the skin incisions, the underlying muscles are exposed. From a posterior approach *(fig 2)*, the muscles connecting the scapula with the trunk are divided step by step. First the trapezius muscle is divided, followed by the detachment of the omohyoid muscle, the levator scapulae muscle, the rhomboideus minor and major muscles and the latissimus dorsi muscle at the inferior angle of the scapula. For detachment of the serratus anterior muscle, the scapula is retracted forward.

Winfried Winkelmann, Professor Dr. med, Department of Orthopaedic Surgery, Westfälische Wilhelms-Universität, Münster, Germany.

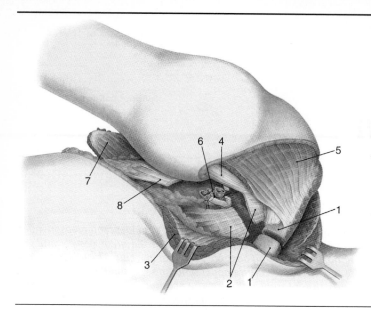

3 *Anterior approach. 1. Clavicle; 2. pectoralis minor m.; 3. pectoralis major m.; 4. biceps brachii, short head; 5. deltoideus m.; 6. axillaris vessels (ligated and divided) and brachial plexus (divided); 7. subscapularis m.; 8. latissimus dorsi m. (Reproduced with permission from Winkelmann W. Interscapulothorakale Amputation. In Bauer R, Kerschbaumer F, Poisel S eds. Orthopädische Operationslehre 3; Schulter und obere Extremität. © Georg Thieme-Verlag, 1997.)*

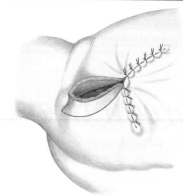

4 *Wound closure. The overlying skin must be resected. (Reproduced with permission from Winkelmann W. Interscapulothorakale Amputation. In Bauer R, Kerschbaumer F, Poisel S eds. Orthopädische Operationslehre 3; Schulter und obere Extremität. © Georg Thieme-Verlag, 1997.)*

The patient is changed to a more supine position *(fig 3)* for the anterior approach and the clavicle is exposed subperiostally.

The clavicle is then osteotomised in the medial third and elevated, and the subclavius muscle is divided. The coracobrachialis and pectoralis minor short head of the biceps muscles are exposed and divided.

The subclavian vessels are separated, individually clamped, double ligated and divided. The nerve cords of the brachial plexus are individually ligated and divided. The amputation is finished by the detachment of the pectoralis, latissimus dorsi and subscapularis muscles.

After deep coverage with the retained muscles and insertion of two Redon drains, the wound is closed. The overlying skin must be resected *(fig 4)*. A compression dressing is applied to prevent deep haematoma.

This amputation is very mutilating and fitting the prosthesis is difficult. Most patients do not wear a prothesis.

References

[1] Winkelmann W. Interscapulothorakale Amputation. In: Bauer R, Kerschbaumer F, Poisel S eds. Orthopädische Operationslehre 3; Schulter und obere Extremität. Stuttgart : Thieme-Verlag, 1997 : 576-578

Index
Volume 3 - Shoulder
Surgical Techniques in Orthopaedics and Traumatology

A

Acromioclavicular dislocation......................55-160-E-10
– : reconstruction.......................................55-160-E-10
Acromioplasty
– : open anterior...55-190-D-10
– : surgical approach...................................55-190-D-10
Amputation
– : forequarter...55-210-E-10
Arm
See: Humeral head
Arthritis
See: Rheumatoid disease
Arthrodesis, shoulder..............................55-200-D-10
– : after failed arthroplasty.........................55-200-D-10
– : rheumatoid arthritis...............................55-200-B-10
Arthroscopy, shoulder
– : arthroscopic acromioplasty....................55-190-C-10
– : arthroscopy, general..............................55-160-C-10
– : in multidirectional instability................55-190-A-10
– : in recurrent anterior instability............55-180-A-10
– : rotator cuff tears....................................55-190-E-10
– : subacromial decompression....................55-190-C-10

B

Bankart defect, shoulder..............................55-180-D-10
Bankart procedure, shoulder.........................55-180-B-10
Bone, graft
– : humeral head reconstruction...................55-190-B-10
Brachial plexus
– : obstetrical palsy, early sequelae.............55-210-A-10
– : obstetrical palsy, late sequelae................55-200-E-10
– : palsy, shoulder arthrodesis.....................55-200-D-10

C

Classification
– : AO/ASIF, extra and intra-articular
  fractures...55-170-B-10
– : clavicle, fractures...................................55-160-D-10
– : Duparc, fractures and vascularisation.....55-170-B-10
– : Enneking, tumour, shoulder...................55-210-D-10
– : Malawar, tumour, shoulder resection......55-210-D-10
– : Neer, fractures.......................................55-170-B-10
– : Rockwood, acromioclavicular injuries....55-160-E-10
– : shoulder dislocations, humeral lesions...55-190-B-10
Clavicle
– : fracture...55-160-D-10
Congenital anomalies
– : elevation of scapula.................................55-210-C-10
– : Sprengel's deformity...............................55-210-C-10
Copeland repair, shoulder instability............55-180-B-10

D

Debreye-Patte approach, shoulder..............55-160-B-10
Dislocation
– : acromioclavicular....................................55-160-E-10
– : chronic shoulder.....................................55-190-B-10
– : posterior, shoulder..................................55-200-E-10
– : sternoclavicular......................................55-170-A-10
Dujarrier's approach, shoulder.....................55-160-B-10

E

Eden-Lange technique..............................55-210-B-10

F

Fixation, internal, upper extremities
– : plate, shoulder arthrodesis......................55-200-D-10
Fracture, arm
– : dislocations of the humeral head..............55-190-B-10
– : proximal humerus...................................55-180-A-10
Fracture, clavicle....................................55-160-D-10

G

Glenoid
– : bone tumour resection..............................55-210-D-10
– : implant...55-170-C-10
– : resurfacing..55-170-E-10

H

Hill-Sachs deformity..............................55-180-B-10
Humeral head
– : prosthesis..55-170-D-10
– : reconstruction of....................................55-190-B-10
– : removal of..55-180-A-10
– : replacement..55-170-D-10
Humerus, proximal
– : arthroplasty, fractures proximal
  humerus...55-180-A-10
– : bone tumour resection.............................55-210-D-10
– : fracture and hemi-arthroplasty...............55-170-D-10
– : fracture, intra-articular...........................55-170-B-10
– : fracture, Neer classification.....................55-170-B-10
– : implant...55-170-C-10
– : prostheses for fractures...........................55-180-A-10

I

Instability, shoulder
– : recurrent anterior, arthroscopic
  techniques..55-180-D-10
– : recurrent anterior, Bankart procedure.....55-180-E-10
– : recurrent anterior, capsuloplasties..........55-180-C-10

K

Kocher's procedure, shoulder......................55-160-B-10

L

Latarjet-Bristow procedure..........................55-180-C-10

N

Necrosis
– : avascular, proximal humerus....................55-170-B-10
Neer
– : classification...55-170-B-10
– : prosthesis..55-180-A-10
– : total shoulder arthroplasty......................55-170-C-10
Nerve
– : entrapments, shoulder.............................55-210-B-40
– : quadrilateral space syndrome..................55-210-B-40
– : serratus palsy...55-210-B-40
– : trapezius palsy..55-210-B-40
– : winging scapula......................................55-210-B-40
Nerve, palsy
– : axillary nerve..55-210-B-40
– : entrapments, shoulder.............................55-210-B-40
– : musculocutaneous nerve.........................55-210-B-40
– : quadrilateral space syndrome..................55-210-B-40

– : serratus palsy...55-210-B-40
– : shoulder, external rotation......................55-210-A-10
– : shoulder, obstetrical, early sequelae........55-210-A-10
– : suprascapular nerve................................55-210-B-40
– : trapezius...55-210-B-10
Nerve, peripheral
– : shoulder paralysis...................................55-210-B-10

O

Osteoarthritis, shoulder
– : arthrodesis..55-200-D-10
Osteosynthesis
– : proximal humerus...................................55-170-B-10
– : shoulder arthrodesis................................55-200-D-10
Osteotomy
– : acromion...55-160-B-10
– : coracoid..55-160-A-10
– : glenoid in multidirectional instability....55-190-A-10

P

Palsy
– : obstetrical, late sequelae, shoulder..........55-200-E-10
– : shoulder, external rotation......................55-210-A-10
– : shoulder, obstetrical, early sequelae........55-210-A-10
– : shoulder, trapezius..................................55-210-B-10
Plate
– : shoulder arthrodesis................................55-200-D-10
Prosthesis, shoulder
– : arthrodesis..55-200-D-10
– : classification...55-170-C-10
– : Neer...55-180-A-10
– : replacement, humeral head......................55-170-D-10

R

Rheumatoid disease
– : rotator cuff...55-200-B-10
– : shoulder, arthrodesis...............................55-200-B-10
– : shoulder arthroplasty..............................55-200-B-10
– : shoulder, hemi-arthroplasty....................55-170-D-10
– : shoulder, synovectomy............................55-200-B-10
– : shoulder, total arthroplasty.....................55-170-E-10
Rotator cuff
– : rupture in total shoulder arthroplasty.....55-170-E-10
– : tears, arthroscopic technique...................55-190-E-10
– : tears, musculo-tendinous transfer...........55-200-C-10
– : tears, open surgery..................................55-200-A-10

S

Scapula, adult
– : bone tumour resection.............................55-210-D-10
Scapula, children
– : congenital elevation of............................55-210-C-10
Shoulder, adults
– : acromioplasty..55-190-D-10
– : approach, anterior...................................55-160-A-10
– : approach, deltopectoral............................55-160-A-10
– : approach, posterior..................................55-160-B-10
– : approach, superior...................................55-160-A-10
– : arthrodesis..55-200-D-10
– : arthroplasty..55-200-B-10
– : arthroscopic acromioplasty......................55-190-C-10
– : arthroscopy...55-160-C-10
– : capsuloplasty...55-180-E-10
– : coracoid transfer.....................................55-180-C-10
– : dislocation, acromioclavicular.................55-160-E-10

– : dislocation, chronic posterior.................... 55-190 -B-10
– : dislocation, sternoclavicular..................... 55-170-A-10
– : fracture, clavicle...................................... 55-160-D-10
– : Hill-Sachs deformity .... 55-180 -B-10
– : impingement syndrome............................ 55-190-C-10
                                                              55-190-D-10
– : instability, anterior .... 55-180 -B-10
– : instability, multidirectional..................... 55-190-A-10
– : instability, recurrent anterior,
    arthroscopic techniques 55-180-D-10
– : instability, recurrent anterior, Bankart
    procedure.. 55-180 -B-10
– : instability, recurrent anterior,
    capsuloplasty.. 55-180 -E-10
– : instability, recurrent anterior,
    Latarjet-Bristow procedure 55-180-C-10
– : musculo-tendinous transfer 55-200-C-10
– : nerve entrapments................................... 55-210 -B-40
– : open surgery for rotator cuff tears 55-200-A-10
– : osteoarthritis.. 55-170-D-10
                                                              55-170 -E-10
– : paralysis .... 55-210 -B-10
– : prosthesis 55-170-C-10
– : quadrilateral space syndrome................... 55-210 -B-40
– : resection 55-170-A-10

– : rheumatoid arthritis .... 55-200 -B-10
                                                              55-170-D-10
                                                              55-170 -E-10
– : rotator cuff tears, arthroscopic
    techniques .... 55-190 -E-10
– : rotator cuff tears, open technique............. 55-200-A-10
– : Rowe repair.. 55-180 -B-10
– : subacromial decompression...................... 55-190-C-10
– : suture anchor method .... 55-180 -B-10
– : tumour... 55-210-D-10
– : winging scapula .... 55-210 -B-40
Shoulder, arthroplasty
– : anterior instability.................................. 55-180 -B-10
– : bipolar... 55-170-C-10
– : chronic posterior dislocations .... 55-190 -B-10
– : hemi-arthroplasty 55-170-D-10
– : hemi-arthroplasty, proximal humerus
    fractures... 55-180-A-10
– : Neer 55-170-C-10
– : resection... 55-170-A-10
– : total shoulder... 55-170 -E-10
Shoulder, children
– : obstetrical palsy...................................... 55-210-A-10
– : obstetrical palsy, late sequelae................. 55-200 -E-10
– : posterior subluxation, dislocation............ 55-200 -E-10

– : scapula, congenital elevation of 55-210-C-10
Sprengel's deformity 55-210-C-10
Sternoclavicular
– : dislocation 55-170-A-10
Suture anchor method
– : arthroscopic techniques............................ 55-180-D-10
– : Bankart procedure.................................... 55-180 -B-10
– : rotator cuff tears .... 55-190 -E-10

T

Tendon
– : shoulder, paralysis................................... 55-210 -B-10
– : shoulder, transfer in obstetrical palsy 55-210-A-10
– : shoulder, transfer in rotator cuff
    deficiency... 55-200-C-10
Tumour
– : amputation, forequarter............................ 55-210 -E-10
– : scapula resection 55-210-D-10
– : shoulder.. 55-210-D-10